MEDICAL RADIOLOGY
Diagnostic Imaging

Editors:
A. L. Baert, Leuven
K. Sartor, Heidelberg

Springer

Berlin
Heidelberg
New York
Barcelona
Hong Kong
London
Milan
Paris
Tokyo

D. Caramella · C. Bartolozzi (Eds.)

3D Image Processing

Techniques and Clinical Applications

With Contributions by

W. Backfrieder · I. Baeli · R. J. Bale · E. Balogh · I. Bargellini · C. Bartolozzi · A. V. Bartrolì
S. Berrettini · E. Bichi Secchi · W. Birkfellner · A. Blum Moyse · P. Boraschi · D. Brennan
J. Bruzzi · G. Gampori · C. Cappelli · D. Caramella · M. Cartellieri · C. Catalano · D. Cioni
M. Citardi · A. Cotten · L. Crocetti · M. Danti · H. M. Fenlon · F. Fraioli · M. P. Fried
C. Gianni · R. Gigoni · E. Gobbetti · R. Hanel · F. Iafrate · R. Iannaccone · S. Iochum
G. Israel · A. Jackson · N. W. John · F. A. Jolesz · J. Kettenbach · R. Kikinis · D. Kovacevic
A. Laghi · P. F. La Palombara · R. Lencioni · M. E. Leventon · S. Lodovigi · S. Loncaric
W. E. Lorensen · M. Macari · A. Malvisti · M. Marcacci · L. Martí-Bonmatì · V. M. Moharir
A. Napoli · E. Neri · L. Nofrini · W. L. Nowinski · L. G. Nyùl · K. Palágyi · M. Panconi
V. Panebianco · R. Passariello · F. Pediconi · M. Perri · S. Picchietti · H. Ringl · L. Salvolini
R. Scateni · A. G. Schreyer · S. Sellari Franceschini · R. Shahidi · E. Sorantin · C. Spinelli
M. Subasic · N. A. Thacker · P. Vagli · S. K. Warfield · G. Zanetti

Foreword by

A. L. Baert

With 216 Figures in 411 Separate Illustrations, 185 in Color

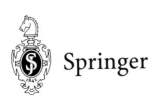
Springer

Davide Caramella, MD
Carlo Bartolozzi, MD
Diagnostic and Interventional Radiology
Department of Oncology, Transplants, and Advanced Technologies in Medicine
University of Pisa
Via Roma 67
56100 Pisa
Italy

Medical Radiology · Diagnostic Imaging and Radiation Oncology
Series Editors: A. L. Baert · L. W. Brady · H.-P. Heilmann · F. Molls · K. Sartor

Continuation of
Handbuch der medizinischen Radiologie
Encyclopedia of Medical Radiology

ISBN 3-540-67470-5 Springer-Verlag Berlin Heidelberg New York

Library of Congress Cataloging-in-Publication Data

3D image processing : techniques and clinical applications / D. Caramella, C. Bartolozzi
(eds.) ; with contributions by W. Backfrieder ... [et al.] ; foreword by A. L. Baert.
    p. ; cm. – (Medical radiology)
  Includes bibliographical references and index.
  ISBN 3540674705 (alk. paper)
    1. Three-dimensional imaging in medicine. 2. Image processing. I. Caramella, D. II.
Bartolozzi, C. (Carlo), 1947- III. Series.
    [DNLM: 1. Image Processing, Computer-Assisted. 2. Diagnostic Imaging–methods.
WN 180 Z999 2002]
  R857.T47 A125 2002
  616.07'54–dc21
                                                    2001049859

Springer-Verlag Berlin Heidelberg New York
a member of BertelsmannSpringer Science+Business Media GmbH

http//www. springer.de
© Springer-Verlag Berlin Heidelberg 2002
Printed in Germany

The use of general descriptive names, trademarks, etc. in this publication does not imply, even in the absence of a specific statement, that such names are exempt from the relevant protective laws and regulations and therefore free for general use.

Product liability: The publishers cannot guarantee the accuracy of any information about dosage and application contained in this book. In every case the user must check such information by consulting the relevant literature.

Cover-Design and Typesetting: Verlagsservice Teichmann, 69256 Mauer

SPIN: 107 657 09   21/3130 – 5 4 3 2 1 0 – Printed on acid-free paper

Foreword

The introduction of computer applications in medical imaging has had a tremendous impact on routine radiological practice in recent years. The possibilities for image processing, presentation and transmission of digitally acquired radiological data are now almost without limits.

This book sets out to provide a sorely needed update of our knowledge of the diagnostic potential of 3D imaging and the virtual rendering of images and constitutes a welcome addition to our series Medical Radiology, which aims to cover all important aspects of clinical imaging in modern diagnostic radiology.

The editors and the contributing authors have striven to focus not only on the theoretical foundations of digital imaging but also on the clinical value of these new methods. Therefore this volume should be of great interest not only to diagnostic radiologists but also to surgeons.

Davide Caramella and Carlo Bartolozzi have been involved in digital radiological techniques for many years, and the department of radiology of the University of Pisa has played a leading pioneer role in exploring the clinical potential of this new technology. Their own excellent knowledge and expertise has enabled them to engage a very distinguished group of internationally known experts in digital imaging as contributors. I would like to congratulate them most sincerely for this outstanding volume, its comprehensive contents as well as its superb illustrations.

I trust this book will meet with the same great success as previous volumes in the series.

Leuven   ALBERT L. BAERT

Preface

In recent times, few fields in medicine have witnessed such impressive progress as the application of computers to radiology: digital acquisition, display, management and processing of diagnostic images have revolutionized the practice of radiology and have determined a growing interest in this field on the part of other medical professionals also.

In particular, post-processing and 3D reconstruction of diagnostic images not only satisfy an aesthetic requirement of radiologists: they have become a necessary tool for the representation of complex anatomical structures and for the understanding of pathological changes in terms of both morphology and function. This is crucial if we consider that the volume of native images produced with new-generation cross-sectional techniques has become increasingly large.

Also the requirements of referring physicians have changed accordingly. Today they not only ask for the "simple" radiological diagnosis accompanying a series of native images; they also request the availability of reconstructed images that allow better appreciation of the disease process, appropriate selection of treatment options, and accurate planning of procedures.

This book, written by leading experts worldwide, provides a comprehensive and up-to-date overview of the role of 3D image processing, covering the introductory technical aspects and then providing in-depth analysis of the main clinical applications. Final chapters discuss the evolutionary aspects of this challenging new area of the radiological sciences, by focusing on recent developments in functional imaging and computer-aided surgery.

We hope that this book, which is the expression of the enthusiastic commitment of many distinguished colleagues, will fulfil the expectations of all medical professionals who are interested in this very important field.

Finally, we would like to express our deep appreciation to the Medical Radiology series Editor, Prof. Albert Baert, and thank most sincerely all the authors for having spent so much time and effort in preparing truly outstanding contributions.

Pisa   DAVIDE CARAMELLA
                                                             CARLO BARTOLOZZI

Contents

Technique

1 US Image Acquisition

Riccardo Lencioni, Marzio Perri, Dania Cioni

CONTENTS

1.1 Introduction

Three-dimensional (3D) ultrasonography, even though it has recently been gaining great popularity, is a relative new tool compared with 3D reconstructions obtained by CT and MR imaging. Ultrasonography offers unique qualities including real-time imaging, physiological measurements, use of non-ionizing radiation and non-invasiveness. Sonographic image quality has benefited from increasingly sophisticated computer technology: to date several systems able to generate 3D ultrasound images have been introduced.

Volume sonographic imaging has sparked interest in the academic community since the 1961. At that time Baum and Greenwood obtained serial parallel ultrasound images of the human orbit and created a 3D display by stacking sequential photographic plates with the ultrasound images (Baum and Greenwood 1961). During the early 1970s industry also became interested in 3D ultrasound imaging: in 1974 the Kretztechnik group, in order to achieve 3D images, developed a cylindrical-shaped transducer incorporating 25 elements mounted on a drum. This equipment performed a volume scan consisting of 25 parallel slices. The next step consisted of a more convenient end-fire transducer producing a fan scan. However, at that time the display and storage technology was not suitable for 3D ultrasound imaging. In 1989 in Paris, at the French Congress of Radiology, Kretztechnik presented the first commercially available ultrasound system featuring the 3D Voluson technique. It is only in the last few years that computer technology and visualization techniques have progressed sufficiently to make 3D ultrasound viable. Nowadays, 3D ultrasound imaging methods allow the presentation, in few seconds, of the entire volume in a single image (Brandal et al. 1999). The success of 3D ultrasound will depend on providing performance that equals or exceeds that of two-dimensional (2D) ultrasonography, including real-time capability and interactivity.

In this chapter, we review the various approaches that investigators have pursued in the development of 3D ultrasound imaging systems, with emphasis on the three steps into which, at present, the process of making 3D sonographic images is divided: data acquisition, data processing and reconstruction, and data visualization.

1.2 Data Acquisition

Various techniques have been described for acquiring a sequence of sonograms and reconstructing them into a final 3D result. Acquiring the sequence is the critical step in the process for two main reasons. First, because the sequence of acquired tomographic images will be assembled into a 3D image, the acquisition geometry must be known exactly to avoid distortions, and the images must be acquired rapidly to avoid patient motion. Second, the mechanism that manipulates the transducer or localizes its position

R. Lencioni, MD, M. Perri, MD, D. Cioni, MD
Diagnostic and Interventional Radiology, Department of Oncology, Transplants, and Advanced Technologies in Medicine, University of Pisa, Via Roma 67, 56100 Pisa, Italy

in space must not interfere with the performance of the sonographic examination. To meet these requirements, various solutions have been proposed. At present the main types of 3D data acquisition systems are: (a) mechanical scanning systems, (b) tracked freehand systems, (c) untracked freehand systems, and (d) 2D transducer arrays.

1.2.1
Mechanical Scanning Systems

Mechanical scanning systems are based on a commercially available linear or annular transducer array mounted on a mechanical assembly that allows precise movement of the transducer by a motor under computer control. Two types of mechanical assemblies have been developed: external transducer fixation drive devices and, more recently, integrated volume transducers.

External transducer fixation drive devices represent the first implementation of mechanical scanning systems. In this approach the transducer is mounted on a special external device (mechanical arm) that holds the transducer firmly, offering precise movement during scanning. The device is then held in a fixed position and a motor drive system on the device moves the transducer in a controlled and well-defined fashion to sweep out a volume. This system provides a high accuracy in locating the position of the transducer relative to the scanned planes. In the past it has been used for vascular (Downey and Fenster 1995a), prostate (Downey and Fenster 1995b) and obstetric (Steiner et al. 1994) imaging. Because of the constraints imposed by a rigid mechanical device that can be cumbersome for the operator and may interfere with the usual sonographic examination, these external devices are not in clinical use. In order to overcome these limitations, integrated volume transducers have been introduced.

The integrated volume transducer consists of a conventional annular array transducer mounted on a hand-held assembly that allows the translation or rotation of the transducer by a motor drive computer system. Integrated volume transducers acquire a volume as a series of slices at slightly different orientations. After each slice the transducer plane is moved, by the stepping motor, to the next location. In this way, the relative angle between slices is exactly known, eliminating distortion in the resultant scan. Integrated volume transducers tend to be relatively larger than standard transducers, but they eliminate most of the issues related to external position sensors with respect

to calibration and accuracy. As a result the sonographer can use the transducer in the same manner as a conventional 2D ultrasonography system, needing only to immobilize the probe during image acquisition. Only a few seconds are required for obstetric studies and approximately 1 min for cardiac-gated studies. Volumes can be acquired and reconstructed rapidly without registration artefacts. Such systems have a relatively small field of view that, although not posing problems for imaging small structures, may represent a significant limitation for large ones. Integrated volume transducers have been produced for both transabdominal and intracavitary probes. This approach has been described for several applications: abdomen (Hamper et al. 1994), prostate (Elliot et al. 1996; Tong et al. 1996; Hamper et al. 1999), heart (De Castro et al. 1998) and obstetrics (Nelson et al. 1996; Johnson et al. 2000). A particular application of this approach is the use of a motorized rotating transducer mounted on the end of a catheter and introduced into the vasculature for intravascular imaging (Klein et al. 1992; Thrush et al. 1997). Withdrawal of the catheter and transducer through a vessel allows collection of a series of 2D images for forming a 3D volume.

The different types of mechanical assemblies used to produce 3D images can be divided into three basic types of motion: linear, tilting, and rotation (Fenster and Downey 2000).

Linear scanning requires that the transducer is moved by the stepping motor in a linear fashion along the surface of patient's skin so that the 2D images obtained are parallel to each other (Fig. 1.1).

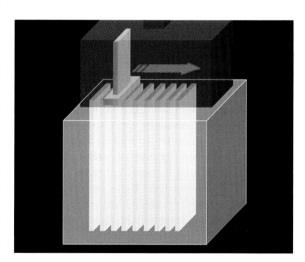

Fig. 1.1. Linear scanning. The transducer is translated linearly over the patient area of interest. A series of parallel 2D images are collected, and then reconstructed into a 3D image

The 2D images are acquired at a regular spatial interval that is adjusted to ensure appropriate sampling of the anatomy. Because the 2D images are parallel and the spatial sampling interval is predetermined, the majority of the parameters required for the reconstruction can be precomputed, and the reconstruction time can be shortened. With this approach, a volume image can be obtained immediately after performance of a linear scan.

With tilt scanning the transducer is tilted about its face, and images are digitized at a predetermined angular interval (Fig. 1.2). The main advantage of this approach is that the scanning device is usually quite small, which allows easy hand-held manipulations. The major problem related to the use of the tilt scanning approach is that the 2D images are acquired in a fan-like geometry, and as a consequence the space between them increases and the resolution decreases with increasing depth.

In rotational scanning the transducer is rotated around an axis that is perpendicular to the transducer array (Fig. 1.3). The 3D image data are then acquired by collecting a series of 2D B-mode images as the probe is rotated at constant speed. As a result, the sampling distance increases and the resolution decreases as distance from the rotational axis increases. In addition, the digitized images intersect along the rotational axis, so that any motion creates artefacts at the centre of the 3D image.

1.2.2
Tracked Freehand Systems

The freehand approach is very attractive: the transducer can be moved freely and without any restriction introduced by mechanics. The examination is performed in the same way as a standard ultrasound study. With tracked freehand systems, the operator holds an assembly composed of the transducer and a position-sensor device and manipulates it over the anatomical area being evaluated. During the acquisition of 2D images the tracking device attached to the probe monitors the spatial position and orientation of the ultrasound transducer. The tracking device has a limited size and weight and does not influence the movement of the transducer, the freedom or the usual working procedure of the physician. This system provides flexibility in selecting the best image plane sampling of the tissue volume from which data are acquired. In addition, it eliminates the need for more complex, dedicated 3D probes which contain a mechanism to move the transducer through a pre-

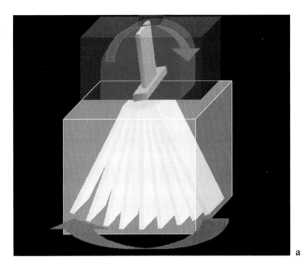

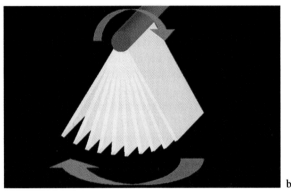

Fig. 1.2a, b. Tilt scanning. a The transducer is tilted about its face. 2D images are acquired and used to generate a volume image. b The tilt scanning approach can also be used with transrectal transducers. The transducer is rotated along its long axis. This approach is being used for 3D ultrasound imaging of the prostate

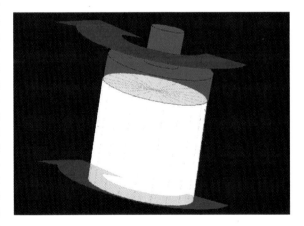

Fig. 1.3. Rotational scanning. The transducer is rotated around an axis that is perpendicular to the transducer array. The 3D image data are acquired by collecting a series of 2D B-mode images as the probe is rotated at constant speed

set field of acquisition. The two principal types of tracking freehand systems are: acoustic tracking and magnetic field tracking.

Acoustic tracking makes use of sound emitters mounted on the transducer and small microphones for sound detection. The microphones must be positioned in different locations above the patient and must be sufficiently near the emitters to be able to detect the sound pulse. As the operator moves the probe the sound emitters are energized in rapid sequence, producing sound waves that are detected by the microphones. The time of flight of the sound impulse from each emitter to each microphone is measured and corrected for environmental conditions, and then used to calculate the position of the transducer and the ultrasound image in a coordinate system defined by the microphone array. The trigger signal that is recorded by the ultrasound system allows coordination of the imaging and positional data. As a consequence, by activating the sound-emitting devices while the probe is moving freely, the position and orientation of the transducer can be continuously monitored and real-time acquisition of images and positional data are obtained (KING et al. 1990; OFILI and NAVIN 1994). A disadvantage of the acoustic system is the requirement of a direct line of sight between the sensing equipment (microphones) and the ultrasound probe. Magnetic field tracking, on the other hand, does not impose any restriction on transducer placement during scanning: magnetic tracking permits free transducer movement, allowing acquisition of arbitrarily oriented 2D images from one or more acoustic windows.

Magnetic field tracking is a relatively new tracked freehand technique which makes use of magnetic localizers to measure the transducer's position and angle in space. At present it is considered the most successful tracked freehand technique. The system includes a magnetic field generator (transmitter), a miniature magnetic sensor (receiver), and a system control unit (Fig. 1.4).

The receiver is small and mounted directly on the ultrasound scan head. Its size does not interfere with standard clinical ultrasound scanning methods. The transmitter, which is usually mounted on the examining table, emits three orthogonal magnetic fields. The control unit measures and compares the relative strengths of all three fields at the receiver. These measurements are used to compute the position and orientation of the receiver relative to the transmitter (Fig. 1.5).

To achieve accurate 3D reconstruction, electromagnetic interference must be minimized, the transmitter must be close to the receiver, and there should

be no ferrous or highly conductive metals in the vicinity (KELLY et al. 1994; DOWNEY et al. 2000). Magnetic field tracking systems can be used with standard and intracavitary transducers. These systems have been used successfully for fetal (KELLY et al. 1994; PRETORIUS and NELSON 1994) and vascular (HODGES et al. 1994) 3D imaging. Recently, there has been some development regarding miniature magnetic position sensors suitable for use with intravascular transducers.

1.2.3
Untracked Freehand Systems

Untracked freehand systems do not require any kind of device added to the probe. The operator has to move the transducer with a uniform and steady motion, in a constant linear or angular velocity. As a result the 2D images are acquired at a regular spatial interval that is adjusted to ensure appropriate sampling of the anatomy. Despite this approach being very attractive for the user, image quality is extremely variable, depending on the regularity of the transducer's movement. Moreover, geometric measurements (distance, volume, area) may be inaccurate. These drawbacks make the tool useless, and in any case unsuitable for accurate clinical applications.

1.2.4
2D Transducer Arrays

Two-dimensional transducer arrays represent the ultimate approach to 3D sonographic acquisition. These arrays are a matrix with a large number of

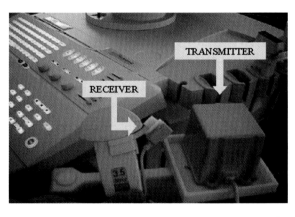

Fig. 1.4. Magnetic field tracking system: components. The system includes a magnetic field generator (transmitter) and a magnetic sensor mounted on the probe (receiver)

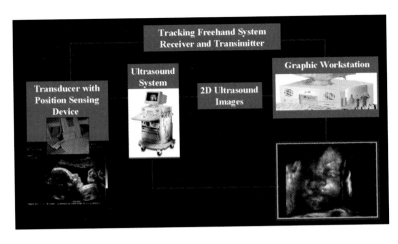

Fig. 1.5. Schematic representation of a 3D magnetic field tracking system. The magnetic field tracking system allows a digitized sequence of 2D ultrasound images to be obtained together with their position and orientation. The data are transmitted to a workstation for 3D image processing. (Courtesy of ESAOTE)

elements arranged in rows and columns which are able, in principle, to achieve unrestricted scanning in three dimensions. A volumetric image is produced without moving the transducer: such an array generates a pyramidal or conical ultrasound pulse and processes the echoes to obtain 3D information in real time. Although the ultimate expectation is that 2D transducer arrays will replace integrated mechanical scanning transducers or other position-sensing transducers, they are still in the research phase. Investigators have described several 2D array systems (TURNBULL and FOSTER 1992; TURNBULL et al. 1992); the one developed at Duke University for real-time 3D echocardiography is the most advanced and has been used for clinical imaging (VON RAMM and SMITH 1990; SMITH et al. 1992; LIGHT et al. 1998). At present the major problem related to the use of 2D transducer arrays consists of the complexity of the system, which requires sophisticated software and huge computer capabilities. In order to reduce system cost and complexity, sparse 2D arrays have been developed (DAVIDSEN et al. 1994; DAVIDSEN and SMITH 1997). Moreover, 2D array transducers are relatively small and, as a result, their field of view also is relatively small: this may be a limitation for large organ imaging (NELSON and PRETORIUS 1998).

1.3
Data Processing and Reconstruction

The 3D reconstruction process involves the generation of a 3D image from a digitized set of 2D images. The 3D reconstruction and processing architecture for 3D ultrasound is critical since it must take advantage of frequent processor, accelerator, and software upgrades to keep up with rapidly changing computer

technology. Two predominant approach have been used thus far: a 3D surface model and a voxel-based volume model (DOWNEY et al. 2000).

1.3.1
3D Surface Model

By the use of the 3D surface model the desired structure is output in the form of a boundary surface that separates the structure from the background. In this approach, the desired features in each acquired 2D image are classified and segmented. The operator outlines the boundaries of the areas of interest on the 2D images manually or with automated computerized methods. Moreover these boundaries can be distinguished from adjacent tissues by assigning a value or colour, and thus a 3D surface model of the anatomy is obtained. The main advantage of this technique is related to the reduction of the amount of 3D data, consisting of only a few boundaries or structure information. Furthermore the contrast between different structures is artificially increased. The major limitation of this approach is the segmentation data process. In fact accurate segmentation of ultrasound data, essential for high-quality rendering, is a difficult problem because, to date, high-performance automatic segmentation systems are not available and the manual approach is tedious and time-consuming. As a consequence this method for 3D ultrasound image reconstruction is not used for clinical applications.

1.3.2
Voxel-Based Volume Model

The voxel-based volume model represents the most common approach to 3D reconstruction techniques.

With this method a volume is generated by placing each 2D image at the proper location in the 3D volume. This approach preserves all the original information during 3D reconstruction: it allows repeated review of the 3D image by a variety of rendering techniques. Using the voxel-based volume model the operator can scan through the data and then choose the most suitable rendering technique. Moreover, this approach allows the use of segmentation and classification algorithms to measure volume and segment boundaries, or to perform various volume-based rendering operations. The major limitation of the voxel-based volume model is that it generates very large data files, requiring large amounts of computer memory and making the 3D reconstruction process slower.

1.4
Data Visualization

Once the volume has been created, it can be viewed interactively by the use of any 3D visualization and rendering software. Visualization of 3D data plays an important part in the development and use of 3D ultrasound, with three predominant approaches being utilized thus far: surface rendering, multiplanar reconstructions, and volume rendering.

1.4.1
Surface Rendering

Surface rendering is the most common 3D display technique. In surface rendering the surfaces of structures or organs are portrayed in the rendition. Surface can be extracted manually or automatically. Manual segmentation methods give the most accurate surface but are a lengthy and laborious task for the operator. Unfortunately, currently available automatic segmentation methods, requiring simple user assistance, cannot be guaranteed always to work correctly in large applications. With this approach the boundaries are represented by a wire frame or mesh, and the surface is texture mapped with an appropriate colour and texture to represent the anatomical structure (FENSTER and DOWNEY 2000; DOWNEY et al. 2000). Echocardiographic (RANKIN et al. 1993; WANG et al. 1994) and fetal (NELSON and PRETORIUS 1992; KELLY et al. 1994; LEE et al. 1995) 3D studies represent the major clinical applications of this rendering technique.

1.4.2
Multiplanar Reconstruction

Two different multiplanar reconstruction techniques have been developed: section display and texture mapping.

Section display allows visualization of multiple sections of the acquired volume scan along three orthogonal planes: the acquisition plane, transverse or sagittal reconstructed plane, and C-plane (parallel to the transducer surface). Computer-user interface tools allows the operator to rotate and reposition these planes so that the entire volume of data can be examined. Because this technique is easy to implement and allows short 3D reconstruction times it has been widely used in clinical applications (HAMPER et al. 1994).

The second technique, called texture mapping, displays the 3D image as a polyhedron with the appropriate anatomy texture mapped on each face. The reconstructed structure can be viewed by slicing into the volume, interactively, to form a cross-sectional image of the volume acquired in any orientation. As a result, this rendering approach provides a good means for visualizing spatial relationships of the entire volume in a readily comprehensible manner (FISHMAN et al. 1991; TONG et al. 1996).

1.4.3
Volume Rendering

Volume rendering methods map voxels directly onto the screen without using geometric primitives. They require that the entire data set be sampled each time an image is rendered or re-rendered. Volume rendering algorithms are attractive tools for displaying an image that synthesizes all the data contained in the numerical volume. The most popular volume visualization algorithm for the production of high-quality images is ray-casting. With the ray-casting approach a 2D array of rays is projected through the 3D image. Shading and transparency voxel values along each ray are then examined, multiplied by factors, and summed to achieve the desired rendering result. A wide spectrum of visual effects can be generated depending on how the algorithm interacts with each voxel encountered by a particular ray. Maximum and minimum intensity projection (MIP) methods are one form of ray-casting where only the maximum (or minimum) voxel value is retained as the ray traverses the data volume. These techniques are quite simple to implement and provide good quality results for several applications (PRETORIUS and NELSON 1994;

NELSON and PRETORIUS 1998; FENSTER and DOWNEY 2000). As a result, volume rendering displays the anatomy in a translucent manner, simulating light propagation in a semitransparent medium. Obviously if the image is complex, with soft tissue structures, interpretation is difficult, even with the addition of depth cues or stereo viewing. Thus, this rendering approach is best suited to simple anatomical structures in which image clutter has been removed or is not present. Volume rendering is been used with excellent results, particularly in displaying fetal (PRETORIUS and NELSON 1995; NELSON et al. 1996; BABA et al. 1997, 1999) and cardiovascular anatomy (SALUSTRI et al. 1995; MENZEL et al. 1997; KASPRZAK et al. 1998).

References

Baba K, Okai T, Kozuma S (1997) Real-time processable three-dimensional US in obstetrics. Radiology 203:571–574

Baba K, Okai T, Kozuma S (1999) Fetal abnormalities: evaluation with real-time-processable three-dimensional US: preliminary report. Radiology 211:441–446

Baum G, Greenwood I (1961) Orbital lesion localization by three dimensional ultrasonography. NY State J Med 61:4149–4157

Brandal H, Gritzky A, Haizinger M (1999) 3D ultrasound: a dedicated system. Eur Radiol 9:S331–S333

Davidsen RE, Smith SW (1997) A two-dimensional array for B-mode and volumetric imaging with multiplexed electrostrictive elements. Ultrason Imaging 19:235–250

Davidsen RE, Jensen JA, Smith SW (1994) Two-dimensional random arrays for real time volumetric imaging. Ultrason Imaging 16:143–163

De Castro S, Yao J, Pandian NG (1998) Three-dimensional echocardiography: clinical relevance and application. Am J Cardiol 18:96G–102G

Downey DB, Fenster A (1995a) Vascular imaging with a three-dimensional power Doppler system. AJR 165:665–668

Downey DB, Fenster A (1995b) Three-dimensional power Doppler detection of prostatic cancer. AJR 165:741

Downey DB, Fenster A, Williams JC (2000) Clinical utility of three-dimensional US. Radiographics 20:559–571

Elliot TL, Downey DB, Tong S (1996) Accuracy of prostate volume measurements in vitro using three dimensional ultrasound. Acad Radiol 3:401–406

Fenster A, Downey DB (2000) Three-dimensional ultrasound imaging. Annu Rev Biomed Eng 2:457–475

Fishman EK, Magid D, Ney DR (1991) Three-dimensional imaging. Radiology 181:321–337

Hamper UM, Trapanotto V, Sheth S (1994) Three-dimensional US: preliminary clinical experience. Radiology 191:397–401

Hamper UM, Trapanotto V, DeJong MR (1999) Three-dimensional US of the prostate: early experience. Radiology 212:719–723

Hodges TC, Detmer PR, Burns PH (1994) Ultrasonic three-dimensional reconstruction: in vivo and in vitro volume and area measurement. Ultrasound Med Biol 20:719–729

Johnson DD, Pretorius DH, Budorick NE (2000) Fetal lip and primary palate: three-dimensional versus two-dimensional US. Radiology 217:236–239

Kasprzak JD, Salustri A, Roelandt JR (1998) Three-dimensional echocardiography of the aortic valve: feasibility, clinical potential, and limitations. Echocardiography 15:127–138

Kelly IG, Gardener JE, Brett AD (1994) Three-dimensional US of the fetus: work in progress. Radiology 192:253–259

King DL, King DL Jr, Shao MYC (1990) 3-D spatial registration and interactive display of position and orientation of real-time ultrasound images. J Ultrasound Med 9:525–532

Klein HM, Gunther RW, Verlande M (1992) 3D-surface reconstruction of intravascular ultrasound images using personal computer hardware and a motorised catheter control. Cardiovasc Intervent Radiol 15:97–100

Lee A, Kratochwil A, Deutinger J (1995) Three-dimensional ultrasound in diagnosing phocomelia. Ultrasound Obstet Gynecol 5:238–240

Light ED, Davidsen RE, Fiering JO (1998) Progress in two-dimensional arrays for real-time volumetric imaging. Ultrason Imaging 20:1–15

Menzel T, Mohr-Kahaly S, Kolsch B (1997) Quantitative assessment of aortic stenosis by three-dimensional echocardiography. J Am Soc Echocardiogr 10:215–223

Nelson TR, Pretorius DH (1992) Three-dimensional ultrasound of fetal surface features. Ultrasound Obstet Gynecol 2:166–174

Nelson TR, Pretorius DH (1998) Three-dimensional ultrasound imaging. Ultrasound Med Biol 24:1243–1270

Nelson TR, Pretorius DH, Sklansky M (1996) Three dimensional echocardiographic evaluation of fetal heart anatomy and function: acquisition, analysis, and display. J Ultrasound Med 15:1–9

Ofili EO, Navin CN (1994) Three-dimensional and four-dimensional echocardiography. Ultrasound Med Biol 20:669–675

Pretorius DH, Nelson TR (1994) Prenatal visualization of cranial sutures and fontanelles with three-dimensional ultrasonography. J Ultrasound Med 13:871–876

Pretorius DH, Nelson TR (1995) Fetal face visualization using three-dimensional ultrasonography. J Ultrasound Med 14:349–356

Rankin RN, Fenster A, Downey DB (1993) Three-dimensional sonographic reconstruction: techniques and diagnostic applications. AJR 161:695–702

Salustri A, Spitaels S, McGhie J (1995) Transthoracic three-dimensional echocardiography in adult patients with congenital heart disease. J Am Coll Cardiol 26:759–767

Smith SW, Trahey GE, von Ramm OT (1992) Two-dimensional arrays for medical ultrasound. Ultrason Imaging 14:213–233

Steiner H, Staudach A, Spinzer D (1994) Three-dimensional ultrasound in obstetrics and gynaecology: technique, possibilities and limitations. Hum Reprod 9:1773–1778

Thrush AJ, Bonnett DE, Elliott MR (1997) An evaluation of the potential and limitations of three-dimensional reconstructions from intravascular ultrasound images. Ultrasound Med Biol 23:437–445

Tong S, Downey DB, Cardinal HN (1996) A three-dimensional ultrasound prostate imaging system. Ultrasound Med Biol 22:735–746

Turnbull DH, Foster FS (1992) Simulation of B-scan images from two-dimensional transducer arrays. II. Comparisons between linear and two-dimensional phased arrays. Ultrason Imaging 14:344–353

Turnbull DH, Lum PK, Kerr AT (1992) Simulation of B-scan images from two-dimensional transducer arrays. I. Methods and quantitative contrast measurements. Ultrason Imaging 14:323–343

von Ramm OT, Smith SW (1990) Real time volumetric ultrasound imaging system. J Digit Imaging 3:261–266

Wang XF, Li ZA, Cheng TO (1994) Clinical application of three-dimensional trans-esophageal echocardiography. Am Heart J 128:380–388

2 CT Image Acquisition: from Single Slice to Multislice

Michael Macari and Gary Israel

CONTENTS

2.1 Introduction

In 1972, EMI introduced the first CT scanner into clinical practice. This unit was specifically engineered to image the brain. The total scan time was approximately 25 min, and produced five images displayed with an 80×80 matrix. These CT scanners, now referred to as conventional CT scanners, involve alternating patient exposure and patient translation (Brink 1995). In this scanner, the X-ray tube and the detector array move in a 360° circle around the stationary table and patient. Currently, it takes approximately 1 s to rotate the tube 360° around the patient and another second to move the patient to the next Z-axis position. Therefore, the scanning efficiency of this system is about 50% (Hu 1998). With conventional CT, a slice thickness and gap between slices are chosen. Furthermore, to increase Z-axis coverage, the slice collimation or interslice gap need to be increased with resultant loss of Z-axis resolution. While conventional CT revolutionized the way medicine was practiced, it is rapidly becoming obsolete.

M. Macari, MD, G. Israel, MD
Department of Radiology, Abdominal Imaging, NYU Medical Center, 560 First Avenue, Suite HW 206 and 207, New York, NY 10016, USA

A major advance in CT technology occurred with the development and implementation of helical CT in 1989, allowing simultaneous patient translation and X-ray exposure (Kalendar et al. 1990; Brink 1995). Helical CT enabled a greater Z-axis distance to be covered in a shorter time period. This reduced artifacts related to patient motion, breathing, and bowel peristalsis and allowed for specific anatomic areas to be covered during peak contrast enhancement. The image quality of helical and conventional CT are equivalent for most parameters with the exception of noise and slice section sensitivity profile. The degree of these differences is dependent on the CT parameters and the reconstruction algorithms used during helical scanning (Polacin et al. 1992). Helical images are noisier. In addition, the helical CT slice broadens during the acquisition since the table and tube are moving simultaneously. As a result, the slice thickness is actually greater than the collimation selected. The degree of slice broadening is related to pitch and limits the speed of table translation with respect to slice collimation (pitch) during helical scanning.

The most recent advance in CT technology has been multidetector row helical CT (Fig. 2.1). Current multislice scanners allow four signals to be acquired

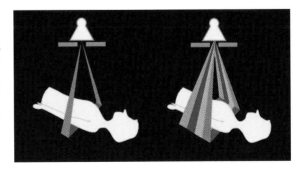

Fig. 2.1. Schematic representation of single-slice acquisition (*left*) and multislice acquisition (*right*). During multislice acquisition up to four signals are acquired with each 360° tube rotation. This allows faster data acquisition, greater anatomic coverage, and thinner slice collimation. (Image courtesy of David Naidich, MD, NYU Medical Center)

with each tube rotation, potentially allowing data to be acquired 4 times faster than with single-slice scanners. As a result, CT data can be obtained faster, with thinner slice collimation and with better contrast utilization than with single-slice helical CT. With the development of multislice CT and current imaging workstations, the radiologist is no longer restricted to axial slice review (Fig. 2.2). Utilizing a single acquisition, thin section (near-isotropic voxel) CT data can be viewed in any orientation (coronal, sagittal, axial and oblique) (Fig. 2.2). Familiarity with this new technology and its capabilities will be critical to optimizing the way radiology is practiced in the new millennium (RUBIN et al. 1996). While many CT applications can be performed adequately with single-slice scanners, multislice CT offers many advantages. This chapter will focus on the transition of CT imaging from single-slice to multislice technology.

duced which allowed four simultaneous slices to be obtained per rotation. As pointed out in a recent article regarding terminology for multislice CT systems, many terms have been used to describe this technology including multidetector row CT, multi-row helical CT, multidetector helical CT, and multislice helical CT, resulting in confusion (SILVERMAN et al. 2001). Since detector elements are set up differently in different machines (matrix detector for GE and adaptive array detector for Siemens) it has been suggested that multislice CT is the most appropriate terminology since multiple slices are being generated per gantry rotation. In the near future CT systems will be available where eight slices are available per gantry rotation. Throughout this paper multislice helical CT will be used to describe the technology whereby multiple CT slices are generated per tube rotation.

2.2
Terminology

In 1989, helical CT was introduced which allowed a single CT slice to be obtained per tube rotation during patient translation. In 1992, a dual-detector helical CT system was introduced by Elscint that allowed two CT slices to be obtained per tube rotation. In 1998, helical CT systems were intro-

2.3
Fundamental Differences Between Single-Slice and Multislice CT

Multislice helical CT refers to a CT system equipped with multiple rows of detectors arranged along the Z-axis (patient orientation) as opposed to the single-row array used with conventional helical CT systems (HU et al. 2000). Depending on the CT manufacturer, the number of detectors along the Z-axis

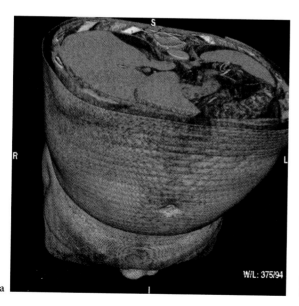
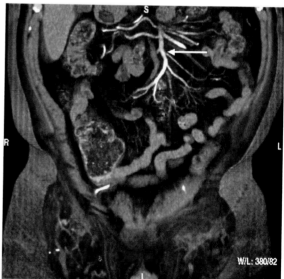

Fig. 2.2a, b. Multislice helical CT data is no longer restricted to axial interpretation. **a** Using multislice CT a 3D volume of data is obtained. **b** Coronal view of the superior mesenteric artery (*arrow*) from the same data set as in **a**. Current workstations allow multislice data to be viewed in any plane, which allows better interpretation and display to clinical colleagues

varies (RYDBERG et al. 2000). In our practice, the GE Light Speed and Siemens Volume Zoom are being utilized. The GE Light Speed detector configuration consists of 16 contiguous 1.25-mm-thick detectors (matrix detector), while the Siemens Volume Zoom scanner consists of two central 1.0-mm detectors with a 1.5-mm, 2.5-mm, and 5.0-mm detector on either side of them (adaptive array detector). In each case the length of the entire detector configuration is 20 mm. Regardless of the detector configuration, four signals must be acquired with each tube rotation with either system. There are potential advantages in the design of each system, which will not be discussed here. The main advantages of multislice CT systems over single-slice systems are increased speed of coverage, decreased scan time, and an opportunity for near-isotropic voxel display. All these factors are interrelated and, depending on the clinical indication, different variations in multislice technology can be used to optimize the examination.

The first advantage of multislice CT is acquisition speed (Fig. 2.3), which is increased for two reasons. First, four signals are acquired for each tube rotation with a multislice CT scanner as opposed to the single-detector systems where a single slice is acquired. For example, if 5-mm-thick sections are required for a particular clinical application, a multislice CT could acquire four 5-mm-thick sections (20 mm coverage/rotation) during a single tube rotation as opposed to a single 5-mm slice (5 mm coverage/rotation) utiliz-

ing single-slice technology. Second, the gantry rotation speed of most multislice CT systems is faster than in single-row systems. In most single-row systems, the X-ray tube completes one rotation every 0.8–1.0 s whereas in many multislice CT systems a 0.5-s gantry rotation speed is available. The increased speed of multislice CT systems allows better utilization the contrast bolus (Fig. 2.4).

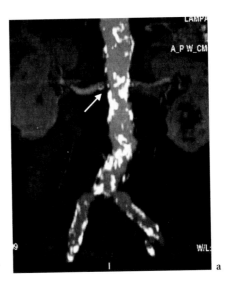

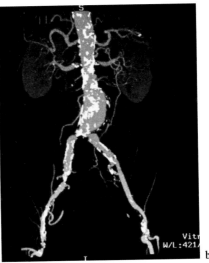

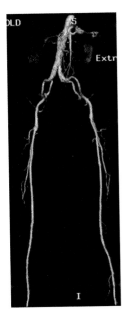

Fig. 2.3. Multislice CT angiogram demonstrating speed and Z-axis coverage of data acquisition. Volume rendered CT angiogram shows the aorta from the supraceliac region to the distal calf runoff. Acquisition was performed with a 4×2.5-mm detector configuration, pitch 1.5 and 0.5 s tube rotation (3 cm coverage/second) in 40 s. Short acquisition time eliminates most breathing and motion artifact and allows the examination to be performed using a single dose of 150 ml of iodinated contrast material

Fig. 2.4a, b. Better utilization of contrast material and improved Z-axis resolution with multislice CT. **a** CT angiography (CTA) performed on a single-slice CT scanner with 3 mm collimation, pitch 2 and 1 s tube rotation time (6 mm coverage/second) shows the abdominal aorta and renal artery stenosis (*white arrow*) with poor opacification of the pelvic runoff vessels. **b** CTA performed on the same patient 1 year later with a multislice scanner using a 4×1-mm detector, pitch 2 and 0.5 s rotation time (16 mm coverage/second) shows improved visualization of runoff vessels and improved Z-axis resolution

The second advantage of multislice is that thinner slice collimation can routinely be obtained (Fig. 2.5). Thin collimation facilitates near-isotropic voxel acquisition enabling useful multiplanar reconstructions of axial data. Using single-slice CT, the X-ray beam collimation affects the volume coverage and the slice thickness (HU 1998). An advantage of multislice CT is that the X-ray beam collimation only partially affects the slice collimation. For example, if we choose 10 mm X-ray beam collimation and a pitch of 1 in a single-slice CT scanner, we cover 10 mm of Z-axis in a single rotation and obtain a 10-mm-thick slice. Utilizing multi-row CT scanning, the same 10 mm X-ray beam can be further divided by the detector row collimation into four 2.5-mm-thick sections. This increases Z-axis resolution by a factor of 4. Alternatively, utilizing multislice CT, a 20-mm X-ray beam collimation can be chosen which can be subdivided into four 5-mm sections by the detector row collimation. Utilizing this scenario (when compared with single-slice CT utilizing a 10-mm X-ray beam) the speed of Z-axis coverage is increased by a factor of 2 (20 mm vs 10 mm) and Z- axis resolution is increased by a factor of 2 (5 mm vs 10 mm). The ability to subdivide the X-ray beam collimation into smaller components is what facilitates thinner slices and near-isotropic voxels.

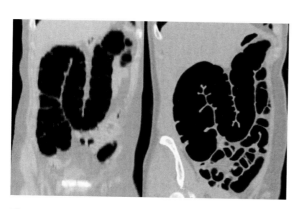

Fig. 2.5. Near-isotropic voxel dimension display is possible using thin collimation with multislice CT. Coronal multiplanar reconstruction (MPR) colonographs of two different patients. The image on the *left* was with single-slice CT using 5 mm collimation, pitch 2 with 2 mm reconstruction overlap. Effective slice thickness in the Z-axis is 6.5 mm. The image on the *right* is with multislice CT using a 4×1-mm detector configuration, pitch 2 and 0.75 mm overlap. Effective slice thickness is 1 mm in the Z-axis, which is only slightly larger than the X and Y pixel dimension

2.4
Pitch, Slice Sensitivity Profile, and Reconstruction Algorithm

The radiologist needs to be familiar with several technical aspects of helical CT in order that data acquisition can be optimized. The first parameter is pitch.

Pitch refers to the table feed (in millimeters) per gantry rotation/slice thickness (HU 1998). Using single-slice helical CT, if the table moves 5 mm per gantry rotation and the slice thickness is 5 mm, the pitch equals 1 (5 mm/5 mm). If the table moves 10 mm per rotation and the slice thickness is 5 mm, the pitch equals 2 (10 mm/5 mm). As pitch increases, Z-axis coverage per unit time is increased. Unfortunately, the penalty for increasing pitch is slice sensitivity broadening (BRINK 1995). The greater the pitch, the faster the table moves during the data acquisition, and the more the slice broadens. At a pitch of 2, the slice sensitivity is broadened by 30% at full width half maximum (FWHM) compared with a pitch of 1. For example, if data are obtained utilizing 3 mm collimation and pitch 2, 6 mm of Z-axis is covered per gantry rotation but the effective slice thickness is not 3 mm but 3.9 mm [3 mm + (3 mm×0.3)]. This still compares favorably with scanning the same Z-axis coverage using 5-mm-thick collimation and pitch 1. Utilizing these parameters, 5 mm of Z-axis coverage is obtained per gantry rotation with an effective slice thickness of 5 mm. In general, a pitch value of greater than 2 should not be used with single-slice spiral CT because of image degradation.

There has been some confusion regarding the precise definition of pitch utilizing multislice CT technology. In fact, there are two definitions. Using multislice CT, pitch has been defined as the table feed per tube rotation/nominal section thickness as determined by the detector row collimation, not the total X-ray beam collimation (HU 1998). Since all current multislice CT systems acquire four signals per tube rotation, the nominal section thickness is defined as the thickness of the detector row collimation that makes up one of the four signals. For example, if the abdomen and pelvis is scanned utilizing a 4×2.5-mm detector configuration (10 mm X-ray beam collimation) and the table feed per rotation is 15 mm the pitch is 6 [15 mm (table feed per rotation)/2.5 mm (nominal section thickness)]. An alternative definition of pitch utilizing a multislice CT system is table feed per gantry rotation/total X-ray beam collimation (RYDBERG et al. 2000; SILVERMAN et al. 2001). In the above example, utilizing this definition, pitch is 1.5 [15 mm (table feed per rotation)/10 mm (total

X-ray beam collimation)]. Both definitions of multislice CT pitch should be understood although some have advocated using the definition of pitch as equal to table feed per gantry rotation/total X-ray beam collimation since it is more consistent with the original definition of pitch for single-slice systems and causes less confusion (McCollough and Zink 1999; Fuchs et al. 2000).

Direct reconstruction of helical images over any 360° segment will result in motion artifact due to patient transport (Polacin et al. 1992). The CT slice profile is broadened over the nominal value by using pitch >1 and by utilizing different reconstruction algorithms (180° vs 360°). One way to limit the broadening that occurs with helical CT is to use a 180° linear interpolation (LI) algorithm as opposed to 360° algorithms. Polacin et al. have shown that all data reconstruction processing algorithms result in slice broadening; however, the effect is much reduced using 180° algorithms compared with 360° algorithms. For example, if one uses a 5-mm section thickness and pitch of 1, the slice profile at FWHM is 6.3 mm and 5.0 mm using 360° and 180° LI algorithms respectively. The effect of slice broadening and choice of reconstruction algorithm is more pronounced at higher pitch levels. If the pitch equals 2, the slice profile at FWHM of that same 5-mm-thick slice is 10.8 mm and 6.4 mm using 360° and 180° LI algorithms respectively. Therefore, it is clear that a higher pitch increases the slice sensitivity profile, and a 180° LI algorithm substantially decreases broadening when compared with a 360° LI algorithm. For almost all single-slice CT reconstructions a 180° LI algorithm is used.

For multislice CT systems, the principles are similar. One hundred and eighty degree LI algorithms are used to reconstruct data but all available points in the Z direction are weighted by a Z filter that helps to reduce data transition artifacts (Fuchs et al. 2000). Utilizing the GE Light Speed unit and 180° LI algorithms, the two standard pitch values available [3 (0.75) and 6 (1.5)] are referred to preferred pitch. Studies performed with the Siemens Volume Zoom unit and 180° LI algorithms have demonstrated no substantial slice broadening over the nominal slice thickness at FWHM up to a pitch value of 8.

2.5
Clinical Advantages of Multislice Relative to Single-Slice CT in the Abdomen

As stated above, the advantages of multislice CT are increased speed, greater anatomic coverage and thinner slice collimation. Utilizing multislice CT, multiple acquisitions within a short period of time are now feasible. This allows dynamic acquisitions through an organ during different phases of intravenous contrast enhancement. This potentially will increase lesion detection and may also allow better characterization as enhancement patterns over time can be studied. The utilization of multiple data acquisitions with multidetector CT has probably been best studied in the liver.

There are many factors that potentially allow increased conspicuity of hypervascular tumors in the liver, including rate and amount of iodinated contrast injection, patient size, slice collimation, window/level settings, and timing of data acquisition. With single-slice CT, dynamic imaging of the liver is limited to just two acquisitions after a bolus of contrast material is injected. These acquisitions generally include an arterial phase performed at between 20 and 25 s and a portal venous phase performed between 70 and 75 s after injection. With multislice scanners, multiple acquisitions are now possible and may allow increased detection of hypervascular lesions (Fig. 2.6). Different investigators have advocated performing multiple acquisitions in patients with hepatic cirrhosis to increase detection of hypervascular tumors. In one study, three acquisitions were advocated including a double arterial (early and late arterial phase) and a portal venous phase to increase detection of hepatocellular carcinoma (Murakami et al. 2001). In this study, double arterial phase imaging showed significantly superior sensitivity to early or late phase arterial imaging alone. Double arterial phase imaging is only possible with multislice systems. A second study showed the benefits of the early arterial, portal inflow (late arterial) and hepatic venous phases when evaluating hypervascular tumors in cirrhotic and non-cirrhotic patients (Foley et al. 2000). In this study, tumor detection was greatest on the late arterial phase images but optimal hepatic arteriograms were obtained during the early arterial phase images. Others have found that by utilizing thinner collimation, which is possible with multidetector CT systems, greater detection of liver lesions is possible. One study found a 46% and 33% increase in the detection rate of hepatic lesions using 2.5-mm sections when compared with 10-mm and 7.5-mm sections respectively (Weg et al. 1998).

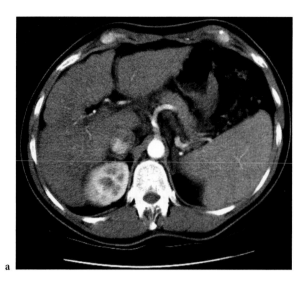
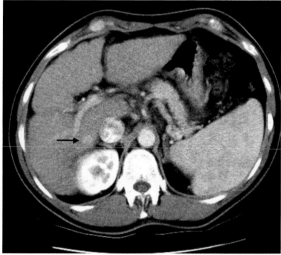

a   b

Fig. 2.6a, b. Utilization of multiple acquisitions to improve lesion detection. **a** Axial CT image in a cirrhotic patient during the arterial phase (23 s after a contrast bolus of 4 ml/s) shows no lesion. **b** Axial CT image in the same patient at 40 s (late arterial phase/portal inflow phase) now shows a hypervascular lesion (*arrow*) in segment VI. Multiple acquisitions potentially allow better depiction of small hypervascular lesions in the liver

In the future, multislice CT may change the practice of medicine. For example, when assessing pancreatic neoplasms, evaluation of peripancreatic vessels has become very important in determining possible resectability (HOUGH et al. 1999). By utilizing multiplanar and volume rendered images, thin section multislice CT will better depict the relationship of the neoplasm to the surrounding vessels (Fig. 2.7). In addition to evaluating the larger vessels such as the superior mesenteric artery and vein, multislice CT will improve assessment of the small peripancreatic vessels that are often dilated in cases of tumor invasion into the superior mesenteric vein (VEDANTHAM et al. 1998).

In assessing the abdominal vasculature non-invasively, multislice CT has become a very important modality in displaying high-quality angiograms (Fig. 2.4). This is especially important with the increasing availability and utilization of bifurcated endovascular stents whose distal ends are deployed in the iliac arteries. This has made the need for longer Z-axis coverage of CT angiography (CTA) necessary. Aside from the aneurysm size, presence of accessory renal arteries and angulation and tortuosity of the aneurysm and aneurysm neck, the presence of iliac and femoral arterial stenoses need to be determined (QANADLI et al. 2000). Traditionally, a combination of conventional angiography and CTA was felt to be necessary to provide all these data. However, multislice technology can reliably provide high-quality CT data sets that may answer all the clinical ques-

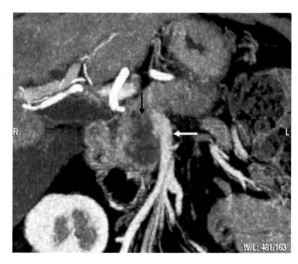

Fig. 2.7. Thin section multislice CT in assessing peripancreatic vascular invasion. Coronal MPR of pancreas during the pancreatic phase of contrast enhancement (40 s after a bolus of iodinated contrast material at 4 ml/s) shows low attenuation mass (*black arrow*) in the head of pancreas consistent with adenocarcinoma. The superior mesenteric vein (*white arrow*) is tethered along its interface with the neoplasm suggesting invasion

tions, and obviate the need for more invasive studies (Fig. 2.8).

With its increased speed of acquisition and thinner slices, multislice CT has replaced single-slice acquisition for CT colonography at our institution. A

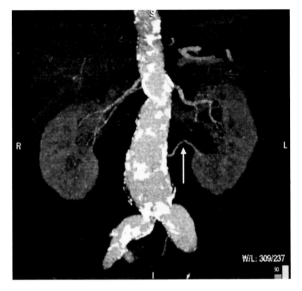

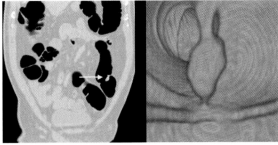

Fig. 2.9. Improved morphologic evaluation at CT colonography with multislice CT. Coronal MPR colonograph (*left*) shows a pedunculated polyp in the descending colon (*arrow*). Three-dimensional endoluminal volume rendered image (*right*) shows a polypoid lesion in the colon

Fig. 2.8. Multislice CT in aortic endograft planning. Coronal maximum intensity projection (MIP) of the abdominal aorta shows an accessory left renal artery (*arrow*) arising from the aneurysm sac and supplying the lower pole of the left kidney. Improved resolution with multislice CT obviates the need for preoperative angiography in many patients

recent study points out the advantages of multislice CT with respect to single-slice techniques in terms of breathing and respiratory artifacts, and degree of colonic distension (HARA et al. 2001). In this study, improved polyp detection with multislice CT compared with single-slice acquisition was not proven. However, the authors had only a small number of significant-sized polyps in each group, and in both single and multislice acquisitions 5-mm-thick slices were used. With thinner slice collimation, improved morphologic evaluation is possible and may improve detection of polyps of all sizes.

Using a single-slice acquisition, our CT colonography protocol consists of 5-mm-thick sections, reconstructed every 2 mm, obtained with pitch of 2 and a 1 s gantry rotation time. This allowed 10 mm coverage per second and an effective slice thickness of 6.4 mm. Currently, using multislice CT, a 4×1-mm detector configuration is used to obtain slices 1.25 mm thick which are reconstructed every 0.75 mm. Pitch is varied between 5 and 7 to allow the data acquisition to occur in a 30 s breath-hold. Because the multislice CT scanner has a 0.5 s gantry rotation time, 10–14 mm is obtained in 1 s with an effective slice thickness of 1 mm. The difference in Z-axis resolution is clear, facilitating multiplanar reconstruction (MPR) and 3D rendering (Fig. 2.9).

2.6
Caution

Does every patient undergoing CT need to be scanned with thin collimation in order to obtain near-isotropic voxels to facilitate MPR and 3D renderings? The answer is no. There are three main reasons for this: an overload of CT data, increased radiation exposure with thinner collimation and, perhaps most importantly, because in many cases the thin collimation is simply not necessary.

Multislice CT may produce extremely large numbers of CT slices. This has been termed a "data explosion" (RUBIN 2000). Current CT workstations are equipped to handle increasingly large data sets and will continue to improve in the future. However, some multislice CT studies such as CTA may produce as many as 1000 transverse axial CT slices (RUBIN et al. 1999). How we interact with these increasingly large data sets is important. Clearly, 1000 transverse axial images cannot be reviewed in the traditional fashion using film. Picture archiving communication systems (PACS) also will be limited when evaluating such large data sets. What will be required is workstations that allow interactive axial, MPR and 3D renderings to be performed in a seamless environment. These workstations are currently available but do slow down when extremely large data sets need to be evaluated. The issue of "CT data explosion" is important, especially since CT manufacturers plan on releasing scanners that will allow up to 8 simultaneous signals to be acquired per gantry rotation.

Not every imaging application needs 2.5-mm-thick sections to be filmed or archived. This will result in too much data. Five-millimeter- or even 7.5-mm-thick sections are usually adequate for data evaluation. Our routine protocol for multislice abdominal and pelvic CT in oncology patients, patients with acute abdominal symptoms, or those undergoing CT for trauma utilizes a 4×2.5-mm collimator detector configuration. Depending on the scanner (GE or Siemens) either 5 mm- or 7-mm-thick sections are reconstructed. When reviewing these thicker images, if there is a question or suspicion of an abnormality, or if multiplanar reconstructed images are required, the initial CT data can be accessed and reconstructed to allow thinner slices and a greater amount of overlap to facilitate optimal evaluation (Fig. 2.10).

The second reason why we should be cautious when performing thin-section multislice CT is the increased radiation dose to the patient which occurs secondary to thinner slices and increased scatter from adjacent slices (HIDAJAT et al. 2001). Special caution should be used with multislice CT since there is a tendency to scan more often and with thinner slices, increasing radiation dose to the patient.

Finally, for some imaging applications the question of significance is important. Is it necessary to obtain the thinnest slices in all patients (BERLAND and SMITH 1998)? For example, is it important to detect a 6-mm low-attenuation lesion that cannot be further characterized at CT? What is the significance of detecting 15 hypervascular lesions versus 10 lesions in a cirrhotic liver? Multislice CT protocols should be tailored to answer the relevant clinical questions.

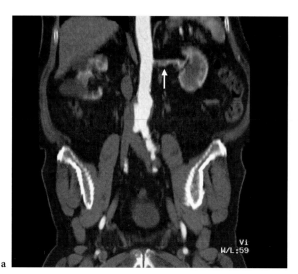

a

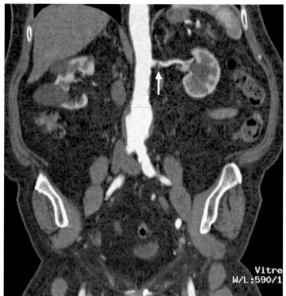

b

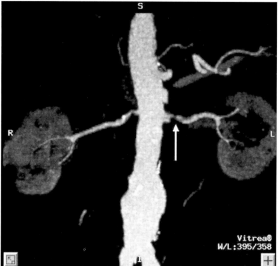

c

Fig. 2.10a–c. Utilization of the ability to reconstruct images at multiple different slice thicknesses and degrees of overlap from a single CTA data set. CTA performed with 4×1-mm detector configuration and pitch 1.5. a Coronal MPR image after data were reconstructed as 3-mm-thick slices overlapped every 2 mm shows blurring of the left renal artery (*arrow*). b With images reconstructed at 1.25 mm thickness and overlapped every 0.75 mm a stenosis is clearly seen at the origin of the left renal artery (*arrow*). c After postprocessing to remove bones, the stenosis is better appreciated (*arrow*)

2.7
Conclusion

Multislice CT offers many advantages over single-slice CT and is clearly the future of helical CT imaging. The increased speed, greater Z-axis coverage, and near-isotropic voxel dimensions are all advantages of multislice relative to single-slice techniques. Caution should be used when performing multislice CT since it is possible to obtain innumerable slices and acquisitions, with a resultant increase in radiation exposure to the patient.

References

Berland LL, Smith JK (1998) Multidetector-array CT: once again technology creates new opportunities. Radiology 209:327–329

Brink JA (1995) Technical aspects of helical CT. Radiol Clin North Am 33:825–840

Foley WD, Mallisee TA, Hohenwalter MD, et al (2000) Multiphase hepatic CT with a multirow detector CT scanner. AJR 175:679–685

Fuchs T, Kachleriess M, Kalendar WA (2000) Technical advances in multi-slice spiral CT. Eur J Radiol 36:69–73

Hara AK, Johnson CD, McCarty RL, et al (2001) CT colonography: single versus multi-detector row imaging. Radiology 219:461–465

Hidajat N, Wolf M, Nunnemann A, et al (2001) Survey of conventional and spiral CT doses. Radiology 218:395–401

Hough TJ, Raptopoulos V, Siewert B, et al (1999) Teardrop superior mesenteric vein: CT sign for unresectable carcinoma of the pancreas. AJR 173:1509–1512

Hu H (1998) Multi-slice helical CT: scan and reconstruction. Med Phys 26:5–17

Hu H, He DH, Foley DW, et al (2000) Four multidetector-row helical CT: image quality and volume coverage speed. Radiology 215:55–62

Kalendar WA, Sesser W, Klotz E, et al (1990) Spiral volumetric CT with single-breath-hold technique, continuous transport, and continuous scanner rotation. Radiology 176:181–183

McCollough CH, Zink FE (1999) Performance evaluation of a multi-slice CT system. Med Phys 26:2223–2230

Murakami T, Tonsok K, Takamura M, et al (2001) Hypervascular hepatocellular carcinoma: detection with double arterial phase multi-detector row helical CT. Radiology 218:763–761

Polacin A, Kalendar WA, Marchal G (1992) Evaluation of section sensitivity profiles and image noise in spiral CT. Radiology 185:29–35

Qanadli SD, Mesurolle B, Coggia M, et al (2000) Abdominal aortic aneurysm: pretherapy assessment with dual-slice helical CT angiography. AJR 174:181–187

Rubin GD (2000) Data explosion: the challenge of multidetector-row CT. Eur J Radiol 36:74–80

Rubin GD, Napel S, Leung AN (1996) Volumetric analysis of volumetric data: achieving a paradigm shift. Radiology 200:312–317

Rubin GD, Shaiu MC, Schmidt AJ, et al (1999) CT angiography: historical perspective and new state-of-the-art using multi-detector-row helical CT. J Comput Assist Tomogr 23:S83–S90

Rydberg J, Buckwalter KA, Caldemeyer KS (2000) Multisection CT: scanning techniques and clinical applications. Radiographics 20:1787–1806

Silverman PM, Kalender WA, Hazle JD (2001) Common terminology for single and multislice helical CT. AJR 176:1135–1136

Vedantham S, Lu DS, Reber HA, et al (1998) Small peripancreatic veins: improved assessment in pancreatic cancer patients using thin section pancreatic phase helical CT. AJR 170:377–383

Weg N, Scheer MR, Gabor MP (1998) Liver lesions: improved detection with dual-detector-array CT and routine 2.5 mm thin collimation. Radiology 209:417–426

3 MR Image Acquisition: From 2D to 3D

Luis Martí-Bonmatí

CONTENTS

3.1 Introduction

In MR imaging, two-dimensional Fourier transformation (2DFT) of the data has been the most commonly used and robust data processing method. Three-dimensional Fourier transformation (3DFT) imaging has been available in MR imaging since its early days (Johnson et al. 1983; Young 1984; Aichner et al. 1994). All the MR pulse sequences used with 2DFT can be also acquired with 3DFT. Initially, the higher acquisition times of these images was responsible for them being little used. However, the interest in three-dimensional (3D) imaging is continuously increasing. Nowadays, the higher quality and gradient power of the MR systems in use, as well as the advances in image processing technologies and computing, are responsible of the increasingly common use of three-dimensional images in the clinical setting.

In routine practice, most of the MR imaging techniques now in use are planar 2DFT, or simply 2D (two-dimensional) imaging, in which only two spatial dimensions have to be encoded. The techniques which spatially encode the whole volume are known as 3DFT, or simply 3D imaging. In 3D reconstruction, in addition to the readout gradient the data are collected with phase encoding pulsed gradients fields in two directions (Johnson et al. 1983; Aichner et al. 1994; Rinck 2001), the reconstruction being done along the three dimensions.

In 2D acquisition, the slice thickness is determined by gradient strength. The individual slices have a limitation in the slice thickness, because of the direct relationship with the signal-to-noise ratio: the lower the slice thickness, the less the signal from a given voxel due to the lower number of protons within the voxel. It is therefore unusual to have a slice thickness lower than 3 mm in 2D acquisition. Also, in 2D acquisition the slices are usually separated by a gap of non-included tissue. Truly cubic voxels are called isotropic, i.e., have the same dimensions in all the three axes. One way to obtain images with isotropic voxels and high spatial resolution is 3D acquisition, which covers the region of interest without any gaps. In 3D sequences, the object can be represented by a 3D array of cubic voxels. This increases the spatial resolution in all the directions of the volume of interest, allowing the use of postprocessing algorithms to increase the diagnostic power of the radiologist.

In this chapter we will cover the basics of 3D image acquisition and discuss the resulting image quality, finishing with some clinical applications.

3.2 Image Acquisition

3.2.1 2D Acquisition

In MR imaging it is possible to encode spatial information by using a magnetic gradient in the slice direction because of the dependence of resonance frequency on local magnetic field strength. In 2D

L. Martí-Bonmatí, MD, PhD
Dr. Peset University Hospital, Unidad de Resonancia Magnetica, Avenida Gaspar Aguilar 90, 46017 Valencia, Spain

imaging a slice defined by the xy coordinates is excited by applying a selective radiofrequency pulse in the presence of the slice selective gradient (Fig. 3.1). The concept of slice selective excitation is related to the creation of a small field gradient along the longitudinal z direction and the application of a radiofrequency pulse covering a specific frequency range. In this way, only the macroscopic magnetization of that particular frequency will be affected and encoded. Thus, a given frequency is related to a position in space of the nuclei emitting that frequency (NITZ 1999). In this way, a set of voxels in an xy plane is defined with a z gradient. The stronger the z gradient, the thinner the slices.

To obtain spatial information for the remaining two dimensions, a combination of phase and frequency encoding is now necessary (Fig. 3.2). The gra-

dients in the frequency encoded x axis and in the phase encoded y axis will give a unique characteristic to each voxel in the xy plane. Encoding in the phase direction will cause a phase shift as a function of location with n voxel rows in the direction of phase encoding. For these n voxel rows, n phase encoding steps are needed, consuming most of the time of the MR sequence (Fig. 3.3). After this second gradient, a third magnetic field gradient is established perpendicular to the direction of slice selection and phase encoding directions. By doing this, the resonance frequencies will be also different for portions along the readout or frequency direction. This magnetic field produces a frequency range over the field of view generating columns of voxels with the same frequency range or bandwidth. Together with the slice encoding Z-axis gradient, all the voxels in the differ-

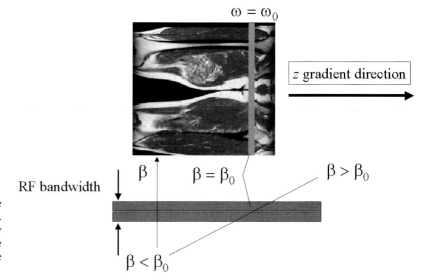

Fig. 3.1. Selection of an axial slice is accomplished by the z gradient. Slice location is determined by the resonance frequency. The slice thickness is determined by the range of frequencies (bandwidth)

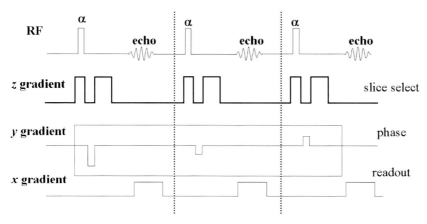

Fig. 3.2. The radiofrequency pulse generates an echo. Within the imaging plane, spatial encoding is generated by phase and frequency encoding gradients

ent slices that constitute the MR acquisition sequence will have a unique characteristic.

The phase encoding preparation gradient is switched on and off while the frequency encoding readout gradient is changed n times for a resolution of n pixels (Fig. 3.3). The 2D data matrix is processed with an inverse 2D technique.

3.2.2
3D Acquisition

Three-dimensional imaging methods are an elaboration of 2D techniques. In 2D techniques, although the data are acquired from a volume, the final result is a set of 2D images. In 3D imaging, the entire sample volume is excited simultaneously by applying the radiofrequency pulse without a slice gradient (Fig. 3.4). To obtain information in the slice encoding direction, a second phase encoding gradient is applied. In 3D imaging, the reconstructed slices should be called partitions. These partitions

are selected by the application of a second phase encoding gradient such that the final voxels will have unique phase angles in two dimensions and a unique frequency of precession in the third dimension. All the digitized data values of the induced currents are stored in a raw data buffer or k space. In 3D, the k space is three-dimensional, with a representation of the x, y and z spatial distribution frequencies (Fig. 3.5). In 3DFT imaging, each measured line contains information on the whole object and all data are recorded from the entire volume of interest, while in 2DFT data are recorded only from the slice selective portion of the volume of interest.

In a graphic representation of a 3D sequence, two phase codifications are simultaneously applied after the initial radiofrequency pulse. The incorporation of a second phase encoding codification in the slice direction (Gz) will notably increase the acquisition time. For every partition in the slice direction, all the phase encoding in the y direction must be repeatedly obtained (Fig. 3.5). Due to the smaller thickness of the partitions in the longitudinal direction, 3D

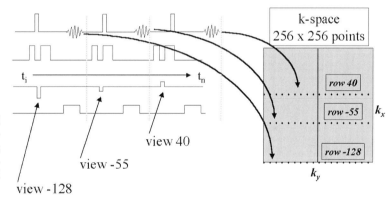

Fig. 3.3. The whole 2D process is repeated n times in the y direction with a different phase encoding gradient. Resolution in the phase encoding direction is proportional to the number of phase steps used to acquire the image

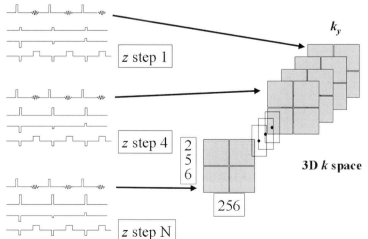

Fig. 3.4. In 3D acquisition, the z gradient is changed after all the y gradient phase encodes have generated an echo, producing a 3D k space

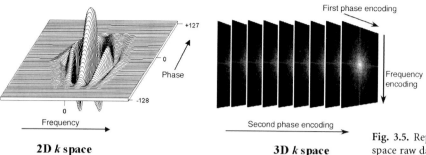

2D k space   **3D k space**

Fig. 3.5. Representation of 2D and 3D k space raw data matrix

sequences usually have an increase in the number of reconstructed images, from tens to hundreds compared with 2D acquisitions. This fact will increase even more the acquisition time compared with 2D images.

Since it is necessary to wait for equilibrium after the acquisition of each profile, the total scan time is very long and proportional to the number of profiles per plane times the number of planes or partitions (JOHNSON et al. 1983; YOUNG 1984; EDELMAN et al. 1990; RINCK 2001). Examination time in a 3D sequence is the result of multiplying several factors: TR (repetition time), matrix size in the phase encoding direction (Ny), number of steps or partitions in the slice direction (Nz) and the number of signal averages (NSA):

Acquisition time: TR · Ny · NSA · Nz

Three-dimensional sequences in clinical use with MR machines need to be obtained within a reasonable measurement time. This can be done mainly with short repetition times [3D gradient recalled echo (GRE) T1-weighted images] or fast imaging sequences. Several options can be used to shorten the acquisition time: (1) shorten the TR, increasing the T1 weighting of the images; (2) do not acquire all the profiles, reducing the matrix size along any or all of the three spatial directions (in the slice direction, reducing the spatial coverage, and in the in-plane encoding steps, reducing resolution); (3) use rectangular or asymmetric fields of view while maintaining the volume of interest within the acquired data set; and (4) partial Fourier methods (PRINCE et al. 1997). The use of fast sequences is based on the utilization of multiple echoes to speed up the filling of the k space [3D turbo spin echo (TSE) and 3D echo planar image (EPI) sequences)] or the acquisition of only half the k space (3D half Fourier imaging). Within these sequences, acquisition time will diminish proportional to these factors.

The slice profile of the 3D data set is nearly rectangular. Due to the phase encoding along the slice selection direction, ringing artifacts can occur producing imperfectly rectangular slice profiles. In 2D imaging, the imperfect slice profiles preclude the use of contiguous slices. When narrow gaps are used in 2D imaging, each slide is contaminated by radiofrequency excitations from the edges of the adjacent slides, a phenomenon called "cross-talk", degrading the resulting images. With 3D images, contiguous partitions will produce high-quality postprocessing reconstruction in any arbitrary plane or orientation.

3.3
3D Images

3.3.1
Signal-to-Noise Ratio

The signal-to-noise ratio (SNR) represents the graininess of an image. In 3D imaging, the SNR is proportional to

$$\frac{B_0^2 \cdot k \cdot PD \cdot f(TR,\alpha) \cdot FOV^2 \cdot \sqrt{CS} \cdot \sqrt{ST} \cdot \sqrt{Nz} \cdot \sqrt{NSA}}{f(TE) \cdot \sqrt{CSV} \cdot \sqrt{N_Y}}$$

where B_0 is the strength of the static magnetic field, k is a constant, PD is the proton density of the tissue, CS the chemical shift, ST the slice thickness and CSV the coil sensitive volume. SNR is directly proportional to the voxel volume, which is related to the acquisition matrix and the field of view in the xy plane. The matrix represents the number of pixels along the frequency (x) and phase (y) encoding axes. The field of view can be defined as the horizontal and vertical distance across the image. Spatial resolution improves as the field of view decreases, within the constraints of signal-to-noise limitations (EDELMAN et al. 1990). The voxel size in the X-axis is the ratio between the length of the field of view in that direction (Lx) and the acquisition matrix in the frequency encoding direction (Nx). Similarly, the voxel size in the y-axis is the ratio between the field of view dimension in that direction (Ly) and the acquisition matrix in the phase encoding direction (Ny). The height of the voxel (Lz) is the slice thickness in 2DFT imaging but the total coverage in the z plane in a 3DFT sequence:

Volume of the voxel = (Lx/Nx) · (Lx/Ny) · Lz

As the number of protons per voxel for a uniform tissue is linearly proportional to the voxel volume, the signal per voxel is also linearly proportional to the voxel volume. Noise, however, is independent of the voxel volume (HENDRICK 1999). Therefore, SNRs in 3D imaging are much higher. In 3D imaging, this large parallelepiped will be divided into several smaller voxels along the z-axis by the application of a second phase encoding step gradient. The number of partitions will be determined by the number of distinct phase encoding steps in this direction. The reconstructed slice thickness in 3D imaging is the ratio between the length of the volume in the longitudinal dimension (Lz) and the number of steps in the second phase encoding dimension (Nz).

The slices in a 3D MR image are resolved by inverse Fourier transforming a collection of k space data samples from MR signals corresponding to every step of the first phase encoding gradient. Each k space data sample contributes to every voxel, increasing the SNR. Each section in a 3D acquisition of S partitions contributes signals S times more often than does the corresponding 2D acquisition (CARLSON et al. 1988), with an advantage of $\sqrt{s}$ in SNR if the other factors are held constant. In this situation, for a constant TR, the imaging time in 3D will be S times longer than in 2D, finally giving similar efficiencies (CARLSON et al. 1988). The SNRs per unit imaging time of 2D multislice and 3D imaging sequences, when optimized, have been proven to be usually similar (JOHNSON et al. 1999). Furthermore, for a fixed imaging time and number of sections, 3D imaging with conventional spin echo sequences had a worse SNR than 2DFT images.

In every phase codification, the signal comes from the whole excited volume and not from only one slice. This advantage is mainly evident only for very thin (<2 mm) section imaging and in combination with partial flip angle and fast MR imaging (CARLSON et al. 1988). With these techniques, the cross-talk or interference among the sections is minimized.

3.3.2
Spatial Resolution

A region of interest is specified by creating a rectangular box that delimits the anatomic region in all dimensions. The region of interest will be constituted by a rectangular array of voxels with assigned values. The achieved in-plane spatial resolution is related to the field of view and matrix size, and to the slice thickness in 2D imaging and partition thickness in 3D imaging. Partition thickness is the thickness of the reconstructed slice in a 3D acquisition. The basic matrix size dictates the size of the pixel and the number of protons involved.

In 3D imaging, the voxel dimensions can be isotropic or near-isotropic (Fig. 3.6). In isotropic voxels the three dimensions of the volume element are equal. In near-isotropic voxels one of the dimensions is larger than the others. This limits the spatial resolution, usually in the slice selection direction. The spatial resolution in the z direction in 3D imaging is further improved by the fact that no gap is left between partitions, with a fully contiguous coverage in all three axes. Isotropic voxels are important in MR imaging in most cases because they allow the reconstruction of postprocessing images with superb quality. In 2D imaging, the gap can be also set to 0, with contiguous slices, by using interleaved slice ordering, usually increasing the acquisition time.

The spatial resolution of an image can be defined as the ability to discern two different points that are close together as separate and distinct. For a given MR sequence, the spatial resolution is given by the SNR and voxel size. Voxel size is related to the pixel size and the longitudinal slice directed z direction.

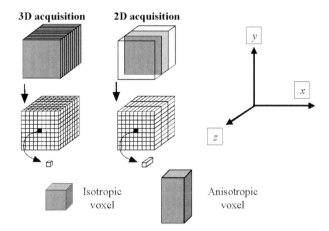

Fig. 3.6. Representation of isotropic and anisotropic voxels. Isotropic voxels have the same dimensions in all the axes

The in-plane resolution is given by the x and y directions, related to the relationship between the field of view (FOV) and the number of phase and frequency encoding codifications. In most 2D images, the higher slice thickness and the presence of a gap between slices limit the longitudinal z resolution.

Three-dimensional methods use a weak slice selection gradient for a given partition thickness, allowing the acquisition of very thin sections and limiting partial volume effects (EDELMAN et al. 1990). The number and thickness of these slices will be proportional to the excited volume of interest and to the number of steps in the second phase encoding direction. As an example, if a volume of interest has 50 mm in the z direction, 50 phase encoding steps will give 50 reconstructed images each 1 mm high. The individual source images in 3D images are reconstructed from the volume data and not from the excitation of individual 2D slices. In 3D imaging the slices are always contiguous or even overlapped.

3.3.3
Artifacts

Resolution power is an image quality characteristic that can be defined as the ability to discriminate an object from its surroundings. Resolution power is proportional to the square root of the SNR, but inversely related to the presence and severity of image artifacts. To obtain a high resolution power, 3D images are well designed because of their higher SNR. However, although the mechanisms are multifactorial, 3D images are prone to motion artifacts that will limit image quality.

Artifacts can be defined as any signal intensity, or void, that does not have an anatomic basis in the image. This factor is related to a poorer image quality and tissue contrast. Elimination of motion artifacts is important in order to obtained better-quality MR images. In 3D imaging, each k space data sample contributes to every voxel. This fact increases the SNR ratio but makes 3D images vulnerable to artifacts. This is due to the fact that in 3D imaging, for each phase encoding step in one direction, all the encoding steps in the other perpendicular direction have to be repeated in order to distinguish two orthogonal phase encoding directions. Elimination of motion artifacts is done mainly by limiting the source of movement. In 3D imaging, it is important that the area of interest remains immobilized.

Apart from motion artifacts, there is an increase in aliasing in the slice select direction, especially in 3D contrast-enhanced MR images. This effect is due to the Ernst angle on unenhanced background tissue occurring on the falling edges of the set flip angle profile (WESBEY et al. 1990). Also, truncation artifacts or Gibbs artifacts can occur in the slice selective direction due to the phase encoding of the data. Furthermore, due to the imperfect slab profile produced by the radiofrequency pulse and the warp along the slice selection direction, there is some data degradation at the outer part of the volume in the z phase encoding direction. This effect is minimized by obtaining partitions only from a thick slab within the volume of interest.

3D GRE images reduce T2* effects and show fewer susceptibility artifacts compared with 2D GRE acquisitions. This is due to the compensation of the local field inhomogeneities by the increased number of phase encoding steps along the z direction (WESBEY et al. 1990). With enough partitions, certain strengths of the z gradient will cancel focal field inhomogeneities produced by the susceptibility variations. Furthermore, susceptibility artifacts decrease with slice thickness, and 3D techniques can produce very thin slices. As an example, this will produce a better delineation of the interface between the brain and the air-containing skull base structures in 3D than in 2D GRE images.

3.3.4
Display

In 3D imaging, extensive anatomic regions can be covered with high resolution in all three directions. True 3D imaging is becoming more accessible with the continued development of instrumentation. The quantity of data and images is greatly increased with these techniques. The display modes of the acquired 3D images can be broadly classified into 2D display (image-by-image, cine mode), surface display and volume display. Although printing thousands of images is very impractical, this number can be limited by photographing only one of every two or three images or fusing two or even more partitions to make hard copies. In this way, the number of hard copies will be reduced. In practical use, 3D data should be visualized on the monitor of the workstation. Cine mode, surface and volume displays are used to increase the diagnostic power of these images. Volume display takes fully advantage of the nature of the 3D data matrix, allowing visualization with volume rendering and maximum intensity projection modes. Three-dimensional data also allow the reconstruction of high-quality multiplanar reconstruction (MPR), precise tissue segmentation and quantification, volume registration and virtual endoscopic views.

3.3.5
Clinical Applications

In certain applications it is advantageous to perform a 3D data acquisition. Most applications of 3D imaging involved the use of TSE or EPI sequences with large TE (echo time) values for T2 weighting and short TR short TE GRE sequences for T1 weighting. Therefore, high-resolution imaging can be obtained in short scanning times in any desired weighting. The following are some areas where 3D imaging has been proven to be clinically useful.

MR Angiography. Three-dimensional GRE sequence with very short TE and TR will produce a very short acquisition time, catching the peak of the arterial enhancement after contrast administration throughout the region of interest. This technique has been validated as a very useful diagnostic tool in the evaluation of the supra-aortic, abdominal and peripheral vessels (Prince 1994; Prince et al. 1997; Remonda et al. 1998; Glockner 2001).

Abdomen. Three-dimensional GRE sequences afford comparable and usually better image quality than 2D images, increasing the conspicuity and confidence for focal lesions (Kim et al. 2001). Breath-hold contrast-enhanced very thin 3D GRE T1-weighted images can be obtained at the arterial, portal and delayed phases after the administration of a contrast agent (Fig. 3.7). This technique has been proven useful in the analysis of different vascular and non-vascular processes affecting the liver and kidneys (Rofsky et al. 1999; Heiss et al. 2000). The superb spatial, temporal and contrast resolution allow studies to be performed in multiple vascular phases, increasing the diagnostic accuracy of both vascular and parenchymal abnormalities.

Biliary, Pancreatic and Renal Tube System. Although these tubes can be visualized by heavily T2-weighted

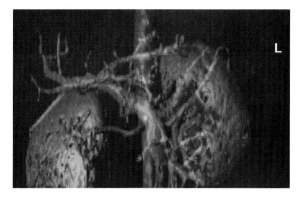

Fig. 3.7. Volume rendering of a 3D T1-weighted GRE breath-hold sequence (TR/TE/flip angle, 4/1.2/20°, 2×1.4×2 mm voxel) showing the aorta, renal arteries and portal vein

3D images and with maximum intensity projections and even virtual endoscopy, the use of very fast single-shot T2-weighted acquisitions is usually preferred to obtain MR cholangiopancreatography and MR urography images.

Brain. Three-dimensional GRE T1-weighted images are very important in the analysis of congenital malformations and cortical dysplasia and to perform brain volume quantification (Fig. 3.8). Three-dimensional T2-weighted images are useful in the analysis of the cranial nerves and tumor volume measurements (Yamada et al. 2000; Yousry et al. 2000). Also, these T2-weighted 3D images with maximum intensity projections produce very detailed examinations of inner ear anomalies. Dynamic 3D GRE T1-

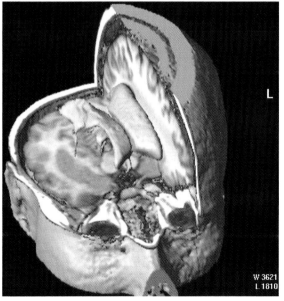

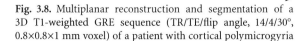

Fig. 3.8. Multiplanar reconstruction and segmentation of a 3D T1-weighted GRE sequence (TR/TE/flip angle, 14/4/30°, 0.8×0.8×1 mm voxel) of a patient with cortical polymicrogyria

weighted angiography is more efficient than 2D MR angiography techniques in the evaluation of intracranial aneurysms (METENS et al. 2000).

Spine. Two- and three-dimensional images give a similar tissue contrast, although 3D TSE T2-weighted images may demonstrate lesions less clearly than 2D images (SWAINSON et al. 1997).

Musculoskeletal. In 3D imaging of both temporomandibular joints, a 3D multislab method can be used to selectively excite the slabs at different times during the TR cycle. This method will provide 3D images of both joints in the same acquisition time as a single joint examination. The 3D images can be also used to quantify cartilage volume and analyze its surface (Fig. 3.9).

Colonoscopy. 3D GRE T1-weighted images after the filling of the colon with a gadolinium-water mixture (1:100) allow the evaluation of colonic polyps with great accuracy, either by direct inspection of the source images or by virtual colonoscopy (LUBOLDT and DEBATIN 1998).

Thorax. The use of gadolinium-enhanced 3D GRE T1-weighted sequences improves the quality of the

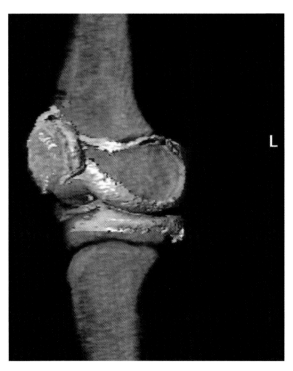

Fig. 3.9. Surface reconstruction of a 3D EPI GRE proton density weighted sequence, showing cartilage segmentation

MR examination in the evaluation of infiltrates, lung cancer, and pulmonary metastases (SEMELKA et al. 2000).

3.4
Conclusions

Three-dimensional Fourier transformation, or simple 3D acquisition, is a MR data acquisition method in which a thick volume is excited and thin slices, or partitions, are resolved by phase encoding along the slice selection direction. In 3D the phase encoding is done along the y and z directions. A variety of methods to increase the speed of 3D acquisitions will improve the clinical utility of these sequences even further. This novel imaging will allow faster acquisition or improved resolution.

In 3D acquisition, the excitation pulse of every cycle will affect the whole volume of data, making the sequence sensitive to motion.

3.4.1
Advantages

For thinner slices with smaller pixels acquired within an acceptable time, the SNR is higher in 3D images than in 2D images (for the same voxel size, the SNR increases as the square root of the number of slices). The slice profile of the 3D data set is rectangular. Slices are contiguous without any gap between them, allowing high-quality image processing, such as multiplanar and surface reconstructions. The 2D technique has the disadvantage of usually leaving small gaps between the slices. Three-dimensional images suffer fewer susceptibility artifacts.

3.4.2
Disadvantages

The acquisition times in 3D acquisition are longer than in similar 2D acquisitions. A number of techniques to decrease acquisition times are used to decrease the scan duration: very short repetition times, different k space samplings, and fast imaging can be used. The susceptibility to motion is higher in 3D acquisition, due to the fact that every echo has information on the whole volume of data. There is an increase in aliasing in the slice select direction, especially in 3D contrast-enhanced MR images.

Acknowledgements. Thanks go to Han Rademaker, Philips Sistemas Médicos, and Javier Lafuente, H.G. Gregorio Marañón, for their help in the preparation of the illustrations.

References

Aichner FT, Felber SR, Muller RN (1994) Three-dimensional magnetic resonance imaging. Blackwell Scientific Publications, Oxford

Carlson J, Crooks L, Ortendahl D (1988) Signal-to-noise ratio and section thickness in two-dimensional versus three-dimensional Fourier transform MR imaging. Radiology 166:266–270

Edelman RR, Kleefield J, Wentz KU (1990) Basic principles of magnetic resonance imaging. In: Edelman RR, Hesselink JR (eds) Clinical magnetic resonance imaging. Saunders, Philadelphia

Glockner JF (2001)Three-dimensional gadolinium-enhanced MR angiography: applications for abdominal imaging. Radiographics 21:357–370

Heiss SG, Shifrin RY, Sommer FG (2000) Contrast-enhanced three-dimensional fast spoiled gradient-echo renal MR imaging: evaluation of vascular and nonvascular disease. Radiographics 20:1341–1352

Hendrick RE (1999) Image contrast and noise. In: Stark DD, Bradley WG (eds) Magnetic resonance imaging, 3rd edn. Mosby, St Louis

Johnson G, Hutchison JMS, Redpath TW (1983) Improvements in performance time for simultaneous three-dimensional NMR imaging. J Magn Reson 54:374

Johnson G, Wadghiri YZ, Turnbull DH (1999) 2D multislice and 3D MRI sequences are often equally sensitive. Magn Reson Med 41:824–828

Kim MJ, Mitchell DJ, Ito K (2001) Hepatic MR imaging: comparison of 2D and 3D gradient echo techniques. Abdom Imaging 26:269–276

Luboldt W, Debatin JF (1998) Virtual endoscopic colonography based on 3D MRI. Abdom Imaging 23:568–572

Metens T, Rio F, Baleriaux D (2000) Intracranial aneurysms: detection with gadolinium-enhanced dynamic three-dimensional MR angiography: initial results. Radiology 216:39–46

Nitz W (1999) Principles of magnetic resonance imaging and magnetic resonance angiography. In: Reimer P, Parizel PM, Stichnoth FA (eds) Clinical MR imaging. Springer, Berlin Heidelberg New York, pp 1–36

Prince MR (1994) Gadolinium-enhanced MR aortography. Radiology 191:155–164

Prince MR, Grist TM, Debatin JF (1997) 3D contrast MR angiography. Springer, Berlin Heidelberg New York

Remonda L, Heid O, Schroth G (1998) Carotid artery stenosis, occlusion, and pseudo-occlusion: first-pass, gadolinium-enhanced, three-dimensional MR angiography – preliminary study. Radiology 209:95–102

Rinck PA (2001) Magnetic resonance in medicine. Blackwell Wissenschafts-Verlag, Berlin

Rofsky NM, Lee VS, Laub G (1999) Abdominal MR imaging with a volumetric interpolated breath-hold examination. Radiology 212:876–884

Semelka RC, Cem Balci N, Wilber KP (2000) Breath-hold 3D gradient-echo MR imaging of the lung parenchyma: evaluation of reproducibility of image quality in normals and preliminary observations in patients with disease. J Magn Reson Imaging 11:195–200

Swainson CJ, Hutchinson CE, Watson Y (1997) A comparison of 2-D and 3-D FSE imaging in MR of the cervical spine. Clin Radiol 52:194–197

Wesbey G, Edelman RR, Harris R (1990) Artifacts in MR imaging: description, causes, and solutions. In: Edelman RR, Hesselink JR (eds) Clinical magnetic resonance imaging. Saunders, Philadelphia

Yamada I, Tsunoda A, Noguchi Y (2000) Tumor volume measurements of acoustic neuromas with three-dimensional constructive interference in steady state and conventional spin-echo MR imaging. J Magn Reson Imaging 12:826–832

Young SW (1984) Magnetic resonance imaging: basic principles, 2nd edn. Raven Press, New York

Yousry I, Camelio S, Schmid UD (2000) Visualization of cranial nerves I–XII: value of 3D CISS and T2-weighted FSE sequences. Eur Radiol 10:1061–1067

4 Surface Rendering

Andreas G. Schreyer, Simon K. Warfield

CONTENTS

4.1
Principles of Visualization

Surface rendering represents a visualization technique which is well established for three-dimensional imaging of sectional image data. This chapter describes image acquisition and data preparation for surface shaded rendering. Additionally the basics of the computational approach are described.

Three-dimensional (3D) visualization of sectional two-dimensional (2D) radiological data appears to be very helpful for diagnosis, as an interdisciplinary communication tool or for surgical planning.

Sectional images such as CT or MR acquisitions are not really 2D. These images always represent a slice of a particular volume with a certain thickness. Thus the pixels visualized on CT or MR images are called voxels because of their 3D nature. Because of the 3D character of the slices, 3D visualization can be achieved fairly straightforwardly.

A.G. Schreyer, MD
Department of Radiology, University Hospital Regensburg, Franz-Josef-Strauss Allee 11, 93053 Regensburg, Germany
S.K. Warfield, PhD
Surgical Planning Laboratory, Department of Radiology, Brigham and Women's Hospital Boston, 75 Francis Street, Boston, MA 02115, USA

First we should try to define the term "visualization". *Collins English Dictionary* describes it as "to form a mental image of something incapable of being viewed or not at that moment visible". Visualization is essentially a mapping process from reality into numbers (computer representation) into graphic display (pictures) into perceptual interpretation by the viewer. The main issue in visualizing volume data is how to display 3D data as a 2D image without losing too much information. There exist several well-developed techniques for displaying data cubes of sectional volume data. Slicing, volume rendering and surface rendering represent the most important techniques applied for 3D visualization. In slicing, a 2D plane, or slice, is extracted from the 3D data volume and displayed as a 2D image. The slice may be either parallel to one of the axes of the volume or at an arbitrary orientation. While a slice will show detailed information about the plane being displayed it does not give an impression of the entire volume. An effective way of visualizing the entire volume is to generate an animation showing a sequence of slices being swept through the volume parallel to one of the axes. Nevertheless this technique does not provide 3D visualization; the slices have to be connected to a 3D image mentally. To "escape flatland" 3D (or higher-dimensional) data have to be projected onto a 2D surface. There are basically two different techniques to represent a data volume with a 3D model. One of them is surface rendering, which is the topic of this chapter. This method basically involves constructing polygonal surfaces in the data sets and rendering these surfaces. On the other hand there is volume rendering, which involves assigning a color and opacity value to each data element and projecting the elements directly onto the image plane without the use of polygons. This technique is described in Chap. 5. There are certain advantages and disadvantages of both methods, which will be discussed later. The following section describes the work flow and techniques for creating surface shaded rendered 3D models.

4.2
Shaded Surface Rendering

4.2.1
Image Acquisition

Principally volume data have to be acquired for surface rendered models. In radiological imaging CT or MR imaging are suitable for 3D postprocessing. Three-dimensional ultrasound is a recently introduced modality which is capable of creating 3D models. Nevertheless, for surface rendering CT and MR imaging are the two main modalities. The quality and accuracy of 3D models is always dependent on the resolution of the original 2D acquisitions. To obtain optimal 3D models the dimensions of the voxels should be isotropic, which means that the voxel data cube is of similar lengths in all three room axes.

In CT imaging there is a high resolution of image data within the axial slice. In spiral CT an entire volume is acquired and the axial slices are computed with a certain slice thickness. Volume acquisition is a prerequisite for 3D postprocessing. Especially in the thorax and abdomen organ position is breath-dependent. The acquisition has to be performed within one continuous breath-hold to avoid different positions of the scanned organ. In spiral CT there is always a trade-off between volume coverage and resolution along the body axis (Z-axis). The recently introduced multislice scanners can at least improve the Z-axis resolution by covering the same volume with thinner slices. With a fixed length which covers the organs of interest for 3D imaging the slice thickness should always be as thin as possible to achieve near-isotropic voxels. For MR imaging so-called 3D sequences are achieving near-isotropic voxel resolution. Resolution in all three room axes should be as good as possible to avoid "stair step artifacts". A good contrast of a surface on the desired object is extremely helpful for automated segmentation. Thus, for example, bones in CT imaging are very easy to segment for surface rendering.

4.2.2
Image Enhancement and Filtering

After an image stack has been acquired it may be preprocessed to improve image quality prior to 3D reconstruction. The preprocessing typically involves application of image filters (mathematical algorithms implemented in software) to the entire data set to remove noise and artifacts, smooth or sharpen the images, or to correct for problems with contrast or brightness (SCHREYER 1998; STOLL 1999). Median and Gaussian filters have the general effect of smoothing images. These are used to eliminate noise and background artifacts and to smooth sharp edges, but also tend to remove some of the detail in small objects. Sharpening filters can be used to accentuate details in the image stack, but also have the effect of highlighting noise and other small artifacts. The application of sharpening filters is most useful when the image stack consists of fine structural components or when edge enhancement is desired. It is important to realize that the application of filters to the data set can ultimately affect quantitative measurements of 3D reconstructions produced from it. Therefore in some instances filters are only used for display purposes, and quantitative measurements are made on the unprocessed data.

4.2.3
Segmentation

To create a shaded surface 3D model the surface of the desired object has to be defined on every 2D sectional image. The term *segmentation* refers to the process of extracting the desired object of interest from the background in an image or data volume. There exist multiple techniques that are used to do this. A simple but time-consuming approach is to outline the desired structure on every image slice manually. But there are semiautomatic methods ranging from the simple, such as thresholding and masking, to the complex such as boundary detection, region growing and clustering algorithms. Moreover there are extremely subtle and computationally challenging automated approaches such as the adaptive template moderated (ATM) approach in combination with spatially varying statistical classification (SVC) (WARFIELD 2000).

Thresholding is a commonly used segmentation method suitable for high-contrast structures. Thresholding involves limiting the intensity values within an individual image or the entire image stack to a certain bounded range. It may be decided that all pixels below a certain value do not contribute significantly to the object of interest and hence can be eliminated. This can be done by scanning the image one pixel at a time, and keeping that pixel if it is above the selected intensity value or excluding it if it is below that value. In a similar manner, thresholding can also be used to eliminate non-consecutive ranges of intensities while preserving the regions containing the intensities of interest. Especially in CT imaging with defined Hounsfield units for voxel intensity it is possible to segment certain structures within particular density values. Consequently bones in CT imaging can be segmented very easily by including all voxels above a certain density. Again for this example contrast-enhanced vessels or a contrast-filled bowel lumen have to be excluded by time-consuming and arduous manual fine editing.

Masking is a procedure whereby an enclosed region of an image or image stack is defined for processing. This can be done either by manually tracing around the regions of interest (e.g., with a mouse in a graphics application) or by an automated routine. A mask can be formed by either manually tracing around the boundaries of the object of interest in the stacked projection or by absolute thresholding, which means making all intensities above a certain value part of the segmentation and excluding all voxels below this value. The mask can then be applied to the entire image stack, such that regions falling within the mask selection area are preserved whereas areas outside this region are eliminated. After the mask has been applied, thresholding and image filtering methods can be used to aid in removing the remaining undesired regions.

Using *connectivity*, connected voxels with similar intensity can be segmented in a volume stack. Applying seed-growing algorithms a seed within the desired object is set. The algorithm tries to find similar connected voxels within the slice itself and on the adjacent image slices. A problem arising from this approach is the spatial nearness of different tissues with similar density. For example, a contrast-enhanced aorta can be connected with the spine. In addition to manual fine tuning, an alternative solution to this problem is *erosion* and *dilatation*. Applying an erosion tool the outer row of pixels of the segmented area is removed. This can help to avoid seed-growing to undesired structures. Dilatation adds pixels again after segmentation has been performed. Thresholding and seed-growing are currently the most common approaches for semiautomatic segmentation. More sophisticated automated segmentation tactics are based on statistical classification of tissue intensity. Another fascinating technique for automated segmentation is the use of anatomical templates. By matching deformable models directly into the image data automated anatomical identification can be achieved (WARFIELD 2000).

4.2.4
3D Visualization

After segmentation on sectional data has been done, the surface of the volume data is generated by approximating and connecting the shape of inter-data boundaries. These visualization pipelines generate a triangle-based wire frame model, which represents the surface of the segmented data. Most commonly a marching cubes algorithm is used, which basically decides whether a surface passes through a data element or not. By "marching" through all the cubic cells intersected by the isosurface the algorithm calculates the intersection points along the edges and produces a triangular mesh to fit to these vertices. Smoothing and triangle count reduction can also be applied as a part of the visualization pipeline. The wire frame model can be covered by a virtual surface by assessing surface properties, reflection and color. In addition a virtual light source can be placed arbitrarily to accentuate the 3D impression.

4.3
Surface Rendering Versus Volume Rendering

Volume rendering is a computer graphics technique whereby the object of interest is sampled into many cubic building blocks, called voxels (volume elements). A voxel is the 3D counterpart of the 2D pixel and is a measure of unit volume. Each voxel carries one or more values for some measured or calculated property of the volume such as intensity value, and is typically represented by a unit cube. The 3D voxel sets are assembled from multiple 2D images, and are displayed by projecting these images into 2D pixel space where they are stored in a frame buffer. In surface rendering, the volumetric data must first be converted into geometric primitives by segmentation. These primitives (such as polygon meshes or contours) are then rendered for display using conventional geometric rendering techniques.

There are some advantages and pitfalls in both methods. An advantage of volume rendering is that the 3D volume can be displayed without any knowledge of the geometry of the data set and hence without intermediate conversion to a surface representation. This conversion step in surface rendering can sometimes be quite complex and can require major user intervention. On the other hand, because the 3D data set is reduced to a set of geometric primitives in surface rendering, this can result in a significant reduction in the amount of data to be stored, and can provide fast display and manipulation of the 3D reconstructions produced by this method. By contrast, since all the image stack data is used for volume rendering, computers with lots of memory and processing power are required to handle volumes rendered in this manner. Because the entire data set is preserved in volume rendering, any part, including internal structures and details, which may be lost when reducing to geometric structures with surface rendering, may be viewed. Thus in surface rendering information on the interior of the surface is lost. Even when semitransparent surfaces are rendered, detail is lost between the layers.

To summarize, volume rendering does not need major manual time-consuming postprocessing. Three-dimensional models can be generated immediately but visualization needs advanced and expensive computer hardware. Surface rendering needs time-consuming postprocessing and segmentation. The 3D models are dependent on the subjective segmentation process, which can be prone to individual error. Because of the segmentation process the 3D models are accurate and can be used for quantitative purposes or precise surgical planning. There are much lower requirements for expensive computer hardware than in volume rendering.

4.4
Clinical Applications

Most clinical applications which involve 3D visualization can be done with surface rendering. Most of these applications are covered in this book. Virtual endoscopy (Jolesz 1997) and surgical planning (Kikinis 1996) are typical applications of this technique. Especially in surgical planning, accurate segmentation with detailed surface rendered 3D models are necessary. For quantitative purposes and precise surgical planning such as that used in neurosurgery, segmented surface rendered models are superior to volume rendering. An interesting approach could be the combination of volume and surface rendering for

surgical planning: surface rendered models provide the detailed anatomical model while the volume rendered volume data provide the surrounding tissue and landmarks.

4.5
Conclusion

Surface rendering offers detailed 3D visualization of sectional image data. Fast 3D interaction and presentation can be done on less advanced computer workstations. The segmentation process is time-consuming and prone to individual error. In addition to semiautomatic segmentation routines such as thresholding and connectivity, which are commonly used in clinical environments, some subtle advanced segmentation algorithms such as adaptive, template-moderated statistical classification can be done. However, these approaches are very challenging and not yet commercially available. Although the usability of volume rendering seems to surpass that of surface rendering algorithms in most 3D visualization applications, there is still a need for surface rendering: accurate surgical planning needs segmentation to assign certain structures for visualization.

References

Jolesz FA (1997) Interactive virtual endoscopy. AJR 169:1229–1235

Kikinis R (1996) Computer-assisted interactive three-dimensional planning for neurosurgical procedures. Neurosurgery 38:640–651

Schreyer AG (1998) 3D modeling of the chest in patients with implanted cardiac defibrillator for further bioelectrical simulation. Computer Assisted Radiology and Surgery – CAR 1998, Tokyo. Elsevier Science, Amsterdam

Stoll E (1999) A new filtering algorithm for medical magnetic resonance and computer tomography images. J Digit Imaging 12:23–28

Warfield S (2000) Adaptive, template moderated, spatially varying statistical classification. Elsevier Science, Amsterdam

5 Volume Rendering

Nigel W. John

5.1 Introduction

Volume rendering is a popular technique used to represent and analyze volume data. The techniques employed can be a valuable aid in clinical applications such as diagnosis and preoperative planning, as they allow the user to see the internal structure and topology of the volume data. This chapter provides an overview of the terminology and main algorithms used in volume rendering. It also describes how this functionality is being implemented in real time to provide interactive clinical tools.

The aim of *volume visualization* is to realistically represent and analyze volume data. The resulting images, even though they are of course two-dimensional (2D), are often called 3D (three-dimensional) *images* or *3D reconstructions* to distinguish them

N.W. John, PhD
Deputy Director, Manchester Visualisation Centre, University of Manchester, Oxford Road, Manchester, M13 9PL, UK

from 2D cross-sections or conventional radiographs. The techniques employed allow the user to see the internal structure and topology of the volume data.

The medical field was the first to exploit volume visualization and the first attempts date back to the late 1970s, with clinical applications reported on the visualization of bone from CT in craniofacial surgery and orthopedics. As well as CT, today MR imaging, ultrasound, SPECT (single photon emission computed tomography) and PET (positron emission tomography) are all common sources of data for volume visualization. Figs.5.1 and 5.2 are typical images obtained from medical data. The same principles are also applied to sampled and simulated data from other domains, such as fluid dynamics, geosciences, confocal microscopy, scientific visualization and meteorology.

There are two basic classes of volume visualization algorithms in use today:
- Surface extraction algorithms
- Direct volume rendering algorithms

The key idea of *surface-based* rendering methods is to extract an intermediate surface description of the relevant objects from the volume data. Only this information is then used for rendering. This topic is covered in detail in Chap. 4 of this book.

In *volume rendering*, images are created directly from the volume data, and no intermediate geometry is extracted. This chapter will introduce you to the terminology and basic techniques needed to understand volume rendering, and provide an overview of the main algorithms used. More details can be found in reviews by Brodlie and Wood (2000), and Ezquerra et al. (1999).

5.2 Terminology

This section introduces the basic terminology used in volume rendering.

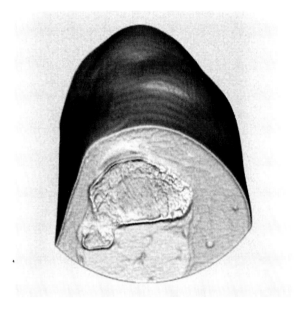

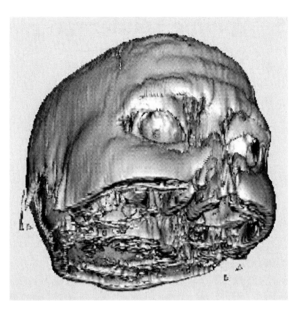

Fig. 5.1. Volume rendered image showing part of a human leg. Source was 58 slices of CT data scanned at a resolution of 512 by 512 pixels

Fig. 5.2. Volume rendering of a human head. Source was 40 slices of MR data scanned at a resolution of 512 by 512 pixels

5.2.1
Volume Grid

A volume is an array of data points arranged in some form of three-dimensional grid. Typically, the grid can be defined as: regular; rectilinear; curvilinear, block structured; unstructured; or some hybrid of these. Curvilinear and unstructured grids are common in numerical simulations and will not be addressed here. Rectilinear grids are by far the most common in medical applications, where data such as CT will have high resolution in the *XY* plane but much sparser resolution in the *Z* plane (the interslice distance). High-resolution medical scanners today can produce a regular grid where the sampling density is equal in all three dimensions, but such data sets are not commonly available to the clinician in a general hospital.

5.2.2
Voxel

Corresponding to the *pixels* (picture elements) of a 2D image, volume elements are called *voxels* (volume elements). The value of a voxel is the average value over the cell grid.[1] Although there is a single value

per voxel, it is recognized that a volume feature may only occupy a part of the voxel – this is called the *partial volume effect*. Common data structures used for voxel models are:
- *binary:* voxel values are either one (object) or zero (no object)
- *gray level:* each voxel holds an intensity value
- *generalized:* in addition to an intensity value, each voxel contains *attributes* describing its membership to various objects, and/or data from other sources
- *intelligent volumes:* an extension of the generalized voxel model, properties of objects (such as color) and their relationships are modeled on a symbolic level. Useful for creating medical atlases.

5.2.3
Resampling Methods

Many algorithms for volume visualization work on *isotropic* volumes, i.e., the data are sampled equally in all three dimensions. The missing information has to be reconstructed in an *interpolation* step. Two simple interpolation methods that can be used are: to select the intensity value of the nearest neighbor; or linear interpolation of the intensities between adjacent images (Fig. 5.3). Higher-order functions such as cubic functions and splines usually give better results

---

[1] Some algorithms will use a point model where data values are given at the vertices of the grid, and the behavior inside the voxel is interpolated from the vertex points.

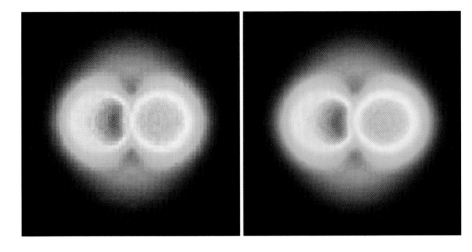

Fig. 5.3. Comparison of nearest neighbor and linear interpolation

for fine details, but are computationally more expensive. For rectilinear data, piecewise trilinear interpolation is common, providing an acceptable compromise between the faster but less accurate nearest neighbor, and the slower but more accurate tricubic interpolation.

5.2.4
Gradient Approximations

Due to the partial volume effect, the gray levels in the 3D neighborhood of a surface voxel represent the relative proportions of different materials inside these voxels. The resulting *gray level gradients* can thus be used to calculate surface inclinations. The gradient of the data set is defined as the rate of change in intensity values and emphasizes gray level differences. The greater the difference, the greater the gradient magnitude. In digital images, the gradient cannot be computed directly – instead we use some discrete approximation. The simplest variant is to calculate the components of a gradient G for a surface voxel at (i, j, k) from the gray levels, f, of its six neighbors along the main axes:

$$G_x = f(i+1,j,k) - f(i-1,j,k)$$
$$G_y = f(i,j+1,k) - f(i,j-1,k)$$
$$G_z = f(i,j,k+1) - f(i,j,k-1)$$

This is known as approximating the gradient by using *central differences*. Scaling G to unit length yields the unit surface vector, which is a good approximation of the surface normal:

$$\vec{N} = \frac{\vec{G}}{|\vec{G}|}$$

The gray level gradient may also be calculated from all 26 neighbors in a 3 by 3 by 3 neighborhood, weighted according to their distance from the surface voxel. Aliasing patterns are thus almost eliminated. The accuracy of this method is not satisfactory for very small objects such as thin bones, however.

5.2.5
Shading

In general, *shading* is the realistic display of an object based on the position, orientation and characteristics of its surface and the light sources illuminating it. The reflective properties of a surface are described with an *illumination model* such as the model developed by PHONG (1975), which uses a combination of ambient light, diffuse reflections (like those from paper) and specular reflections (like those from polished metal). A key input into these models is the local surface orientation, described by a *normal vector* perpendicular to the surface. The gradient approximation technique described above can be used to obtain an approximation of the normal vector at each voxel.

5.2.6
Data Classification

A voxel data set is often treated as a set of different colored transparent gels. This model allows for the concept of being able to see all of the data. Typically then, a voxel is assigned a color value, c, and a transparency value, α. Commonly used terms are:

- Opacity: all light is prevented from passing through the material $\alpha=1$).
- Transparency: all light passes through the material ($\alpha=0$).
- Translucency, or semi-transparency: graded transparency ($0<\alpha<1$).

A composite color is formed by summing the product of the percentage of each material times its color.

DREBIN et al. (1988) developed a probabilistic (fuzzy) scheme to classify air, fat, tissue and bone types in CT data. This method relies on the fact that not more than two tissue type distributions overlap. A voxel therefore contains one of seven possibilities: air; air and fat; fat; fat and tissue; tissue; tissue and bone; bone. Each voxel is assigned a material percentage, either directly or by using probabilistic classification such as the maximum-likelihood classifier. Given any material property and the material percentage models, a composite model for that property is calculated by multiplying the percentage of each material by the property assigned to each material. This method is not suitable if different structures have mostly overlapping or even identical gray level ranges. This situation frequently occurs! Here more sophisticated techniques such as multidimensional segmentation is needed (POKRIC et al. 2001).

5.3
Direct Volume Rendering

Direct volume rendering keeps all the gray level information originally acquired during the scanning process. This makes it an ideal technique for interactive data exploration. Threshold values and other parameters that are not clear from the beginning can be changed interactively. Furthermore, volume-based rendering allows a combined display of different aspects such as opaque and semi-transparent surfaces, cuts and maximum intensity projections. Compared with surface rendering techniques, direct volume rendering:
- renders the volume directly without recourse to intermediate geometry;
- allows the display of weak and fuzzy surfaces;
- relaxes the condition that a surface is either present or not.

Fig. 5.4 demonstrates the different results obtained by using volume and surface rendering techniques on the same data set, an MR scan of the inner ear.

A variety of software and hardware approaches are possible to implement direct volume rendering. Overviews of the main solutions in use today are presented below. We do not cover domain-based techniques, however, where the spatial volume data is first transformed into an alternative domain, such as the Fourier domain, and then a projection is generated directly from that domain.

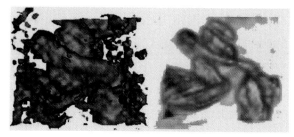

Fig. 5.4. Volume visualization of MR data of the inner ear (20 slices). *Left image* uses surface rendering. *Right image* uses direct volume rendering

5.3.1
Traversing the Volume

There are two basic scanning strategies for traversing the volume:
- *Feed-backward projection* or *image order traversal*. The pixels in the image plane are traversed and imaginary rays are cast through each pixel into the volume. The path of the ray determines the pixel value.
- *Feed-forward projection* or *object order traversal*. The data volume is traversed and each voxel in the volume is projected onto the image plane.

These strategies correspond to the image and object order rasterization algorithms used in computer graphics.

5.3.2
Volume Rendering Integral

For any ray, amount of light received at the image plane is:

$$I_\lambda = \int_0^L C_\lambda(s)\mu(s)e^{-\int_0^s \mu(t)dt} \, ds$$

where λ is wavelength, μ is density, L is length of ray, and $C_\lambda(s)$ is light of wavelength λ reflected at s in the ray direction. The volume rendering integral accumulates intensity over the length of a ray through the volume, attenuating it (the exponential term) according to the density of the material through which it passes. $C_\lambda(s)$ can be based on the Phong reflection model. The weighting by $\mu(s)$ reflects the density at the point – the greater the intensity, the greater the intensity of reflected light. Through a number of steps (BRODLIE and WOOD 2000), this integral can be approximated as:

$$I_\lambda = \sum_{i=0}^{n} C_\lambda(i)\alpha(i)\prod_{j=0}^{i-1}(1-\alpha(j))$$

Basically, this is a sum over intensities of individual samples, each intensity attenuated by the product of intensities accumulated as the light passes from sample to observer. The values of C and α are only known at data points, so interpolation is needed to calculate values at sample points $i\Delta s$.

5.3.3
Ray Casting

Ray casting is an image order traversal technique. Most implementations are based on the method developed by LEVOY (1988). The algorithm proceeds as follows:
- Shade the acquired data to obtain a volume of color values:
  a) Calculate the Normal for each voxel using a local gradient approximation, e.g., using central differences.
  b) Using an appropriate shading model, calculate a color/intensity value for each voxel, creating a volume of colors. Classify the data to obtain an opacity value for each voxel. Use a classification technique to assign opacity for each sample location. The optimum classification technique depends on the data type.
- At each sample point along the ray (Fig. 5.5), calculate the color and opacity using trilinear interpolation. The *Over* operator (PORTER and DUFF 1984) is typically used to composite the intensity values from back to front for all voxels along each ray.

The main disadvantage with ray casting is that it is computationally expensive – cost is proportional to the volume size. Several techniques have been proposed to speed up ray casting algorithms, including: early ray termination (LEVOY 1990); hierarchical spa-

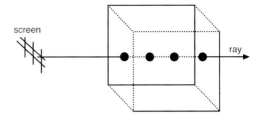

Fig. 5.5. Casting a ray through the volume grid. Composite color and opacity values at sample points to calculate the final pixel value

tial enumeration (LAUR and HANRAHAN 1991); templates (YAGEL 1992); space leaping (YAGEL 1993); and shear warp (LACROUTE and LEVOY 1994). Another alternative is to parallelize the ray casting code so that it can be used on multiprocessor systems. Many approaches have been implemented, covering shared memory (NIEH and LEVOY 1992; CHALLINGER 1992) and distributed memory architectures (ELVINS 1992; MA and PAINTER 1993).

5.3.4 Splatting

Splatting (WESTOVER 1991) is a good example of an object order traversal technique. The algorithm proceeds as follows:
- *Determine in what order to traverse the volume.* Voxels are projected in the order of their distance from the image plane a slice at a time. Therefore you need to calculate which slice is nearest the image plane, and ensure that close voxels obscure distant voxels.
- *Classify and shade the voxels in each slice.* Classify the voxels according to some opacity transfer function or look-up table. Calculate the gradient using central differences and use this information in the shading formula.
- *Project each voxel in a slice onto the image plane.* A reconstruction filter, usually a Gaussian distribution, is used to determine the extent of the splat (its footprint) on the image plane.
- *Attenuate according to the filter.* The classified, shaded voxels are then attenuated according to where they fall within the footprint. Voxels projected into the middle of the footprint will have the highest contribution.
- *Merge the attenuated splats.* Composite the attenuated (r,g,b,α)- tuples that fall within footprint to give a pixel value for the image buffer.

Splatting can be likened to throwing a snowball onto a glass plate.

5.4
Hardware Implementations

Due to the computationally intensive nature of direct volume rendering, hardware implementations are necessary to obtain interactive performance. Two widely used solutions are described below.

5.4.1
VolumePro Volume Rendering Board

The VolumePro 500 volume rendering board is a cost-effective hardware implementation of object order ray casting. This PCI (personal computer interface) accelerator card is based on the Cube-4 architecture (PFISTER and KAUFMAN 1996) and uses the shear warp algorithm. The current version can render a 256^3 volume and perform gradient estimation in real time. It can process 500 million interpolated, Phong-lit, composited samples per second. However, it cannot yet integrate volume and polygonal data, or provide perspective projections.

5.4.2
Texture Mapping Hardware

CABRAL et al. (1995) proposed a novel technique for using texture mapping hardware to implement volume rendering. The technique is often called *volume slicing* and has been used successfully in several clinical applications. The best performance is obtained on high-performance workstations where 3D texture hardware is available. Hardware look-up tables can be used to apply color and opacity. For gradients, multiple passes of the graphics pipeline are needed, however. Images can also be "fuzzy" compared with those generated by conventional methods.

The texture mapping technique can also be adapted for 2D hardware. In this case, three copies of the voxel data are required – sampled across the three orthographic projections. Only one data set is used for the rendering stage at any one time, and as the volume rendered data are rotated it is necessary to swap between which of the three data sets are used in the rendering calculation. The Silicon Graphics O2 workstation provides hardware 2D texture maps and similar functionality is becoming common on PC Graphics cards. Work has also been carried out to implement this technique as a web-based application using VRML (virtual reality modeling language) and JAVA (HENDIN et al. 1998).

OpenGL Volumizer is an API (application programming interface) that can be used to develop applications using texture hardware. Volumizer uses voxels and tetrahedrons as volume primitives. Any 3D shape can be tessellated into a finite number of tetrahedra and so the renderer only needs to be optimized for this simple shape. Volumizer decouples geometry from appearance and supports modeling capabilities such as volume deformation, co-registration and arbitrary shaped volumes of interest.

5.5
Conclusions

Volume rendering of medical images can bring real added value to a clinician. Applications range from diagnostic use, to preoperative planning on patient-specific data. This chapter has presented an overview of the main algorithms and techniques used to achieve volume rendering. The ever-improving algorithms, and increasing availability of hardware solutions, will dramatically increase the use and acceptance of volume rendering as a valuable clinical tool.

References

Brodlie K, Wood J (2000) Recent advances in visualization of volumetric data: state of the art report. Eurographics 2000, Interlaken, Switzerland, pp 65–84

Cabral B, Cam N, Foran J (1995) Accelerated volume rendering and tomographic reconstruction using texture mapping hardware. Proceedings of the ACM/IEEE symposium on volume visualization, pp 91–98

Challinger J (1992) Parallel volume rendering on a shared memory multiprocessor. Technical report UCSC-CRL-91-23, University of California, Santa Cruz

Drebin RA, Carpenter L, Hanrahan P (1988) Volume rendering. Comput Graph 22:65–74

Elvins T (1992) Volume rendering on a distributed memory parallel computer. Proceedings of IEEE Visualisation 1992

Ezquerra N, Navazo I, Morris TI (1999) Graphics, vision, and visualization in medical imaging: a state of the art report. Eurographics, 1999, pp 21–80

Hendin O, John NW, Shochet O (1998) Medical volume rendering on the WWW using JAVA and VRML. In: Westwood J, Hoffman H, Stredney D, Weghorst S (eds) Medicine meets virtual reality. IOS Press, Amsterdam, pp 34–40

Laur D, Hanrahan P (1991) Hierarchical splatting: a progressive refinement algorithm for volume rendering. Comput Graph 25:285–288

Lacroute P, Levoy M (1994) Fast volume rendering using a shear-warp factorization. Computer Graphics Annual Conference Series 1994, pp 451–458

Levoy M (1988) Display of surfaces from volume data. IEEE Comput Graph Appl 8:29–37

Levoy M (1990) Efficient ray tracing of volume data. ACM Trans Graph 9:245–261

Ma K, Painter J (1993) A data distributed, parallel algorithm for ray traced volume rendering. Proceedings of the 1993 parallel rendering symposium. IEEE, San Jose

Nieh J, Levoy M (1992) Volume rendering on scalable shared memory MIMD architectures. Proceedings of the 1992 workshop on volume visualization

Pfister H, Kaufman A (1996) Cube-4 – a scalable architecture for real-time volume rendering. Proceedings of the ACM/IEEE symposium on volume rendering, pp 47–54

Phong B (1975) Illumination for computer-generated pictures. Comm ACM 18:311-317

Pokric M, Thacker N, Scott MLJ (2001) The importance of partial voluming in multi-dimensional medical image segmentation. Submitted to MICCAI 2001. Technical report of IERAPSI Project, University of Manchester

Porter T, Duff T (1984) Composing digital images. Comput Graph 18:253–259

Westover L (1990) Footprint evaluation for volume rendering. Comput Graph 24:367–376

Yagel R (1992) Template based volume viewing. Comput Graphics Forum 4:153–157

Yagel R (1993) Accelerating volume viewing by space leaping. OSU-CISRC-3/93 TR10. Department of Computer Science, Ohio State University

6 Virtual Endoscopy

Emanuele Neri, Paola Vagli, Cheti Spinelli

CONTENTS

6.1
Introduction

Virtual endoscopy is a computer-generated simulation of the endoscopic perspective obtained by processing CT, MR or US datasets (Rubin 1996; Yuh 1999) and is one of the applications of virtual reality in medicine (Geiger and Kikinis 1994).

The first presentations of virtual endoscopy in the radiological field were given by Vining in 1993 and 1994, who reported its application in the study of bronchi and colon respectively. The idea of flying through anatomical structures was followed by many investigators who experienced the use of virtual endoscopy. Initial studies aimed to demonstrate the feasibility of the technique in the exploration of the entire human body (Lorensen 1995; Hara 1996; Rubin 1996), but soon focused investigations were being carried out for specific clinical problems. Nowadays virtual endoscopy reports on the colon, stomach, bronchial tree, larynx and trachea, middle and inner ear, paranasal sinuses, brain ventricles, vessels, biliary tract, urinary tract and joints. The terminology used to describe the technique has been adapted to the anatomical district being examined, i.e. virtual colonoscopy, bronchoscopy, cholangioscopy, uretero-

E. Neri, MD, P. Vagli, MD, C. Spinelli, MD
Diagnostic and Interventional Radiology, Department of Oncology, Transplants, and Advanced Technologies in Medicine, University of Pisa, Via Roma 67, 56100 Pisa, Italy

renoscopy, angioscopy, etc. Most investigators agree that colon exploration represents the main clinical impact of virtual endoscopy.

6.2
Technical Approach to Virtual Endoscopy

6.2.1
Image Acquisition

The unique difference between virtual endoscopy and other 3D (three-dimensional) imaging methods is the type of perspective. In virtual endoscopy the typical perspective of fibre-optic endoscopes is reproduced by a dedicated computer program; one can freely fly through or around 3D objects that are produced by common 3D processing techniques based on surface or volume rendering. As consequence the properties of the data that are used to generate virtual endoscopy are the same as for any data used for other image processing techniques: volumes that respect the spatial relationships of the human body. However, in virtual endoscopy there are specific requirements of image acquisition related to the scope of the virtual endoscopic examination.

An obvious question regarding image acquisition is whether the acquisition should be tailored specifically to virtual endoscopy or whether virtual endoscopy is a technique that can be applied on any dataset. In many situations virtual endoscopy is proposed as additional tool to the standard examination and imaging is performed using routine protocols, e.g. a general survey of the abdomen. In such cases many parameters of the acquisition in CT or MR imaging can influence the quality of virtual endoscopy.

6.2.1.1
Large Bowel

A typical example is the study of the colon with pneumocolon. Prior to examination the patient must

undergo adequate colon cleansing in order to avoid
the presence of faecal residues that can simulate
polyps or block their visualization. During the CT
acquisition a muscle relaxant is administered intravenously to reduce large bowel movement and increase
distension of the lumen. A standard scout view in lateral and anterior-posterior projections is acquired to
verify the distension of the entire colon (Fig. 6.1). The
patient is asked to cooperate in the phase of acquisition by holding the breath as much as possible to
permit maximum coverage of the abdomen. Using
single-slice CT a collimation of 3–5 mm can be used to
encompass the entire colon with pitch 2 and reconstruction spacing 1–2.5 mm; with a multi-row detector CT system the collimation can be further reduced
to 1 mm and the scanning time can be shortened
accordingly (LAGHI 2000; RUST 2000; ROGALLA et al.
2000; HARA 2001). The use of intravenous contrast is
still under debate but it seems to increase the detection of polyps, although it is not a requisite for endoluminal views (MORRIN et al. 2000; Lovenstein 2001).

Data for exploring the colon can also be produced
by MR imaging (LUBOLDT 1999, 2000). To obtain
valuable datasets the patient should have the same
preparation as required for CT, but before the examination a gadolinium or barium enema is performed. The volumetric acquisition is obtained by T1-
weighted SPGR (spoiled gradient recalled) sequences
in the coronal plane, with 5-mm partition thickness
and the use of phased-array coils at high field strength
(1.5 T). Similarly to CT colonography, the use of
pneumocolon has recently been proposed also for
MR imaging (MORRIN 2001).

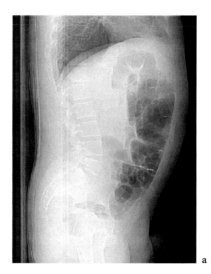
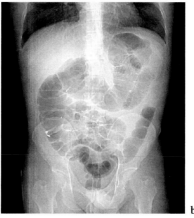

Fig. 6.1. CT scout views obtained after pneumocolon, in supine position, lateral (**a**) and anterior-posterior (**b**) projections; both demonstrate the complete distension of the colon

6.2.1.2
Vessels

As in the case of the colon, the study of vessels with
virtual endoscopy requires the use of contrast in
order to opacify the lumen and permit adequate
segmentation with surface or volume rendering.
The acquisition of data on the aorta can be performed with the traditional CT angiographic technique (BARTOLOZZI 1998) or with MR angiography
(HANY 1998). In CT angiography of the aorta, image
acquisition is performed after selection of the appropriate scan delay (generally performed with a bolus
timing test) from contrast administration. Our scanning protocol with single-slice CT includes collimation 3 mm, pitch 2 and reconstruction spacing 1 mm
for the study of the abdominal aorta, and 5 mm collimation for the study of thoracic aorta (NERI 1999b).
RUBIN (2000) performed CT angiography with mul-

tidetector CT in 48 patients with aortic aneurysm or
dissection, using the following parameters: 2.5 mm
nominal section thickness, a pitch of 6.0, and a table
speed of 15 mm per rotation (18.75 mm/s); they compared the study with single-slice CT. In summary
the authors observed that using multirow detector
CT, CT angiography was 2.6 times faster, scanning
efficiency was 4.1 times greater, contrast efficiency
was 2.5 times greater, dose of contrast material
was reduced without a significant change in aortic
enhancement and sections were thinner. The better
resolution of images acquired suggests a subsequent
better quality for virtual endoscopy.

The optimal MR angiography datasets for virtual
endoscopy are those obtained with a contrast-
enhanced technique. A bolus of intravenous gadolin-

ium (20–30 mg/ml at 2 ml/s) is administered to the patient, and in the same fashion as for CT angiography, the acquisition starts with the appropriate scan delay for the arterial phase (20–30 s). The imaging sequence is similar to that for the study of the colon, and involves a SPGR sequence in the coronal plane with 3 mm partition thickness (HANY 1998; WILDERMUTH and DEBATIN 1999). Previous and preliminary work reported the use of time-of-flight (TOF) sequences, but this technique is no longer proposed for such a purpose (DAVIS 1996).

6.2.1.3
Bronchi

Virtual endoscopy of the bronchial tree is done by processing spiral CT datasets (FERRETTI 1995; VINING 1996; SUMMERS 1996; AQUINO and VINING 1999). The study of this region is dependent on two main critical factors: patients should hold their breath as long as possible in order to minimize movement artefact, and images should be acquired at a very high resolution to detect even segmental branches of the bronchi. NEUMANN (2000) reported that the best results of virtual endoscopy were obtained using an examination protocol with a small beam collimation and a maximum pitch. The author concludes that the performance of virtual bronchoscopy strongly depends on the applied CT examination protocol and the observer's experience with the software used for 3D imaging.

LEE (1997) proposed the following single-slice spiral CT protocol for virtual endoscopy of the bronchial tree: thickness 3 mm, pitch 1, reconstruction interval 1.5 mm. The technique has a limited scan distance of 9 cm, but the pitch can be increased to 2 to achieve 18 cm coverage (enough for the trachea and major airways). FISHMAN (2000) proposed the following protocol for virtual endoscopy with multidetector CT: detector collimation 1 mm, slice thickness 1.25 mm, reconstruction spacing 1 mm, pitch 6 (time per rotation 0.5 s). In both cases no oral and intravenous contrast agents are needed.

6.2.1.4
Biliary and Urinary Tract

In our experience, as well as that of other authors, biliary and urinary tract imaging with MR imaging has been used to generate virtual endoscopy of this anatomical district (DUBNO 1998; NERI 1999a, 2000a). Datasets were obtained with MR cholangiopancreatography and MR urography techniques, producing

so-called water images. These methods exploit the presence of stationary fluids within the biliary and urinary tracts that are therefore used as endoluminal contrast. Imaging sequences includes heavily T2-weighted acquisitions in the axial, sagittal and coronal planes. As an alternative method to MR imaging in exploring the biliary tract, preliminary studies with CT cholangiographic datasets have been done by our group (NERI 1997) and PRASSOPOULOS (1998).

6.2.1.5
Larynx

The study of the larynx is another important application of virtual endoscopy, and the use of high-resolution spiral CT images is recommended. RODENWALDT (1997) evaluated the image quality of virtual endoscopy performed in a cadaver phantom, scanned with single-slice spiral CT and varying the scanning collimation from 1 to 10 mm, and the pitch from 0.5 to 3. The best correlation between virtual endoscopy and the anatomical findings, in terms of diagnostic quality of the axial slices and useful longitudinal coverage of the examination, was observed with a collimation of 3 mm and a pitch of 1.5. In the larynx the complex anatomy requires the use of thin collimations (1–3 mm), but also the movement of the glottic plane in the course of phonation is a potential source of artefacts. This factor suggests the need for a fast scanning technique; MAGLI et al. (2001) report their experience with multi-row detector CT carried out in the evaluation of 22 patients (10 normal, 12 with pathology), using slice thickness 1.3 mm, increment 0.6 mm, pitch 0.875, rotation time 0.75 s.

To obtain virtual endoscopy of the larynx, image acquisition is performed with the patient supine on the CT table with moderate extension of the neck. The patient is asked to phonate the vowel sounds "ee" or "ay"; this allows the true vocal cords to be parallel and more clearly visible since they are aligned in the midline of the glottis.

6.2.1.6
Nose and Paranasal Sinuses

The study of nasal cavity and paranasal sinuses with virtual endoscopy can be performed by processing spiral CT datasets (Fig. 6.2). ROGALLA (1998) carried out virtual endoscopy in 45 spiral CT examinations of the paranasal sinuses at a low radiation dose and compared the virtual view with endoscopic images obtained during sinus surgery. DE NICOLA (1997) applied virtual endoscopy with a surface reconstruc-

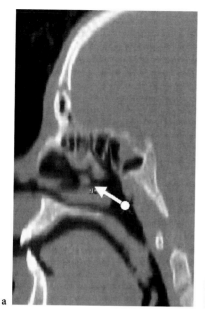

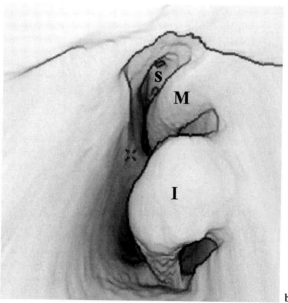

a

b

Fig. 6.2. CT virtual endoscopy of the nasal cavity created with a perspective positioned in the rhinophar-ynx (**a**). The *arrow* indicates the orientation of the virtual endoscope. The right superior (*s*), middle (*M*) and inferior (*I*) turbinates are shown (**b**)

tion to spiral CT datasets in a wide range of paranasal sinuses pathologies; GILANI (1997) tried the same thing with a volume rendered reconstruction. Spiral CT is the method of choice in 3D imaging of the paranasal sinuses. The spiral CT acquisition proto-col includes an axial thin section helical scan with 1–3 mm collimation, variable pitch and 1–2 mm reconstruction spacing, bone reconstruction algo-rithm and 16 cm field of view. However, excellent results of virtual endoscopy of the nose and parana-sal sinuses in defining anatomy were also obtained by MORRA (1998), who performed the study with a conventional CT scanner and proposed the follow-ing protocol: axial and coronal scan with 1.5–3 mm collimation, 1.5–3 mm table feed, 120 kV, 140 mA, 2 s scan time, bone reconstruction algorithm and 14–16 cm field of view.

Although MR imaging plays an important role in diagnostic imaging of paranasal sinus pathologies, to date there are no data concerning the application of virtual endoscopy. The main reason is probably the inherent difficulties of obtaining suitable 3D MR datasets.

6.2.1.7
Middle and Inner Ear

POZZI MUCELLI (1997), who was the first to gen-erate virtual endoscopic images of the tympanic

cavity, used conventional CT with high-resolution acquisitions (1 mm collimation) and obtained excellent results in visualizing the ossicular chain (Fig. 6.3).

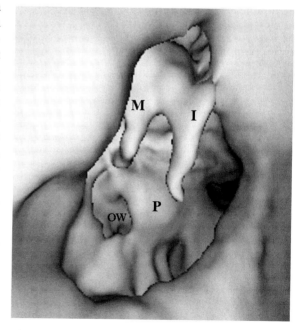

Fig. 6.3. CT virtual endoscopy of the middle ear, generated from a point located in the external auditory canal, shows the incus (*I*), malleus (*M*), promontory (*P*) and oval window (*OW*)

In the study of the middle and inner ear we have proposed the following single-slice spiral CT protocol: axial and coronal acquisitions, beam collimation 1 mm, pitch 1 and 0.5 mm reconstruction spacing (see Chap. 10 for details) (NERI 2000b). In this study all components of the middle ear could be visualized, but also endoluminal views of the bony labyrinth were created. TOMANDL (2000) applied the same acquisition protocol, and used a volume rendered technique to reconstruct the labyrinth with excellent results in terms of anatomical definition of the labyrinthine components.

No substantial difference between spiral CT and conventional CT in generating virtual endoscopy of the middle and inner ear is reported; however, the anatomical details of the middle ear seem to be better displayed using multi-row detector CT (see Chap. 10), but again we look forward to the impact of virtual endoscopy, not yet reported.

6.2.2
Image Acquisition in Ultrasound

A brief summary of the use of virtual endoscopy with ultrasound datasets is mandatory, although there are only few preliminary experiences in this field. The image acquisition is discussed in detail in Chap 1. In summary, image acquisition can be performed through direct 3D acquisition with 2D (two-dimensional) US arrays, or 3D reconstruction from a series of 2D images produced with one-dimensional US arrays.

Once the datasets have been acquired they are processed with a volume rendering technique, but for optimal segmentation of the anatomical structures the acquisition should be performed with US techniques that enhance the contrast between structures. YUH (1999) used power Doppler to image carotid arteries, but also grey-level ultrasound has been used to study the female pelvis and bladder with virtual endoscopy. Recently, NAKATA (2001) reported preliminary experience in the study of abdominal vessels with power Doppler and virtual endoscopy.

6.2.3
Volume Generation

Each patient's dataset is composed of a definite number of series corresponding to the different phase of acquisition, unenhanced or enhanced. Now-adays, the image format conforms to the DICOM standard, and all available workstations support it (PRIOR 1993; ACKERMAN 1994). Thus, potentially any CT or MR scanner can send images to any workstation for image processing. CT image resolution is 512×512×12 bit (corresponding to 0.5 megabyte); i.e. a dataset for the study of the whole colon with single-slice spiral CT comprises about 150–180 images if 3 mm collimation and 2 mm reconstructions spacing is used, with a consequent volume of about 75–90 megabytes. In case of an MR study the entity and resolution of image produced is approximately one half that of CT, with a consequently smaller computer memory load.

Once the CT or MR datasets have been acquired and transferred to dedicated workstations these are processed by the software to generate the volume. The volume is produced by stacking all the reconstructed slices along the centreline of each slice (Fig. 6.4). The centreline corresponds to the longitudinal axis (Z-axis) in spiral CT, but in the case of MR imaging can be oriented along any other plane (coronal, sagittal). One problem of MR imaging arises when the acquisition plane is oblique; in this case some software does not accept the reslicing of such native images because they are not perpendicular to the centreline.

The volume is in general automatically created by the 3D software, and the radiologist is asked only to select the desired imaging series to be reconstructed (Fig. 6.4). To reduce the image overload a small volume can be reconstructed by selecting the images corresponding to a restricted anatomical area. To do this the start and end points of the acquisition (on the Z-axis) should be annotated and then these values can be changed by the operator at the image processing workstation.

Within the software architecture the volumetric dataset is organized in terms of voxels. These are near-cubic elements that arise from each image pixel. This latter is the basic building block for the voxel, to which a Hounsfield value (in case of CT) or an intensity value (in the case of MR imaging) is assigned; each voxel also has a defined spatial position and dimension in the volume.

The ideal volumetric dataset, which represents precisely the imaged structures, is obtained when all voxels are isotropic and therefore their shape is cubic. Unfortunately conventional CT and spiral CT do not completely fulfil this acquisition requirement. Dedicated MR sequences and multi-row detector CT seem to overcome this limitation.

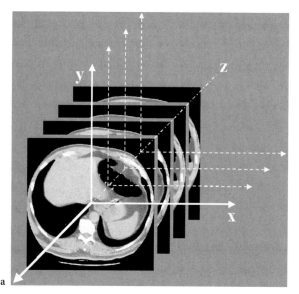
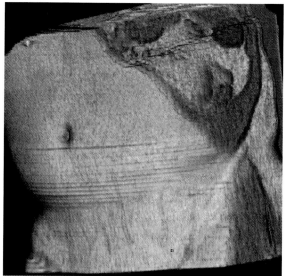

Fig. 6.4. CT axial slices are aligned along the Z-axis (a) to generate the final volumetric dataset (b). The entire process is performed automatically by 3D rendering software

6.2.4
Volume Segmentation

Surface and volume rendering are the methods used to virtually represent the human body in three dimensions. Each has a specific principle of dataset segmentation in order to select the anatomical structure to display from the inside. For details on the technical basis of segmentation in surface and volume rendering see Chaps. 4 and 5 (Fig. 6.5).

Most available software for virtual endoscopy allows the radiologist to interact with the volumetric sample and segment it in real time. By using surface rendering the change in visible structure is made by the selection of a threshold which defines the edge line of a surface to display and represents effectively the boundary between two different density or intensity values (e.g. the colonic mucosa and the colonic lumen filled with air). Thus, before starting the inner visualizations with this method the operator should be aware of the different threshold values used. For example the colonic surface in a CT study with pneumocolon can be optimally represented with thresholds ranging from –800 to –700 HU, the middle ear –500 HU, while the threshold for displaying aortic lumen depends on the degree of contrast enhancement (in both CT and MR angiography).

In the volume rendering technique the generation of an endoscopic view is quite flexible and interactive when the computer used is powerful enough. However, volume rendering requires high computa-

tional power and specific hardware capabilities (see Chap. 5). Almost all commercially available software has been implemented with predefined volume rendering protocols that produce an endoluminal view of specific organs. To simplify the concept, in volume rendering the use of a threshold is strongly smoothed by the use of transfer opacity functions (Fig. 6.1); therefore the boundary between structures with different voxel properties is attenuated and progressively increased or decreased by a linear scale of values.

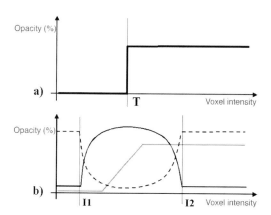

Fig. 6.5. Surface rendering (a) and volume rendering (b) principles of dataset segmentation. *I1–I2* voxel intensity interval, *T* threshold value

6.2.5
Perspective Generation

The typical endoscopic view is generated by a ray casting algorithm (Roth 1982). In ray-casting, parallel rays are virtually generated by a point source (the eye of the observer or the point at which the endoscope is positioned); the rays traverse the acquired volume in a divergent direction and by applying surface or volume rendering algorithms the encountered voxels are classified by the attribution of opacity values. In surface rendering the voxels located above or below a specific threshold that are encountered by the rays cast are fixed and transformed in a mesh of polygons reflecting each ray. The algorithm used to perform the surface extraction is called a "marching cube" algorithm (Lorensen and Cline 1987). This transforms the cubic shape of a voxel into a mesh of triangles (triangulation), and the final composition of the transformed voxels constitutes an isosurface.

In volume rendering the classification of voxels is by linear opacity functions that attribute different opacity values to particular voxel intensities. The advantages of this approach are the optimization of the dynamic range and the ability to change tissue opacities to produce 3D renderings which maintain surface details and which represent the entire dataset.

The final image of surface or volume rendered ray casting will have a conic field of view (as in endoscopy). The field of view can be changed by the viewing angle. Most software uses a large viewing angle, but increasing this value causes a certain distortion of the surface morphology, and affects the possibility of recognizing pathological findings. This approach seems to have other limitations that also apply to real endoscopy, i.e. when exploring the colon from rectum to caecum, even using the widest viewing angle not all haustral folds are entirely visualized (Fig. 6.6). For maximum diagnostic confidence backward navigation is recommended, from caecum to rectum, in order to explore hidden corners not visible with a single navigation. This is a time-consuming approach and many investigators are trying to set up different viewing perspectives that can display the entire colonic wall in a single navigation. Paik (2000) proposed a map projection of the colon based on both Mercator and stereographic techniques and compared this approach with the conic view. This showed that the percentage of mucosal surface visualized by map projection (98.8%) could only be achieved by the conic view at a very high viewing angle, which causes

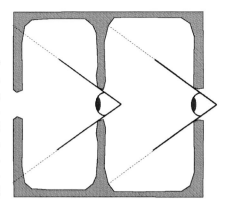

Fig. 6.6. Effects of conic view in virtual endoscopy of the colon. The exploration can be obscured by colonic folds; if a restricted viewing angle is used some hidden corners of the colonic wall are not visualized

viewing distortion of the mucosal details. Moreover, when polyps >7 mm were analysed the map projection showed a significantly higher sensitivity (87.5%) than axial images (62.5%) and conic views (67.5%).

One similar and interesting approach to colon visualization, called "unfolding", has been proposed by Sorantin (2001). The technique is based on non-linear ray-casting of polyps, and non-linear 2D scaling to compensate the distortions due to the unfolding (Vilanova Bartroli 2000). Effectively the colon is completely unfolded and projected on a bi-dimensional plane. A similar approach has been proposed by Wang (1996, 1998) in multiple applications.

6.2.6
Fly Through Path

Fly-path planning is a critical issue in virtual endoscopy. Navigation through tubular structures is quite difficult, especially if these are tortuous and have sharp curves or a major calibre increase or decrease along their path (Fig. 6.7). The calculation of the shorter and central navigation path is required to help the radiologist. The ideal assisted navigation should allow the radiologist to stay comfortably in front of the computer display and view a movie of the complete fly-through the structure during the examination. This is easy to perform in a structure that is fairly straight, such as the abdominal aorta or trachea, but difficult when examining the colon.

The requirements of assisted navigation are: automatic path planning, collision detection and direct interaction with the objects displayed. The last point should consist of the following steps: stop the naviga-

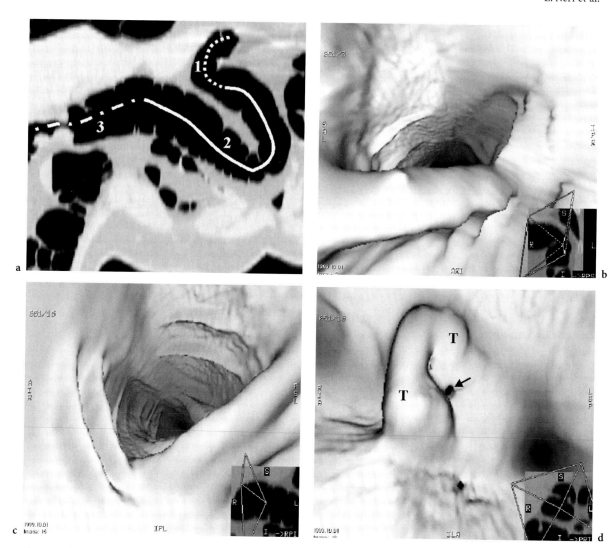

Fig. 6.7a–d. Navigation from the left to right flexure in a patient with right-sided colon cancer. The colon is manually unfolded by using a curved planar reconstruction traced on axial native images (**a**) and the centreline is traced at three steps: left flexure (*1*), transverse colon (*2*) and right (*3*) flexure, and each virtual endoscopic view is generated accordingly (**b, c, d**). The final perspective demonstrates an interruption of the lumen caused by a stenosing tumour (*T*); a residual lumen (*arrow*) can be observed in the central part of the mass. In all virtual endoscopic views the position and direction of the endoscope can be monitored by a cross-reference image located in the right inferior corner

tion, look at the object, touch the object and cross-correlate the image with other images [axial, multiplanar reconstruction (MPR), external 3D models].

The calculation of an automatic path has been proposed by various authors. JOLESZ (1997) proposed a method in which the endoscopic camera is considered as a robot and the walls of the organs as obstacles. The obstacles are identified as ranges of threshold values or tissue labels and the path planner labels all voxels within the 3D dataset with a distance to a goal. Then, from a given starting point, the path planning algorithm finds the shortest path to the goal and

the voxel coordinates for each point in the path are recorded.

PAIK (1998) proposed a method based on the medial axis transform. The method calculates the centreline of hollow organs by iterative thinning of the segmented structure and path correction. A similar method is the cylindrical approximation of tubular organs, proposed by VILANOVA BARTROLI (2000).

However, any given automatic path is not free of errors in calculation and collision with the organ's surface is possible. Collision detection algorithms exist, such as the JOLESZ (1997) method. The surface is identified as a variation in threshold value and therefore when the endoscope find it, it changes direction.

A collision detection algorithm is also used in VRML (virtual reality modelling language), where surface rendered models represent different objects in a virtual world that can be explored through Internet browsers. We have created and used VRML to fly-through abdominal aortic aneurysms. The fly-through path was created after segmentation of CT angiography datasets by calculating the centreline of consecutive sections of the aorta obtained along planes perpendicular to the main axis of the vessel (Fig. 6.8) (NERI 2000c).

Direct interaction with objects displayed in the endoscopic views is an absolute requirement of virtual endoscopy. The main criticism of this technique is that it can wrongly represent objects of the real world. To overcome this problem most software allows one to visualize the target object, click on it with the computer mouse and obtain the corresponding axial or MPR image intersecting it. On the other hand it must be remembered that virtual endoscopy is not a stand-alone technique, but is one of the possible ways in which volumetric datasets can be represented. Therefore constant correlation with native data should be always performed, especially to confirm endoscopic findings.

6.3
Conclusion

Virtual endoscopy is an emerging technique in radiology. It can be used for visualizing CT, MR and US datasets, and even if in each case the technical approach is quite similar, the image acquisition strongly affects the final 3D image. In most cases image acquisition is performed with specific proto-

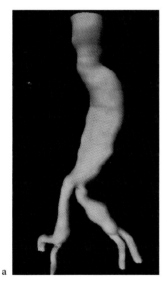

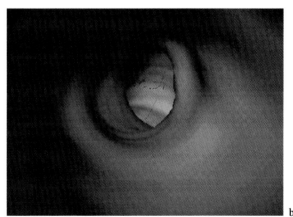

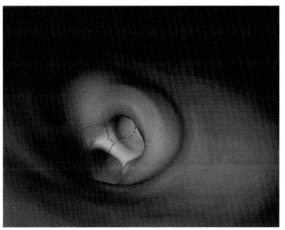

Fig. 6.8. VRML model of the abdominal aorta in a patient with an infrarenal aneurysm (**a**). The endoluminal assisted navigation is obtained from the aneurysm's neck (**b**) to the bifurcation (**c**) by calculating the centreline of the vessel

cols for characterizing pathologies that are not compliant with 3D reconstructions. On the other hand developments in image acquisition are oriented to generate volumetric data much more compatible with this purpose. Thus, in future virtual endoscopy in radiology will be less affected by image acquisition; the real issue is whether or not it will be clinically relevant in all its possible applications.

References

Ackerman LV (1994) DICOM: the answer for establishing a digital radiology department. Radiographics 14:151–152

Aquino SL, Vining DJ (1999) Virtual bronchoscopy. Clin Chest Med 20:725–730

Bartolozzi C (1998) CT in vascular pathologies. Eur Radiol 8:679–684

Davis CP (1996) Human aorta: preliminary results with virtual endoscopy based on three-dimensional MR imaging data sets. Radiology 199:37–40

De Nicola M (1997) Virtual endoscopy of nasal cavity and paranasal sinuses. Eur J Radiol 24:175–180

Dubno B (1998) Virtual MR cholangiography. AJR 171:1547–1550

Ferretti G (1995) Endoluminal 3D reconstruction of the tracheo-bronchial tree (virtual bronchoscopy). J Radiol 76:531–534

Fishman EK (2000) Spiral and multidetector CT of thoracic pathology: techniques and clinical applications. Radiology 217:618

Geiger B, Kikinis R (1994) Simulation of endoscopy. AAAI spring symposium series: applications of computer vision in medical images processing, Stanford University, pp 138–140

Gilani S (1997) Virtual endoscopy of the paranasal sinuses using perspective volume rendered helical sinus computed tomography. Laryngoscope 107:25–29

Hany TF (1998) Diagnostic impact of four postprocessing techniques in evaluating contrast-enhanced three-dimensional MR angiography. AJR 170:907–912

Hara AK (1996) Detection of colorectal polyps by computed tomographic colography: feasibility of a novel technique. Gastroenterology 110:284–290

Hara AK (2001) CT colonography: single- versus multi-detector row imaging. Radiology 219:461–465

Jolesz FA (1997) Interactive virtual endoscopy. AJR 169:1229–1237

Laghi A (2000) Optimization of the technique of virtual colonoscopy using a multislice spiral computerized tomography. Radiol Med 100:459–464

Lee KS (1997) Evaluation of tracheobronchial disease with helical CT with multiplanar and three-dimensional reconstruction: correlation with bronchoscopy. Radiographics 17:555–567

Lorensen WE (1995) The exploration of cross-sectional data with a virtual endoscope. In: Morgan K, Satava RM, Sieburg HB, Mattheus R, Christensen JP (eds) Interactive technology and the new paradigm for healthcare. IOS Pres /Ohmsha, Amsterdam, pp 221–230

Lorensen WE, Cline HE (1987) Marching cubes: a high resolution 3D surface reconstruction algorithm. Comput Graph 21:163–169

Lovenstein T, Holtmann G, Schoenfelder D (2001) MR colonography without colonic cleansing: a new strategy to improve patient acceptance. AJR 177:823–827

Luboldt W (1999) MR colonography: optimized enema composition. Radiology 212:265–269

Luboldt W (2000) Colonic masses: detection with MR colonography. Radiology 216:383–388

Magli T, Fella R, Scialpi M, Lorenzini E (2001) Virtual laryngoscopy with multislice volumetric spiral CT: preliminary study. Eur Radiol 11 (Suppl 1):399-400

Morra A (1998) Virtual endoscopy of the nasal cavity and the paranasal sinuses with computerized tomography: anatomical study. Radiol Med 96:29–34

Morrin MM (2001) MR colonography using colonic distention with air as the contrast material: work in progress. AJR 176:144–146

Morrin MM, Farrell RJ, Kruskal JB, Reynolds K, McGee JB, Raptopoulos V (2000) Utility of intravenously administered contrast material at CT colonography. Radiology 217:765–771

Nakata N (2001) Ultrasound virtual endoscopic imaging. Semin Ultrasound CT MR 22:78–84

Neri E (1997) Spiral CT, three-dimensional reconstructions and virtual endoscopy of the biliary tract. Eur Radiol 7:311

Neri E (1999a) MR virtual endoscopy of the pancreaticobiliary tract. Magn Reson Imaging 17:59–67

Neri E (1999b) Virtual CT intravascular endoscopy of the aorta: pierced surface and floating shape thresholding artifacts. Radiology 212:276–279

Neri E (2000a) MR virtual endoscopy of the upper urinary tract. AJR 175:1697–1702

Neri E (2000b) Virtual endoscopy of the middle and inner ear with spiral computed tomography. Am J Otol 21:799–803

Neri E (2000c) Virtual reality modeling language: applications to the study of abdominal aortic aneurysms. Radiology 217:486–487

Neumann K (2000) Real-time interactive virtual endoscopy of the tracheo-bronchial system: influence of CT imaging protocols and observer ability. Eur J Radiol 33:50–54

Paik DS (1998) Automated flight path planning for virtual endoscopy. Med Phys 25:629–637

Paik DS (2000) Visualization modes for CT colonography using cylindrical and planar map projections. J Comput Assist Tomogr 24:179–188

Pozzi Mucelli RS (1997) Virtual endoscopy of the middle ear with computed tomography. Radiol Med 94:440–446

Prassopoulos P (1998) Development of virtual CT cholangio-pancreatoscopy. Radiology 209:570–574

Prior FW (1993) Specifying DICOM compliance for modality interfaces. Radiographics 13:1381–1388

Rodenwaldt J (1997) 3D virtual endoscopy of the upper airway: optimization of the scan parameters in a cadaver phantom and clinical assessment. J Comput Assist Tomogr 21:405–411

Rogalla P (1998) Virtual endoscopy of the nose and paranasal sinuses. Eur Radiol 8:946–950

Rogalla P, Meiri N, Ruckert JC (2000) Colonography using multislice CT. Eur J Radiol 36:81–85

Roth SD (1982) Ray casting for solid modelling. Comput Graph Image Proc 18:109–144

Rubin GD (1996) Perspective volume rendering of CT and MR images: applications for endoscopic imaging. Radiology 199:321–339

Rubin GD (2000) Aorta and iliac arteries: single versus multiple detector-row helical CT angiography. Radiology 215:670–676

Rust GF (2000) Virtual coloscopy with multi-slice computerized tomography. Preliminary results. Radiologe 40:274–282

Summers RM (1996) Virtual bronchoscopy: segmentation method for real-time display. Radiology 200:857–862

Tomandl BF (2000) Virtual labyrinthoscopy: visualization of the inner ear with interactive direct volume rendering. Radiographics 20:547–558

Vining DJ (1993) Virtual bronchoscopy: a new perspective for viewing the tracheobronchial tree. Radiology 189:438

Vining DJ (1994) Virtual colonoscopy. Radiology 193:(P)446

Vining DJ (1996) Virtual bronchoscopy. Relationships of virtual reality endobronchial simulations to actual bronchoscopic findings. Chest 109:549–(P)553

Vilanova Bartroli A (2000) Cylindrical approximation of tubular organs for virtual endoscopy. In: Hamza MH (ed) Computer graphics and imaging, October 25–27,1999, Palm Springs, Calif, USA. IASTED/ACTA, pp 283–289

Wang G (1996) Unwrapping cochlear implants by spiral CT. IEEE Trans Biomed Eng 43:891–900

Wang G (1998) GI tract unraveling with curved cross sections. IEEE Trans Med Imaging 17:318–322

Wildermuth S, Debatin JF (1999) Virtual endoscopy in abdominal MR imaging. Magn Reson Imaging Clin North Am 7:349–364

Yuh EL (1999) Virtual endoscopy using perspective volume-rendered three-dimensional sonographic data: technique and clinical applications. AJR 172:1193–1197

7 Pitfalls and Artefacts in Virtual Endoscopy

Emanuele Neri, Paola Vagli, Silvia Picchietti

CONTENTS

7.1
Introduction

Artefacts can be defined as false features in the image that significantly alter the interpretation of the patient anatomy and pathology. For the radiologist, the recognition of artefacts is important to avoid incorrect diagnoses, and therefore precise knowledge of them is mandatory. Artefacts as well as other 3D (three-dimensional) representation methods affect virtual endoscopy. The appearance of artefacts in endoluminal views may add further difficulties to the interpretation of virtual endoscopy images (Bode et al. 2001). Artefacts can be grouped into two types, in relation to the phases of virtual endoscopy generation: image acquisition and image processing.

7.2
Artefacts Related to Image Acquisition

Image acquisition is the key process for obtaining valuable endoluminal perspectives. In this phase the choice of parameters determines the spatial and contrast resolution of the images; in most cases a trade-off is necessary between imaging parameters for the

E. Neri, MD, P. Vagli, MD, S. Picchietti, MD
Diagnostic and Interventional Radiology, Department of Oncology, Transplants, and Advanced Technologies in Medicine, University of Pisa, Via Roma 67, 56100 Pisa, Italy

specific acquisition method (MR imaging, CT, US, digital subtraction angiography), and patient characteristics and clinical conditions (Whiting et al. 2000; Laghi et al. 2000).

7.3
Imaging Parameters

CT is ideally suited to the acquisition of volumetric data. Initial applications of 3D image processing were oriented to the study of bone structures; with conventional scanners these were limited to the study of skeletal structures in which the acquisition process could not be influenced by body movements. However, since the introduction of spiral scanners this limitation has been overcome and both thorax and abdomen have been effectively imaged with a significant reduction in movement artefacts. Such artefacts, which slightly affect the quality of axial slices, become clearly visible in 3D images, where continuity of the volume acquired is essential to reproduce a reliable 3D model. Single-slice spiral CT, and nowadays multislice CT scanning, of the thorax and abdomen are performed during a single breath-hold. In this way the patient is able to hold the same position for the entire acquisition time. In axial scanning the patient performs a breath-hold for each acquisition, but this cannot guarantee continuity between slices since breaths can differ significantly from each other. In summary, for 3D bone studies conventional scanning can be still considered effective, but when the thorax or abdomen are to be imaged, spiral scanning is required. Spiral scanning is not exempt from pitfalls. The greatest possible coverage of the patient's body should be acquired in the shortest possible time. Collimation and pitch are the parameters involved in this issue. A wider collimation permits larger volume coverage but reduces the spatial resolution and moreover influences the quality of 3D images. Various authors have emphasized the use of 2–3 mm collimation in the study of small arterial structures (such as the renal arteries) in order to reduce partial volume artefacts. Initial experiences in the study of the renal arteries with CT angiography compared different collimation and pitch values; in general most investigators suggested the use of the thinnest collimation with a variable pitch to increase the scan velocity. To reduce partial volume averaging the reconstruction spacing should be reduced as much as possible. A typical artefact that arises from the use of a large collimation and high pitch is the stair-step artefact. This is highlighted in 3D images (multiplanar or shaded surface display) representing anatomical structures that have an oblique main axis with respect to the longitudinal axis of the scan (Fig. 7.1). In CT 3D imaging a further element which influences the quality of

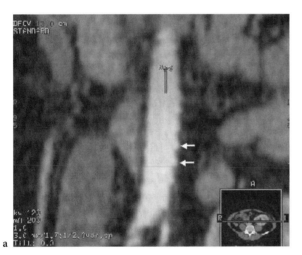

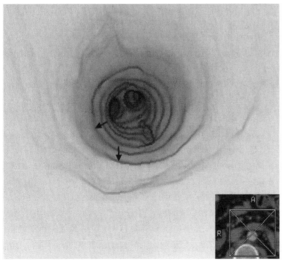

Fig 7.1a, b. Stair-step artefacts at CT angiography. **a** Multiplanar reconstruction of the abdominal aorta in the coronal plane shows multiple stair-step artefacts (*arrows*). **b** The same artefacts are visible in the endoluminal view created from the level of the renal arteries looking toward the aortic bifurcation (*arrows*)

reconstructions is contrast enhancement. The brightest contrast is obtained in the arterial system, which is thus the easiest area in which to apply the 3D imaging process. In fact, to permit 3D representations of the arterial or venous system, dedicated CT angiographic protocols are required. In fact, to selectively image vessels, dedicated CT angiography combines the amount of contrast administered (quantity and flow rate) to the patient with the scan delay. If the optimal combination is reached the patient will be scanned during maximum enhancement of the vessel. This will be reflected in the final 3D reconstruction, where the vessels will be clearly distinguished from the surrounding structures.

In MR imaging also, the appropriate scanning parameters are essential to produce suitable images for 3D processing. These parameters are basically determined by the imaging sequence. A 3D sequence in MR imaging is generally too long for imaging those parts of the body which have physiological movements. For example, a 3D conventional spin echo sequence for imaging the abdomen can have a duration of 10–20 min, and even if respiratory triggering is used, movement artefacts are still present in the final volume. One partial solution is to use fast spin echo imaging or gradient echo imaging where the MR study is limited to the evaluation of specific structures or to the entire abdomen or thorax. Valuable examples are MR angiography oriented to study the vessels, or MR cholangiography and urography for the study of the bile ducts and urinary tract respectively. In such studies the quality of the 3D image is influenced by the brightness of the imaged structures. In MR angiography scan delay and contrast quantity play almost the same role as in CT angiography. However, the power of gradients, magnetic field, as well as the use of dedicated coils for the abdomen or thorax (phased-array), allow an increase in the spatial resolution and a reduction in the scanning time.

7.4
Patient Factors

The patient represents a critical factor in 3D imaging. If the skeletal structures are imaged, no artefacts occur in the scanned volume, but if the neck, thorax and abdomen are to be imaged deglutition, respiration and peristalsis are significant enough to influence the quality of reconstructions.

The study of the larynx represents a specific situation where deglutition influences imaging. The movements of the glottis in consensus with the opening of the oesophagus cause artefacts in CT and MR imaging. In scanning the larynx, therefore, the patient should be requested to avoid deglutition. Moreover, if the study is dedicated to the evaluation of the vocal cords, phonation should be performed during acquisition. Phonation of the vowels "i" or "e" causes the adduction of the true vocal cords, the free border of which becomes clearly visible in the midline of the glottis plane. Since patient cooperation is essential, imaging patients with a cough adds further problems to this difficult task (RODENWALDT et al. 1997; GUAZZARONI et al. 2001).

As mentioned above, thoracic scanning is significantly influenced by respiration. Movements of the thoracic inlet cause discontinuity between slices, which are presumed to be continuous, and are reflected in the final 3D reconstruction. However, such artefacts can be avoided if the patient cooperates enough to permit scanning during a single breath-hold. Another artefact that occurs in scanning the thorax concerns the thoracic aorta, and can be defined as a pulsation artefact. This is caused by the transmitted pulsation of the heart to the entire thoracic aorta, which significantly affects the ascending part. The vessel wall has an appearance similar to a stair-step artefact, but in this case the obliquity of the vessel with respect to the longitudinal plane is not the cause. Pulsation artefacts mimic the presence of intimal flaps in the proximal portion of the ascending aorta (BATRA et al. 2000). The use of multiplanar reconstructions and virtual endoscopy can obviate this incorrect diagnosis by demonstrating that the false flap does not extend beyond one or two slices in the longitudinal plane.

In the study of the abdomen the presence of artefacts depends on the anatomical structure being evaluated. The study of the aorta with CT angiography requires the accurate selection of scanning parameters such as collimation, pitch and reconstruction algorithm, while slice thickness, acquisition plane, bandwidth, etc., play a significant role in MR angiography. However, given the proper imaging parameters the major factor influencing the examination is the circulation time. This reflects a patient's specific cardiovascular setting and for each patient should be calculated using a circulation time test; after the test the appropriate scan delay can be selected to achieve the optimal aortic enhancement. An inappropriate scan delay results in inadequate enhancement of the arterial system (scan delay too short) or the simulta-

neous enhancement of arterial and venous systems (scan delay too long). The resulting volumetric data will be inadequate for an optimal reconstruction. In the first case the aorta will be represented as an inhomogeneous structure with alternate areas of high and low enhancement. The low contrast will influence maximum intensity projections (MIPs) and volume renderings aimed at demonstrating a stenosis (of the superior mesenteric or renal arteries). In the second case, the same enhancement of aorta and vena cava will add difficulties to MIP , volume renderings and virtual endoscopy in distinguishing the lumen of one vessel from another (Fig. 7.2). If the target structure of abdominal imaging is the colon, as in the case of

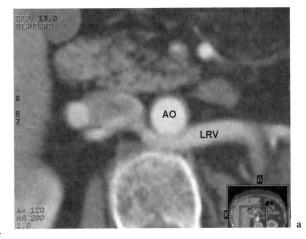

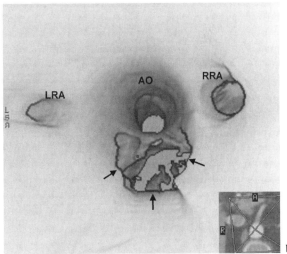

Fig 7.2a, b. Incorrect selection of the scan delay at CT angiography. a The left renal vein (*LRV*) posterior to the aorta (*AO*) is opacified by the contrast medium. b Virtual endoscopy shows a false hole (*arrows*) in the posterior wall of the aorta due to difficulty in the segmentation process in separating the aorta from the renal vein. *RRA* right renal artery, *LRA* left renal artery

CT or MR colonography, patient factors involved in determining the quality of the examination are bowel cleansing and the presence of peristalsis. Faecal residues and fluid levels represent an obstacle to the complete evaluation of the colonic lumen (Fig. 7.3). In endoluminal views, where the unique element displayed by the algorithm is the surface of the colon, polyps and faecal residuals have the same appearance; only the use of axial native images allows polyps to be recognized, even if their detection is not always precise. In fact despite the fact that density (polyps are parenchymal structures) and contrast enhance-

ment (a significant uptake of contrast can be documented if polyps are large enough) are the most sensitive criteria for detecting polyps, these are not always precise (MORRIN et al. 2000). In MR the "faecal tagging" solution has been proposed but the lower spatial resolution of the technique limits the visualization of small polyps (SCHOENFELDER and DEBATIN 2000; LAUENSTEIN 2001).

As mentioned there are many patient variables which affect the quality of 3D imaging; most are due to physiological factors, but in some cases there are external elements that affect imaging, i.e., when patients have metallic prostheses or surgical clips. A typical example is a patient with a femoral head prosthesis: the beam hardening caused by the prosthesis on CT imaging obstructs the visualization of the rectum and sigmoid colon on CT colonography, while on MR imaging the paramagnetic effects of the prosthesis cause a complete absence of signal in the pelvis. Another example of beam hardening artefacts is those caused by an aortic endoprosthesis. However, even small surgical clips can be a problem in 3D imaging; in patients who have undergone laparoscopic cholecystectomy the visualization of bile ducts can be altered in MR cholangiography.

7.5
Artefacts Related to Image Processing

In many cases, although the imaging method and patient factors are optimal, artefacts can arise from the incorrect selection of the parameters used in a specific rendering method. The first rendering method introduced in 3D imaging was based on visualization of the surface of 3D models; the surface is commonly represented by a web of polygons that connect and normalize the external surface of voxels (see Chap. 4). If this process, called "triangulation", is not sufficiently applied the surface still displays the voxels and appears coarse. Such an appearance alters the visualization of thin structures, as in the case of the renal arteries. However, the major critical factor influencing surface rendering is the segmentation phase. This method requires the selection of thresholds, lower and upper, to identify a range of density or signal intensity (thus the brightness of voxels) to select the anatomical structure to be visualized. A typical example is virtual endoscopy of the aorta. In this case, the incorrect setting of thresholds produces artefacts. On the one hand, if the lower threshold is set to include more than one anatomical structure

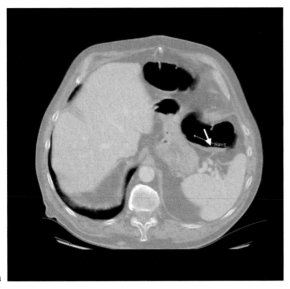

a

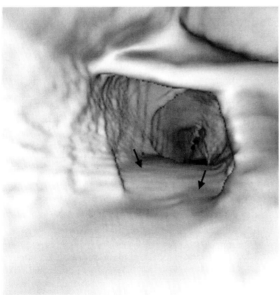

b

Fig 7.3a, b. Residual fluid at CT colonography. **a** The presence of a fluid level can be appreciated in the left flexure (*arrow*). **b** The residual fluid (*arrows*) covers part of the colonic wall

(i.e., aorta and vena cava), these will be represented as a continuous environment communicating through one or multiple "holes". Alternatively if the density range is too small (as a result of increasing the lower threshold or decreasing the upper threshold), inhomogeneities of the contrast material within the lumen of the aorta will be represented as floating bodies (Fig. 7.4). Moreover, a change in threshold can produce a significant alteration of the morphology of the anatomical structure to be represented. In the case of the renal arteries or bronchi, the restriction of the density range results in a false stenosis.

Although surface rendering is limited by artefacts, it is still used effectively, and similar problems affect volume rendering. In fact the dramatic changes in opacity and transparency can alter the visibility of

the internal wall of hollow organs. In the study of the colon, the use of high transparency effects and consequent reduction of wall shading effects reduce sensitivity in detecting polyps.

7.6
Conclusions

Virtual endoscopy is extremely sensitive to multiple parameters that affect the entire process needed to generate the final endoluminal view, from the acquisition to the inner navigation. Radiologists using such technology should know the methods for avoiding artefacts, and be able to recognize artefacts in endoluminal views.

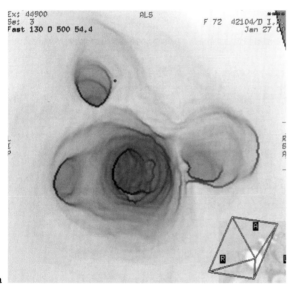

a

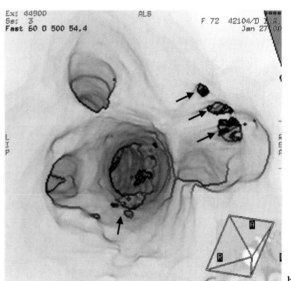

b

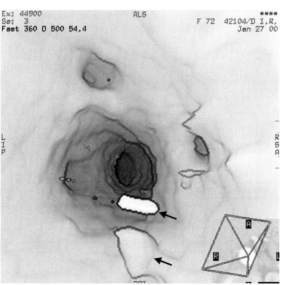

c

Fig 7.4a–c. Incorrect selection of the segmentation threshold at surface rendered CT virtual endoscopy of the aorta. **a** Endoluminal view of the aorta with a threshold range 130–500 HU. No artefact is visible. **b** Threshold range 60–500 HU; the lower threshold shift from 130 to 60 allows the software to include external voxels in the display which appear as holes (*arrows*). **c** Increasing the lower threshold to 360 HU displays inhomogeneities of the contrast medium, which appear as floating bodies or shapes within the aortic lumen (*arrows*)

References

Batra P, Bigoni B, Manning J (2000) Pitfalls in the diagnosis of thoracic aortic dissection at CT angiography. Radiographics 20:309–320

Bode A, Dammann F, Pelikan EH (2001) Analysis of artifacts by virtual endoscopy visualization of spiral CT data. Rofo Fortschr Geb Rontgenstr Neuen Bildgeb Verfahr 173:245–252

Guazzaroni M, Turchio P, Di Rienzo L (2001) Virtual laryngoscopy of neoplastic pharyngeal and laryngeal pathology. Radiol Med 101:265–269

Laghi A, Catalano C, Panebianco V (2000) Optimization of the technique of virtual colonoscopy using a multislice spiral computerized tomography. Radiol Med 100:459–464

Lauenstein T, Holtmann G, Shoenfelder D (2001) MR colonography without colonic cleansing: a new strategy to improve patient acceptance. AJR 177:823–827

Morrin MM, Farrell RJ, Kruskal JB (2000) Utility of intravenously administered contrast material at CT colonography. Radiology 217:765–771

Rodenwaldt J, Kopka L, Roedel R (1997) 3D virtual endoscopy of the upper airway: optimization of the scan parameters in a cadaver phantom and clinical assessment. J Comput Assist Tomogr 21:405–411

Schoenfelder D, Debatin JF (2000) Virtual reality in MR colonography. Radiologe 40:283–289

Whiting BR, McFarland EG, Brink JA (2000) Influence of image acquisition parameters on CT artifacts and polyp depiction in spiral CT colonography: in vitro evaluation. Radiology 217:165–172

8 3D Image Fusion

Alan Jackson and Neil A. Thacker

CONTENTS

8.1 Introduction

The routine production of 3D (three-dimensional) imaging data from modern imaging systems has led to a rapid growth in image post-processing methods. As described in previous chapters many of these can be applied to single 3D data sets to improve data interpretation by producing 3D visualizations of data content, or by allowing automatic identification of specific features using segmentation techniques. However, in many cases the data content of a single 3D image is inadequate to provide all the information required. Under these circumstances a combination of information from two or more separate data sets may be necessary. As practising radiologists we subconsciously perform this type of data fusion when we use images from CT and different MR sequences to attempt to better characterize an abnormality. Faced with a cystic mass at the base of the brain we would routinely request T1- and T2-weighted MR images to determine the presence of free fluid in the cyst and the presence and extent of oedema. We would use MR angiography to determine the spatial relationship of the lesion to the major vessels and CT scanning to determine the presence of bony abnormality. When we perform this type of analysis we are instinctively increasing the information content of our data, using additional examinations to provide complementary information required for our analysis. When we report this type of multi-modality imaging investigation we also instinctively register the anatomical locations of features from the various examinations. A similar process occurs when we compare images from a single case taken at different times to allow monitoring of disease progression.

The increased data content of such multi-parametric data sets can also be used to support a range of sophisticated image analysis techniques with a wide range of both clinical and research applications. However, automated analysis of data from multiple 3D images inevitably assumes spatial coregistration between the data sets. In practice it is extremely unusual to acquire images with these characteristics. Simultaneous collection of two or more data sets will ensure accurate coregistration. This can be exploited by the use of multiple echoes on MR examinations to produce matched proton density weighted and T2-weighted images from the same series of excitations. However, this approach is extremely restrictive and in most cases 3D images will be collected at different times and often on different modalities. In these circumstances separate 3D images must be coregistered in some way to provide absolute spatial alignment.

A. Jackson, MD, Professor of Neurology, Imaging Science and Biomedical Engineering, The Medical School, University of Manchester, Oxford Road, Manchester, M13 9PT, UK
N.A. Thacker, PhD, Imaging Science and Biomedical Engineering, The Medical School, University of Manchester, Oxford Road, Manchester, M13 9PT, UK

8.2 Basic Theory of Image Coregistration

The aim of image coregistration techniques is to ensure that: "each pixel in the various data sets represents exactly the same volume of tissue in the patient." In practice there are many ways in which we can attempt to achieve this and the selection of technique will depend on the imaging modalities involved, the reason for coregistering the images and the accuracy of coregistration required for the analysis technique to be employed.

The simplest approach to coregistration of data sets is to attempt to acquire subsequent images with a spatial geometry identical to that of the original base images. Image registration can be attempted by using a baseline set of images to guide the acquisition of the subsequent acquisitions. In practice this is relatively difficult except with MR imaging, where the ability to produce rapid high-resolution anatomical survey images allows relatively accurate manual prescription of the slice positions. Using this approach allows matching of images with a typical accuracy of only 1–2 voxels, which is inadequate for many applications (HAJNAL and BYDDER 1997).

An alternative and attractive solution has been applied to the problem of providing anatomical localization of isotope images from SPECT (single photon emission computed tomography) and MR scans. These isotope modalities are of relatively low spatial resolution. Additionally they commonly aim to identify very specific physiological targets, such as inflammation, so that little or no anatomical information may be present in the image. This invalidates most coregistration techniques except for the use of small spatial localization markers (fiducials) which can be seen on the isotope study and another anatomical imaging modality such as CT or MR imaging. The use of fiducials is not entirely satisfactory since they may become dislodged or change their relative position to internal tissues as the patient moves. Manufacturers have tackled this specific problem by constructing hybrid scanning systems which allow simultaneous acquisition of CT and SPECT or PET (positron emission tomography) data (Fig. 8.1). These systems

allow accurate identification of the site of isotope uptake even where a single focus of isolated uptake occurs in an image with no anatomical information (Figs. 8.2, 8.3). These systems have the additional advantage that the CT attenuation data can be used to calibrate the tissue attenuation maps required for quantitative analysis of the isotope data. Image acquisition systems, which allow combination of data sets from MR imaging, CT and rotational angiography, are also being developed to support interventional image-guided procedures (Fig. 8.4).

In single-modality imaging, such as CT scans acquired before and after contrast or MR examinations with different sequences, the images are often acquired as part of a single examination and the patient is not moved between acquisitions. Despite this, small amounts of movement commonly occur. If a normal volunteer is asked to keep absolutely still throughout a long examination sequence then movement of several millimetres can be expected in images of the head over a period of 5–10 min, even if the head is supported and partially restrained (Fig. 8.5). In other areas of the body such as the pelvis this movement may be less marked and in others such as the limbs it may be far worse. In addition to this unconscious movement there are also problems associated with physiological movements due to breathing, cardiac motion, vessel pulsation and peristalsis. These movements are also often associated with distortion of the tissues and loss of the spatial relationships between tissues from one image to the next. These physiological sources of movement and tissue deformation introduce special problems into the design of coregistration modalities for many areas of the body and have led most workers to concentrate on the design of coregistration techniques for use in the brain. The rationale for this is twofold. Firstly the brain is protected from movement-related deformation by the skull and can, in many circumstances, be assumed to act as a rigid body, subject

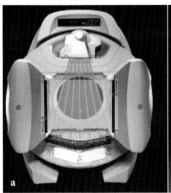
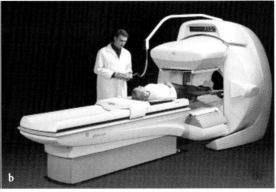

Fig. 8.1a, b. A schematic product photograph of a combined CT and gamma camera system. (Courtesy of GE Medical Systems)

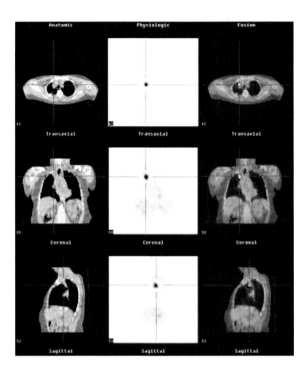

Fig. 8.2. Images of a patient with small cell lung carcinoma imaged using combined CT and fluorodeoxyglucose PET: CT (*left*), PET (*centre*) and fused images (*right*). Images illustrate a tumour in the right upper lobe. (Courtesy of Duke University and GE Medical Systems)

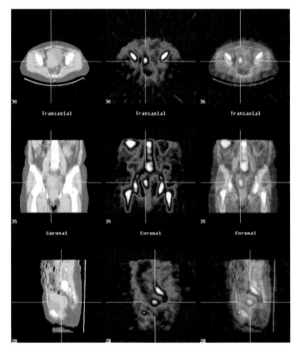

Fig. 8.3. Images acquired using combined CT and Ga[67] SPECT: CT (*left*), SPECT (*centre*) and fused images (*right*). Images illustrate uptake of isotope in a recurrent cervical carcinoma. (Courtesy of Rambam Medical Center and GE Medical Systems)

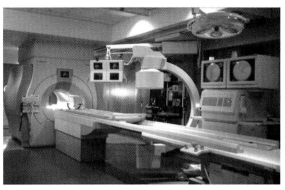

Fig. 8.4. Interventional MR suite combining 1.5 T MR and C-arm angiography systems. (Courtesy of Philips Medical Systems)

only to motion and not to deformation. Secondly, many of the major applications for coregistered data sets have been developed and clinically applied in the brain. In this chapter we will initially concentrate on techniques for coregistration of imaging data from the brain in order to illustrate the concepts and applications of the technique.

In view of the problems of spatially synchronizing image acquisitions it is necessary in the majority of cases to coregister 3D images using post-processing techniques. In principle this is relatively simple to perform, requiring two basic steps: (1) image registration and (2) image reslicing. Image registration is the process of measuring the exact difference in spatial location between the two data sets. Data reslicing is the process of resampling one of the data sets so that it is perfectly spatially coregistered with the baseline image.

8.3
Accuracy of Spatial Location Information in 3D Images

Medical 3D images consist of a matrix of image intensity values which make up a "spreadsheet" of data describing the object. The dimensions of the individual data elements govern the spatial resolution of the images so that smaller voxels will provide a higher spatial resolution. However, these 3D data sets commonly contain information that allows the spatial location of features within the image with accuracy far higher than the spatial resolution. This information is derived from the distribution of image

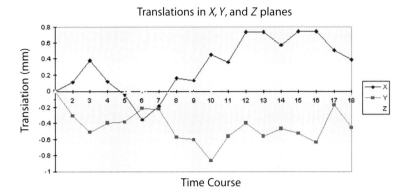

Translations in *X*, *Y*, and *Z* planes

Time Course

Fig. 8.5. Graph of head movement occurring during a functional MR scan. The graph shows translations in the *X*, *Y* and *Z* planes during the collection of 18 dynamic images over a period of just under 2 min

intensities within the data space. The image intensity in each pixel reflects the tissue, or mixture of tissues within it. Variations in tissue content produce intensity gradients across several pixels or well-defined edges where they occur over a small distance. If these gradients and edges are misaligned in two otherwise matched images then subtraction of the images will clearly identify areas of misregistration even where these are less than 1 pixel in magnitude. This occurs because the subtraction process is sensitive to the pixel intensity, which can be affected by even a small spatial misregistration (Fig. 8.6). The magnitude of the pixel in the difference image will be affected by the degree of misregistration and by the relative intensities of the two tissues forming the tissue boundary. Within a large 3D image many of these edges and gradients will be present, varying in extent, orientation and magnitude. The process of coregistration is designed to minimize these differences and accurate coregistration should eliminate them completely (Fig. 8.7). Automated coregistration algorithms work by minimizing these differences on the assumption that the minimum difference between the images will be seen where the images are perfectly coregistered.

8.4
Image Registration

The image registration process produces a description of the difference in spatial location between the two images. In the simplest case this description will contain details of the movements (translations) required in the three ordinal directions (anterior-posterior, right-left and superior-inferior) and of the rotations required in the same three planes (pitch, roll and yaw). The standard mathematical description is called the transformation matrix and can be

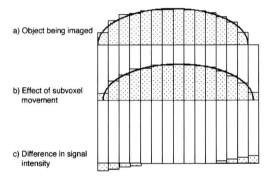

a) Object being imaged

b) Effect of subvoxel movement

c) Difference in signal intensity

Fig. 8.6a–c. Changes in image intensity generated by subvoxel shifts. **a** The intensity profile (histogram) produced by imaging a smooth curved object. **b** The object has moved by a fraction of a pixel. **c** The difference in image intensities generated by the subtraction of **a** from **b**. (Adapted from Hajnal and Bydder 1997)

used to guide resampling of the test data set so that it matches the base images.

Estimation of the appropriate transformation matrix can be performed in a number of ways. In theory the position of a 3D data set can be described by specifying the coordinates of three fixed points or of one fixed point and a plane. The simplest method to coregister two data sets is therefore to define a series of standard registration points or fiducials.

This technique is used in stereotactic brain surgery where the brain is rotated into a standard plane by identification of two points: the centres of the anterior and posterior commissures, and of the horizontal midline plane. The two points are used to define a baseline horizontal plane, the sagittal midline plane forms a vertical baseline and a coronal plane passing through the anterior commissure forms the third. The location of any point in the brain can then be described using a set of *X,Y,Z* coordinates which are defined using the intersection of the three planes as the zero point. To allow for variations in brain

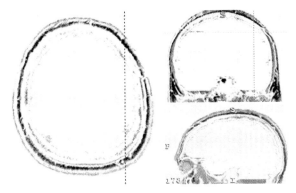

Fig. 8.7. Subtraction images of two 3D MR brain scans performed in a normal individual. The brains in the two scans have been coregistered and subtracted, resulting in complete loss of structural information in the brain. Note that the peripheral tissues are clearly seen since these were removed from one data set prior to coregistration

which is, in turn, directly related to the spatial resolution of the images. Even with high spatial resolution MR imaging this is unlikely to be greater than 1 mm in any direction, which could cause significant potential error in the location of the anatomical landmarks. With other imaging modalities such as SPECT and PET the low spatial resolution and lack of anatomical information in many images may make the identification of anatomical fiducials impossible, or at best highly inaccurate. The effects of these errors on the spatial localization of the data set will be least if the fiducial points are well separated and greater if they lie close together. This has led many workers to develop artificial fiducial markers that can be seen on all the imaging modalities employed (KREMSER et al. 1997; MAURER et al. 1997; ALP et al. 1998; ZYLKA and SABCZYNSKI 1999; WEST et al. 1999). Small samples of radioactive isotope in a lipid solution will provide clear points for identification on both MR and isotope imaging. The design of the fiducial markers can be adjusted depending on the combination of imaging modalities to be employed (Fig. 8.8). The problem with external fiducials is rendering their position fixed with regard to the internal structures being studied. For imaging the brain fixation of fiducial markers to the skin is unsatisfactory since the scalp is highly mobile with respect to the skull. Markers can be fixed in a tooth bar, which is designed to fit accurately into the bite and which considerably reduces the problems of fiducial movement, whilst maintaining the fiducial positions at the periphery of the imaging volume. In some circumstances fiducials may be fixed by attaching them to bone screws fixed into the skull. This may be justified in cases where accurate image-guided surgery is necessary but is inappropri-

size the coordinate system is linearly scaled in all three axes. This stereotactic coordinate system was described by TALAIRACH (TALAIRACH and TOURNOUX 1988) and is commonly referred to as the Talairach system. Assuming that brains have the same shape and differ only in size then any anatomical area can theoretically be described in terms of its Talairach coordinates. This assumption holds true for normal brains, which show remarkably stable stereotactic locations for deep brain structures. The location of cortical areas within the coordinate system is more variable and distortion of brain shape due to pathology can also cause significant changes in the stereotactic locations of anatomical structures.

The use of anatomical fiducials relies on the ability of the images to accurately allow their identification,

Fig. 8.8. Digital subtraction angiogram of a large posterior communicating aneurysm (**a**). Time-of-flight MR angiography (**b**) demonstrates flow within the aneurysm. Data fusion with T2-weighted anatomical MR imaging allows demonstration of intra-aneurysmal clot (*blue*) (**c**). Fiducial-based coregistration allows fusion of the clot and combined MR data set with the original angiogram (**d, e**)

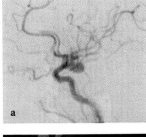
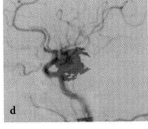
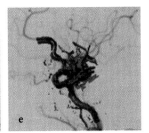
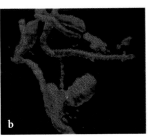
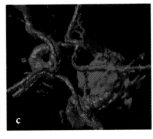

ately invasive in most cases. The use of fiducial markers is therefore limited to specific applications, where automated coregistration algorithms are inappropriate due to inadequate information content in one of the images. Using fiducial-based techniques the coordinates of each fiducial within the each image are measured and the corresponding transformation matrix can be calculated from these coordinate sets. This is a simple calculation which is undemanding of computer power and which can be easily performed by taking measurements on most image analysis workstations and calculating the transformation matrix using a simple program or spreadsheet application.

The most commonly applied technique for image coregistration is to estimate the transformation matrix by direct comparison of the two images (Woods et al. 1998a,b). This approach has been used manually in 2D imaging for many years to produce subtraction angiograms. Prior to digital imaging an exact but inverted copy of a plain skull film was used to mask the bony details from a matching angiogram image. This combination was used to produce a dense composite negative in which the bone details were cancelled out by superimposition of the positive and negative images. This process is still used today in digital subtraction angiogram systems. To optimize the quality of the subtraction the negative and positive images can be moved relative to each other until no edges are seen in the images. Automated coregistration techniques use the same approach by comparing various orientations of the two images and measuring the differences between them. The actual measurement of difference between the images may use one of several difference metrics. These range from relatively simple measures, such as the difference in intensity between the images (Hajnal and Bydder 1997), to more complex metrics, such as the standard deviation of the ratio of the voxel intensities designed (Woods et al. 1998a,b), to optimize the accuracy of the registration technique. Whatever the chosen metric may be, the aim of the program is to find the orientation of the two images that minimizes the cumulative difference between corresponding voxels. A simple example of this is given in the equation below using the chi-squared statistic (χ^2):

$$\chi^2 = \sum_n \frac{(SI_a - SI_b)^2}{n}$$

where SI_a is the intensity of the voxel in image a and SI_b the intensity in image b and n is the total number of voxels. The minimum value for χ^2 is calculated

by moving image a relative to image b until the minimum value is found. This approach is extremely demanding of computing power and can be very time-consuming, especially with large data sets. To reduce the computation time a number of strategies have been employed including using only voxels above a certain threshold, using only voxels with data in both images and performing the minimization iteratively using gradually increasing spatial resolution to allow the software to "home-in" on the correct solution. The exact approach used depends on the specific software package employed and the time taken is also directly related to the image size. Many automated grey-level matching techniques have now been described and most seem capable of estimating the transformation matrix to subpixel levels under ideal conditions.

In practice it is important to be aware that automated grey-scale matching algorithms of this type operate on the basis of a series of essential assumptions and can be expected to perform poorly where these assumptions are incorrect. These assumptions are:

- that the relative grey scale values of structures are the same in both images;
- that the relative spatial relationships of all structures in the imaging volume are identical in both images.

The first assumption is essential if direct comparison of the images is to be used as the difference metric but can be avoided by the selection of alternative appropriate metrics. Even in images where the relative grey-scale values differ considerably it is possible to obtain acceptable coregistration by choice of an appropriate metric such as an image of edge strength or some alternative derived value which will make the image sets more directly comparable.

The second assumption is intrinsic to the technique. We are attempting to accurately coregister two identical volumes which must therefore be identical. In practice we often wish to coregister volumes which actually differ significantly, often to improve the identification of these differences. We can assume that the difference between the images is minimal and will not affect the overall coregistration; however, this is also an assumption and will not always be true. Once again the errors can be reduced by selection of an appropriate metric for minimization and by performing coregistration using only a part of the image set. A classic example of this is the coregistration of head scans, where accurate coregistration is impossible in most cases due to variations in the facial structures, which are highly variable and which dominate the matching process. Coregistration of head images is therefore conducted using one baseline image and a second image which has had the extracerebral tissues edited out to avoid errors. This technique of skull stripping is essential for the acquisition of accurate coregistrations (Fig. 8.7).

An alternative approach to coregistration is to identify a plane in one image and to coregister it to the same plane using a surface matching technique. This approach can be used to coregister the images of the cranial vault by extracting the CSF (cerebrospinal fluid) surface and using this "convex hull" to match to the same surface from another image. The technique tends to be less accurate than grey-scale matching methods but can be extremely useful where these approaches are not appropriate. This method is commonly used to coregister imaging data with an image of the body surface derived from stereo cameras or interferometry, which can allow image guidance of surgical or radiotherapy techniques in theatre.

8.5
Data Reslicing

Once the transformation matrix has been calculated one of the data sets must be resliced so that it matches the baseline image. The aim of the reslicing process is to calculate a value for every voxel that is identical to the value we would have obtained if the image had been acquired in that position. Reslicing is performed by calculating a new value for each voxel from the intensities of the voxels in the original image in which it now lies. This requires us to make an assumption about the relative contribution that each voxel would make to the new voxel value. Once we have decided on this assumption we can use the data from surrounding voxels to synthesize a final value for the new voxel. This process is known as interpolation. The simplest approach to data interpolation is to assume that the contribution to signal intensity from the original voxels will be linearly related to the proportion of the voxel included in the final sample. This approach (known as linear interpolation) is simple to perform, uses linear algebra and requires data only from the voxels which contribute directly to the final pixel. The accuracy of the interpolation process can be improved by the selection of an appropriate nonlinear function. The appropriate function will depend on the imaging modality and the image formation process. This is a particular problem with MR data,

which are acquired as a series of phase/frequency maps in the Fourier domain and reconstructed using an inverse Fourier transform. This results in a complex relationship between pixels and the surrounding image elements. This relationship, described by a sinc function, means that voxels nearest to the reference point will have the greatest effect on the intensity of the interpolated data but that even pixels at the extremes of the image will have some residual effect. To perform a sinc interpolation the contribution of each voxel in the image to the new single voxel value is calculated as the product of the original voxel values and the sinc function (Fig. 8.9). Since the sinc function has significant negative components many voxels will make negative contributions to the final voxel value, which is calculated by summing all the individual voxel contributions.

It would be incorrect to believe that the images interpolated this way are identical to what would have been obtained if the subject had been translated in the spatial domain to the required position. That assumption would be true only if the original data were exactly defined by the truncated Fourier description in the original data set. However, provided the sinc kernel has a size equal to the image, interpolation with a sinc function is at least consistent with the way the image has been acquired and no information which was available at the scanner is lost. Such interpolation would have to be considered optimal.

For computational reasons it is inappropriate to apply a large sinc kernel, but as the kernel itself is quite spatially compact it is possible to truncate it at some level. A common kernel size for medical image

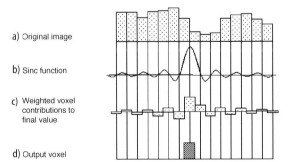

Fig. 8.9a–d. The calculation of a new voxel value following a subvoxel shift using sinc interpolation. **a** The intensity profile of the original image. A new image is to be generated 0.5 pixel to the left. **b** The sinc function aligned on the centre of the new pixel. **c** The product of the sinc function and the corresponding pixels in the original image. **d** The sum of these, which is the final calculated voxel value. (Adapted from HAJNAL and BYDDER 1997)

subtraction work is 13×13×13 (Hajnal et al. 1995a; Freeborough et al. 1996). This is a direct result of the first-order reciprocal scaling and a range of 6 pixels is required for the sinc function to reduce to a negligible level (i.e. less than 1% for a windowed kernel). The computational implications of using large-scale kernels are offset somewhat by the fact that the coefficients required for sinc interpolation can be decomposed (Freeborough et al. 1996), so that the computation is linearly proportional to the kernel size rather than its volume (a "fast sinc"). In addition re-normalizing the sinc function so that it has a constant integral improves interpolation accuracy and allows the use of smaller kernels which increases processing speed (Thacker et al. 1999a). Thus despite its somewhat complicated form, sinc interpolation seems to offer as good a solution as the best techniques in terms of computational requirement on equivalent-sized kernels.

8.6
Complex Coregistration

The techniques we have described in the preceding sections make the assumption that the structure to be coregistered is a "rigid body" so that the relative spatial relationships of all structures in the imaging volume are identical in both images. This would be true for a solid phantom imaged in different positions where the differences between any corresponding structure can be described by the transformation matrix. Such movements of rigid bodies in a coordinate space are the simplest form of affine transform, which also permits linear reslicing along arbitrary axes.

In many applications attempts to coregister data are confounded by deformation of the tissues which has occurred between the data collections. In many cases this distortion will affect the tissues throughout the image. A good example would be an attempt to coregister the abdominal organs on abdominal CT scans obtained in the supine position with scans obtained prone. These images are not simply the same images inverted but will demonstrate a complete change in the spatial relationships of one organ to another and of the internal structures within the organs. An affine or rigid body transformation cannot describe the changes which have occurred in these situations and the coregistration process requires a far more complex "non-affine" transformation, sometimes referred to as image warping. The

problems with non-affine transformation techniques are considerable. Using the brain as an example, many groups have developed methods to improve coregistration results by application of non-affine transformations. These brain warping techniques have been employed to correct for variations between individuals when coregistering images to a computerized brain atlas or to improve spatial coregistration between different individuals to allow transformation of several studies into a standard data space. Unfortunately image warping techniques must be based on a theoretical physical model of the tissues. If such a model were perfect and were able to describe the interplay of physical properties such as flexibility, rigidity and tensile strength in every tissue component then it might be possible to constrain the solutions to the warp sufficiently to provide the correct solution. This approach, called finite element modelling, is widely used in engineering where the physical properties of materials are well documented. However, it can easily be seen that the finite element modelling approach is extremely limited in medical applications due to the extreme complexity of the body and the variability in tissue properties.

An alternative approach to image warping is to assume that the elastic properties of the tissues are constant. This is clearly totally incorrect and no one would suggest that the skull and the brain display identical elastic properties if a force is applied to the head. However, many models assume that this approach is appropriate in a limited tissue such as the brain itself. In these circumstances a degree of distortion detected by noting displacement of specific structures can be "corrected" by application of a linear or other simple image warp. For small regions within a single structure this is often appropriate. However, for whole volume coregistration the problems with this approach are that it makes assumptions about the way in which structures will move relative to one another (Fig. 8.10). These models are based on the assumption that the structures in the two brains have the same spatial relationship which has become distorted by a process described by the warping technique. These assumptions can be confirmed only by observation of the displacements which occur to other structures when the warp field is applied. Several workers have looked at the standard deviation of the spatial coordinates of easily recognized structures following warping of brain images. If the assumptions of the warping process are correct then these should be smaller after warping than when a simple affine transform is applied. One example of such a study used the computerized brain

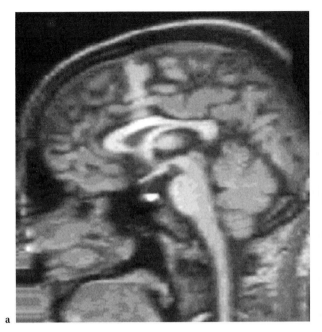 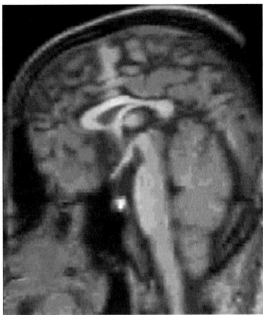

a   b

Fig. 8.10a,b. (a) A sagittal MR image of the head and (b) a warped image. The warp has assumed a linear elasticity in all tissues and has been used to "stretch" the brain below the anterior commissure–posterior commissure line, ventrally by 50%. Note the distortion of the anatomy and that equal degrees of distortion are seen in all tissues

atlas developed at the Karolinska Institute in Stockholm and showed an improvement in registration accuracy when a non-affine process was included in the registration method. Despite this the standard deviations of the coordinates of individual structures varied from 0.9 to 4.5 mm (INGVAR et al. 1994). Interestingly when this same atlas, developed on averaged data from Swedish subjects, was applied to a Japanese population the distribution of the same structures was worse than that obtained with a simple affine transform. This illustrates the problems of generalized image warping techniques which cannot contain sufficient constraints to accurately describe the behaviour of biological systems. Despite this, significant improvements may be seen in specific limited applications such as the coregistration of multiple normal brains for functional MR imaging (ASHBURNER and FRISTON 2000).

The problems of the image warping approach can be easily illustrated with a simple thought experiment. Imagine 3D MR images of two brains are being coregistered into the Talairach coordinate system. In each patient one cerebral hemisphere is smaller than the other so that an affine warp cannot be applied successfully. In one patient the smaller hemisphere demonstrates a diffuse lobar atrophy affecting all areas of the brain; in the other a focal disorder has caused loss of the central basal ganglia and the

peripheral cortical mantle is relatively normal. If we hope to warp these images back into a standard normal brain configuration, perhaps to apply a computerized brain atlas, we will need to include in our warping model specific information about the location and severity of tissue loss and the physical properties displayed in the tissues which have responded to it. The only hope for such an approach is to identify multiple anatomical landmarks which can be used to allow detailed comparison of the distortions between the two images and from which we can derive information about the nature of the distortion which has occurred in different areas. These landmarks may be identified manually. Alternatively a grey-scale coregistration technique similar to the one applied for affine transformations may be used. The technique must be modified to allow non-affine distortions and will generate not a simple transformation matrix but a complex detailed distortion map describing the individual changes in voxel shape which must be applied to produce the minimum difference between the images. This approach can applied successfully if the aims of the experiment are appropriate and if the user realizes the inherent inaccuracies of the technique. Estimations of the warp field required to align normal and pathological brains can be used to indicate the areas of the brain where the majority of tissue loss or gain has occurred (Fig. 8.11). Due to the

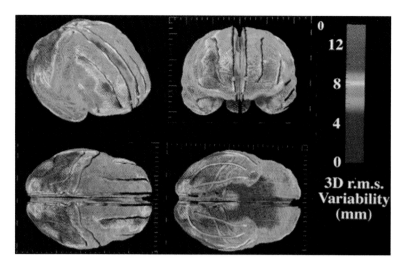

Fig. 8.11. Images showing the differences in the cortical structure between a group of normals and a group of patients with Alzheimer's disease. The patients' brains have been warped into a standard coordinate system and these images show the differences in the amount of deformation needed to make the diseased brains conform to the normals. The colour coding therefore represents the average amount of tissue deformation required, showing considerable atrophy has occurred in the frontal and posterior parietal lobes

limitations of the method the spatial accuracy of the warp information will be lower, often far lower than the spatial resolution of the image, and will be subject to errors where misregistrations have occurred between apparently similar structures.

An alternative approach to this type of image warping is to develop techniques to identify specific anatomical structures within the tissue. These anatomical statistical trained models (STM) are trained using a large sample of images on which specific features are manually identified. The statistical variability of these features is then calculated and the trained STM can the "search" similar images to find the best estimation of the structure. This approach can be applied to the identification of structures such as cerebral gyri, blood vessels or bone edges. The problems with STMs relate to the complexity of the models in 3D data sets and the reliance on the training set of images to accurately describe the variations which may occur in the sample. However, within the limits of their training set STMs can be used to identify target features which could be used to drive a locally focused image warping technique.

8.7
Applications of Data Coregistration

The ability to coregister 3D data sets facilitates a wide variety of post-processing techniques. Some of these are described in brief below. The list is far from exhaustive and serves to illustrate the importance of data fusion in medical applications.

8.7.1
Analysis of Temporal Image Sequences

The techniques of automated image coregistration were first applied to medical data sets to improve the stability of data analysis in functional magnetic resonance imaging (fMR). Functional MR techniques for the measurement of brain activation, cerebral perfusion and capillary permeability rely on the analysis of multiple images collected over a period of 2–60 min. All these analysis techniques perform calculations on a pixel by pixel basis which use the signal intensity changes in the pixel which occur over time. The nature of the changes and of the analysis performed is presented in detail in Chap. 24. In all cases the presence of movement in the data set means that the time course change may represent the movement of structures through the sample space rather than physiologically induced signal changes (ASHBURNER and FRISTON 2000). This is of particular importance in blood oxygen level dependent (BOLD) fMR where data collections tend to be long lasting and the subject is often performing cognitive or motor tasks that produce motion (THACKER et al. 1999b). This motion may be greatest when the subject is performing the task so that the presence of motion correlates with the timing of the test paradigm. This stimulus-correlated motion can produce spurious activations on fMR which are eliminated by appropriate motion correction (Fig. 8.12).

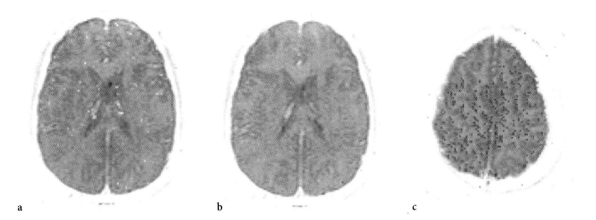

a   b   c

Fig. 8.12a–c. Functional MR experiment using a block paradigm. In this case the subject is at rest throughout the experiment. a Apparent areas of significant activation which disappear after coregistration. b, c Activations in a synthetic data set constructed from multiple identical copies of the baseline image. These copies were then coregistered to mimic exactly the movements made by the subject during the actual experiment. These data appear to generate multiple areas of highly significant activation that are entirely due to coincidental stimulus-correlated motion. The activations axe for greater than seen in the red data only because the noise structure in the synthetic images is identical in each image

8.7.2
Visualization from Multiple Data Sets

The ability to coregister images from multiple modalities or from multiple examinations allows the development of true data fusion to support both 2D and 3D visualization techniques. We have already seen examples of coregistered CT and isotope images acquired simultaneously from dedicated systems (Figs. 8.2, 8.3). Using post-processing coregistration we can produce similar fused images that allow identification of anatomy from CT or MR imaging with overlays of data from PET or SPECT (Fig. 8.13). Since these data acquisitions are 3D in nature we can visualize these fused data using standard 3D visualization techniques to demonstrate separate tissue components from different images. Figure 8.14 demonstrates the relationship between the skull (identified on CT), an acoustic neuroma (identified on

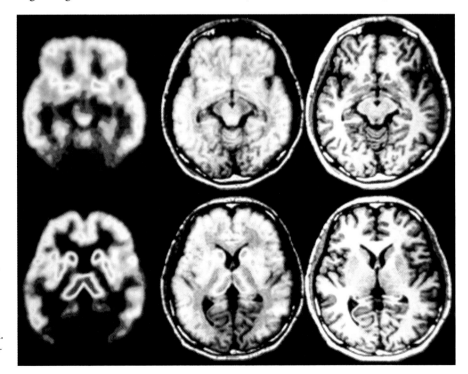

Fig. 8.13. Images of C[11]-buprenorphine binding on PET (left) and MR images of the same brain (right) with fused images shown in the centre. (Courtesy of Dr. A. Jones, Hope Hospital, Salford, UK)

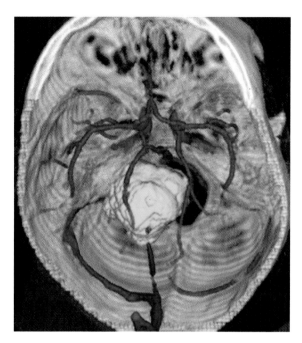

Fig. 8.14. Three-dimensional visualization of an acoustic neuroma patient. The image demonstrates the relationship between the skull (identified on CT), an acoustic neuroma (identified on contrast-enhanced MR imaging) and the adjacent blood vessels (identified on time-of-flight MR angiography)

contrast-enhanced MR imaging) and the adjacent blood vessels (identified on time-of-flight angiography). Such combined images allow improved 3D image interpretation and are of particular use in surgical planning applications.

8.7.3
Computerized Brain Atlases

Several groups have developed computerized atlases of the human brain that can be applied to images from individual patients to improve the identification of structures. This is particularly useful in educational applications and in the identification of structures, such as Brodmann's cortical areas, which are not anatomically defined on the images themselves (GREITZ et al. 1991; INGVAR et al. 1994; NOWINSKI et al. 1997; WOODS et al. 1999; NOWINSKI and THIRUNA-VUUKARASUU 2000). These atlases vary from simple affine transformation systems which assume that the brain is a rigid structure to more sophisticated systems which apply a low-order non-affine warp in order to improve fitting of the data to the atlas. In practice these atlases are extremely useful for the approximate identification of cortical areas in clinical patients and on images from modalities where

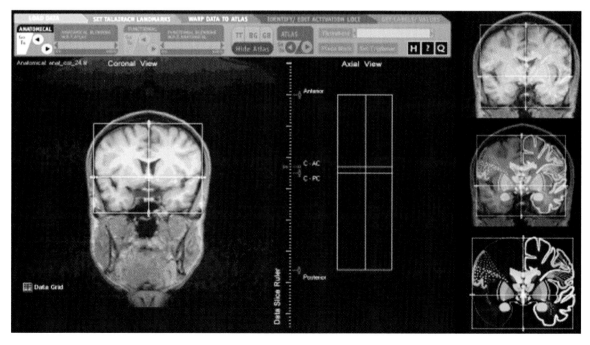

Fig. 8.15. Screenshot from the *Brain Atlas for Functional Imaging* (NOWINSKI and THIRUNAVUUKARASUU 2000) showing the application of a Talairach coordinate system to a coronal image from a 3D brain MR image. After application of the coordinate space the images can be coregistered to the standard Talairach map. The images on the *right* show the coregistered images with varying degrees of opacity to demonstrate the image (*top*), the pure atlas (*bottom*) and a fused version (*middle*)

anatomical content is poor such as isotope investigations or fMR (Figs. 8.15, 8.16).

Atlases can also be used to guide the selection of brain regions for more complex analyses (GARDNER and YAZDANI 1998). We have used a simple coordinate system based on the position and size of the CSF space to allow automatic measurements of the position and severity of cerebral atrophy in patients with dementia. In this case the atlas is deliberately extremely simple and of very low spatial resolution, identifying only the front, middle, back, top and bottom and right and left of the CSF space. Despite this the distribution of CSF in this standard space allows differential diagnosis between dementias of different types with accuracy in excess of 80%. This is illustrated in Fig. 8.17, which shows the separation of patients with different dementing diseases using this technique (THACKER et al. 2000).

8.7.4
Subtraction Imaging

Another application of data coregistration is to allow comparison of apparently similar examinations to improve the detection of small structural changes. The use of an automated coregistration technique

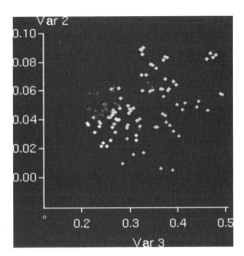

Fig. 8.17. Scattergram of the distribution of cerebrospinal within a simple stereotactic coordinate system. Each point represents a single patient with Alzheimer's disease (*green*), fronto-temporal dementia (*orange*) or vascular dementia (*red*). *Blue* points are normal age-matched controls. Note the excellent separability of the groups, which provides useful support information for diagnosis

will allow generation of matching images with sub-voxel accuracy, which can then be directly compared (Fig. 8.18). This process assumes that the differences between the images will not affect the accuracy of

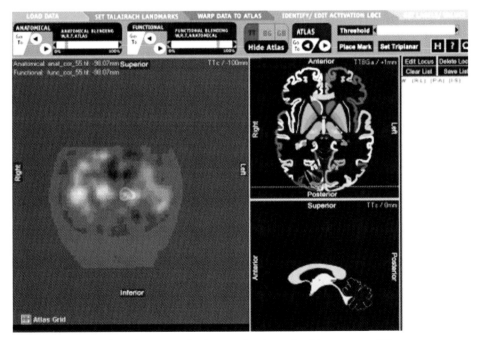

Fig. 8.16. Screenshot from the *Brain Atlas for Functional Imaging* (NOWINSKI and THIRUNAVUUKARASUU 2000). Image shows a coronal image from a functional MR series which has been coregistered into the Talairach coordinate system. The *right* panels indicate the position of the marker point on the atlas and the *far right* panel gives a coordinate description of the areas of activation

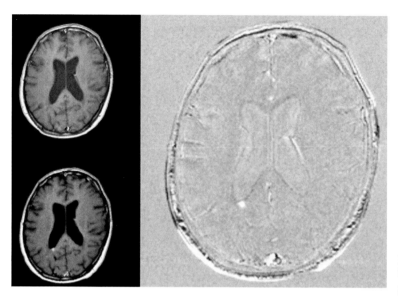

Fig. 8.18. MR images and a subtraction image of an enhancing plaque in a patient with multiple sclerosis

the coregistration process. Where changes are small, affect only a small volume of the data and do not occur in areas of strong edge strength this assumption appears to be true. The beauty of this approach is that is possible to visualize tiny changes in structure of the order of a fraction of a pixel in magnitude (Bydder 1995; Hajnal et al. 1995b; Hajnal and Bydder 1997). This allows visualization of changes due to brain atrophy, tumour growth or other processes where the change between the images is too small to be appreciated by eye (Fig. 8.19).

The interpretation of subtraction images is quite difficult since changes may be caused by either failure of coregistration, changes in intensity or movements of tissue boundaries (Bydder 1995). In addition the magnitude of the differences in the subtraction images can be small, making them difficult to identify. The use of statistical approaches to identify significant differences between the images improves the detection of difference and allows automated identification of the pixels that have changed. The use of statistical subtractive techniques also allows the comparison of images with different grey-scale characteristics that would demonstrate residual signal on standard subtraction images (Fig. 8.20).

8.7.5
Measuring Change in Brain Volume

The accuracy of automated coregistration algorithms has been utilized to allow measurement of the small volume changes that occur due to atrophic brain dis-

eases. Using an accurate coregistration technique will produce images with no features in the brain except in areas where the brain edge has moved due to atrophy. These changes can be seen at the brain edge even when the movement is far less than 1 pixel in magnitude, and form the basis of the subtraction technique described above. Where the signal intensities on each side of the boundary are known the intensity of the voxel in the difference mage can be used to calculate the movement of the edge within the

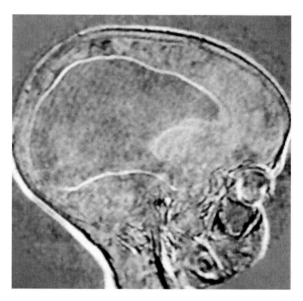

Fig. 8.19. Subtraction image from two MR examinations in a child with hydrocephalus. The white border around the ventricle indicates that the ventricle has shrunk between the examinations

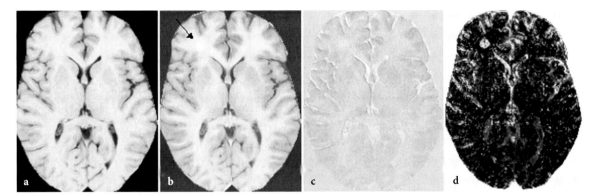

Fig. 8.20a–d. The principles of statistical non-parametric image subtraction in a normal brain. **a, b** Two inversion recovery images which have been acquired with different inversion times to produce small but significant differences in grey-scale structure. In **b** a small phantom area has been inserted (*arrow*). This circle is lighter than the background image by 2× the standard deviation of the background noise and can hardly be detected by eye. **c** A subtraction image of **b** minus **a**. The circle is slightly more visible but the major difference is the intensity of the grey matter due to the difference in image acquisition technique. **d** A statistical subtraction map where the intensity of the pixels indicates the probability that the image structure is different. The circular phantom is clearly seen

voxel that must have occurred. The volume change can then be expressed as the appropriate fraction of the voxel volume. This technique has been applied to the brain of patients with Alzheimer's disease and allows detection of hippocampal atrophy in only 6 months (FREEBOROUGH et al. 1996). The technique can also be used to measure volume changes due to other pathological processes such as tumours.

8.7.6
Segmentation and Classification

One of the main advantages of coregistration is the ability to combine information about a single voxel from images acquired using different modalities. This generates a data-rich multi-parametric data set for each voxel that can be used to characterize the voxel far more accurately than could be achieved with a single image (ALFANO et al. 1997; HOLDEN et al. 1995). This type of data set can be analysed using statistical clustering techniques to separate specific tissue types from the data with great accuracy (Fig. 8.21). The data content of these multi-parametric images can be adjusted by selection of appropriate imaging modalities to add the missing information required for a particular analysis. This allows accurate identification not only of normal tissues but of pathological abnormalities within the data set.

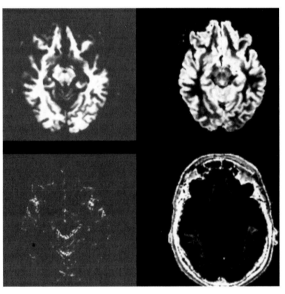

Fig. 8.21. Multi-spectral segmentation of normal tissues from a coregistered series of MR data sets. The images show the probability distribution (tissue maps) for (*clockwise from top left*) white matter, grey matter, cerebrospinal fluid and soft tissues

8.7.7
MR Prescription Guidance

Techniques for 3D image coregistration are becoming far faster as algorithmic improvements are developed. This has led several manufacturers to experiment with systems to allow automated prescription of the scanning geometry in MR imaging based on previous images. The concept is relatively simple. When a patient attends for a follow-up scan the system will perform a relatively detailed survey scan. This survey will be coregistered to the scan performed on the previous visit and the transformation matrix will be used to adjust the scanning parameters. In theory this should allow the follow-up scan to be acquired in a geometry already coregistered to the original examination. In practice there remain some logistical problems with this approach and it is not clear how practical it will be to obtain sub-pixel coregistered examinations of large anatomical data sets. However, in fMR experiments this technique is of considerable benefit, allowing the image prescription to track the movements of the head as the experiment is performed. Although this does not remove the need to coregister the data it does mean that the amount by which the images need to be transposed is minimized and is of similar magnitude for all images. This approach also allows the generation of acceptable fMR images on the scanner console without further coregistration in clinical applications.

References

Alfano B, Brunetti A, Covelli EM (1997) Unsupervised, automated segmentation of the normal brain using a multispectral relaxometric magnetic resonance approach. Magn Reson Med 37:84–93

Alp MS, Dujovny M, Misra FT (1998) Head registration techniques for image-guided surgery. Neurol Res 20:31–37

Ashburner J, Friston KJ (2000) Image registration. In: Moonen CTW, Bandettini PA (eds) Functional MRI. Springer, Berlin Heidelberg New York, pp 285–300

Bydder GM (1995) The MacKenzie Davidson Memorial Lecture: detection of small changes in the brain with serial magnetic resonance imaging. Br J Radiol 68:1271–1295

Freeborough P, Woods R, Fox N (1996) Accurate registration of serial 3D MR brain images and its application to visualising change in neurodegenerative disorders. J Comput Assist Tomogr 20:1012–1022

Gardner JC, Yazdani F (1998) Correlating MR lesions and functional deficits in multiple sclerosis patients: anatomical atlas registration. Phys Med Rehabil Clin North Am 9:569–586

Greitz T, Bohm C, Holte S (1991) Computerized brain atlas: construction, anatomical content, and some applications. J Comput Assist Tomogr 15:26–38

Hajnal JV, Bydder GM (1997) Registration and subtraction of serial magnetic resonance images. I. Technique. In: Bradley WG, Bydder GM (eds) Advanced MR imaging techniques. Martin Dunitz, London

Hajnal JV, Saeed N, Soar EJ (1995a) Registration and interpolation procedure for subvoxel matching of serially acquired MR images. J Comput Assist Tomogr 19:289–296

Hajnal JV, Saeed N, Oatridge A (1995b) Detection of subtle brain changes using subvoxel registration and subtraction of serial MR images. J Comput Assist Tomogr 19:677–691

Holden M, Steen E, Lundervold A (1995) Segmentation and visualization of brain lesions in multispectral magnetic resonance images. Comput Med Imaging Graph 19:171–183

Ingvar M, Bohm C, Thurfjell L (1994) The role of a computerized adjustable brain atlas for merging of data from examinations using PET, SPECT, MEG, CT and MR images. In: Thatcher R, et al (eds) Functional neuroimaging: technical foundations. Academic Press, San Diego

Kremser C, Plangger C, Bosecke R (1997) Image registration of MR and CT images using a frameless fiducial marker system. Magn Reson Imaging 15:579–585

Maurer CR Jr, Fitzpatrick JM, Wang MY (1997) Registration of head volume images using implantable fiducial markers. IEEE Trans Med Imaging 16:447–462

Nowinski W, Thirunavuukarasuu A (2000) Brain atlas for functional imaging. Thieme, Stuttgart

Nowinski W, Bryan R, Raghavan R (1997) The electronic clinical brain atlas multiplanar navigation of the human brain. Thieme, Stuttgart New York

Talairach J, Tournoux P (1988) Co-planar stereotactic atlas of the human brain. Thieme, Stuttgart

Thacker NA, Jackson A, Moriarty D (1999a) Improved quality of re-sliced MR images using re-normalized sinc interpolation. J Magn Reson Imaging 10:582–588

Thacker N, Burton E, Lacey AJ (1999b) The effects of motion on parametric fMRI analysis techniques. Physiol Meas 20:251–263

Thacker N, Bathgate D, Varma A (2000) Automated analysis of the distribution and severity of cerebral atrophy in dementing diseases: diagnostic power in Alzheimer's, frontotemporal and vascular dementia. Proceedings of the 8th annual meeting of the ISMRM, 2000, Denver

West J, Fitzpatrick JM, Wang MY (1999) Retrospective intermodality registration techniques for images of the head: surface-based versus volume-based. IEEE Trans Med Imaging 18:144–150

Woods RP, Grafton ST, Watson JD (1998a) Automated image registration. II. Intersubject validation of linear and nonlinear models. J Comput Assist Tomogr 22:153–165

Woods RP, Grafton ST, Holmes CJ (1998b) Automated image registration. I. General methods and intrasubject, intramodality validation. J Comput Assist Tomogr 22:139–152

Woods RP, Dapretto M, Sicotte NL (1999) Creation and use of a Talairach-compatible atlas for accurate, automated, nonlinear intersubject registration, and analysis of functional imaging data. Hum Brain Mapp 8:73–79

Zylka W, Sabczynski J (1999) Effect of localization devices and registration methods on the accuracy of stereotactic frame systems predicted by the Gaussian approach. Comput Aided Surg 4:77–86

Clinical Applications

9 Electronic Brain Atlases: Features and Applications

Wieslaw L. Nowinski

CONTENTS

Abstracts

This chapter addresses the construction, features, applications, and potential of electronic brain atlases for neuroradiology and neuroeducation. An electronic brain atlas database with complementary atlases containing gross anatomy, subcortical structures, brain connections, and sulcal patterns was constructed. This database contains two-dimensional and three-dimensional, mutually coregistered atlases with about 1000 structures and 400 sulcal patterns.

Six commercial applications have been developed and described here based on this database suitable for neuroradiology, neuroeducation, human brain mapping, and stereotactic functional neurosurgery. Three applications are low-cost CD-ROMs: *The Electronic Clinical Brain Atlas*, *Brain Atlas for Functional Imaging*, and the *Cerefy Student Brain Atlas*. The *Cerefy Neuroradiology Atlas* is a web-enabled application.

The use of the electronic brain atlas as a tool for faster scan interpretation, facilitating communicating information, increasing confidence, and speeding up learning is illustrated. The atlas: (1) reduces time in image interpretation by providing interactive multiple labeling, triplanar display, higher parcellation than the scan itself, multi-modal fusion, and display of underlying anatomy for functional images; (2) facilitates the communication of information about the interpreted scans from the neuroradiologist to other clinicians and medical students; (3) increases the neuroradiologist's confidence; and (4) reduces time in learning neuroanatomy and scan interpretation.

9.1 Introduction

Introduction of new modalities and advanced diagnostic imaging techniques will increase the difficulty of learning how to interpret scans. The continuous increase in contrast and spatial resolutions of scans will also require from the neuroradiologist more advanced knowledge of neuroanatomy. As a result, new approaches for speeding up and facilitating the interpretation of scans as well as reducing neuroradiologists' learning curves will be needed. Model-enhanced neuroradiology may be one of solutions. Increased demand for advanced, fast, and economical image processing and understanding is widening the relevance of electronic brain atlases to neuroradiology.

Making maps and atlases is an ancient art-science. The map represents, organizes, and communicates data on the object of interest. Throughout history man has been producing maps of objects around him; initially the land and sea, later other planets and solar systems, and most recently the human genome and human brain. Our work, which started in the Decade of the Brain, has focused on the construction of electronic brain atlases and the development of

W.L. Nowinski, D.Sc, PhD
Medical Imaging Laboratory, Kent Ridge Digital Labs, 21 Heng Mui Keng Terrace, Singapore 119613

atlas-assisted clinical applications. Electronic brain atlases have numerous research, clinical, and educational applications. Their pioneering applications in neuroeducation include, among others, *BrainStorm* (DEV et al. 1992), *Digital Anatomist* (SUNDSTEN et al. 1994), A.D.A.M. (ADAM 1994), and *Voxel-Man* (HOHNE 1995). Electronic brain atlases are also used in stereotactic functional neurosurgery, neuroradiology, and human brain mapping. In addition, they have potential applications in radiation therapy, drug testing for model-assisted analysis of pharmacological MR imaging, and drug delivery for exact localization of targets.

We have developed a comprehensive electronic brain atlas database with complementary atlases containing gross anatomy, subcortical structures, brain connections, and sulcal patterns. This database was derived from the classic printed brain atlases published by Thieme. These printed atlases were digitized, enhanced, segmented (color-coded or contoured), labeled, aligned, and organized into atlas volumes. The electronic atlases feature high-quality processed atlas images, and fully segmented and labeled structures. The anatomical index has about 1000 structures per hemisphere and more than 400 sulcal patterns. Three-dimensional extensions of the atlases were constructed. In addition, all two-dimensional and three-dimensional atlases were mutually coregistered. This electronic brain atlas database, called the *Cerefy Brain Atlas Database*, is applicable to: neurosurgery (NOWINSKI 1998a; NOWINSKI et al. 2000b), neuroradiology (NOWINSKI et al. 2001a), brain mapping (NOWINSKI et al. 2000a, NOWINSKI and THIRUNAVUUKARASUU 2001), and neuroeducation (NOWINSKI et al. 2001b).

The goal of this chapter is to provide an overview of the brain atlases and their features as well as to describe the Cerefy atlas-assisted applications, and demonstrate their usefulness for neuroradiology and neuroeducation.

9.2
Brain Atlases

9.2.1
Definition of an Electronic Brain Atlas

We define an electronic brain atlas as a set of three major components: *brain model* (these can be images, contours, surface, polygonal or volumetric models), *textual database* (the list of structures with their descriptions and related links), and supporting *tools* (for operations such as registration, labeling, mensuration, or presentation) along with corresponding data (such as labels) (Fig. 9.1).

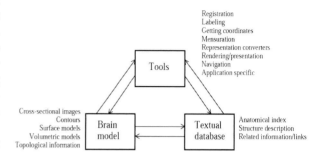

Fig. 9.1. Definition of an electronic brain atlas

9.2.2
Types of Brain Atlases

Numerous types of brain atlases have been constructed varying in material used as well as their functionality and applications.

9.2.2.1
Printed Atlases

A number of excellent printed brain atlases are available including DUVERNOY (1988), NETTER (1991), SCHNITZLEIN and MURTAGH (1980), and others such as DEARMOND et al. (1989), FIX (1987), KRAUS and BAILEY (1994), MARTIN (1989), MCMINN et al. (1993), and NIUWENNHUYS et al. (1981). In addition, several stereotactic brain atlases have been constructed since the 1950s. These include TALAIRACH et al. (1957), SCHALTENBRAND and BAILEY (1959), ANDREW and WATKINS (1969), VAN BUREN and BORKE (1972), SCHALTENBRAND and WAHREN (1977), SZIKLA et al. (1977), AFSHAR et al. (1978), TALAIRACH and TOURNOUX (1988, 1993), and ONO et al. (1990). A major limitation of their use is the difficulty in mapping the printed atlas plates into an individual brain.

9.2.2.2
Electronic Stereotactic Atlases

Deformable electronic atlases overcome some limitations of printed atlases and open new possibilities. In addition to atlas warping, they offer many features not available in printed atlases, such as interactive labeling of scans, flexible ways of presentation in two and three dimensions, defining regions of interest, mensuration, searching capabilities, and integration of information from multiple sources.

To combine the widely accepted stereotactic printed atlases with the capabilities offered by electronic atlases, several popular printed atlases have been converted into electronic form, including: the Schaltenbrand and Bailey atlas (1959), by Kazarnovskaya et al. (1991), Yoshida (1992), and Hardy et al. (1999); the Schaltenbrand and Wahren atlas (1977), by Kall (1992), Niemann et al. (1994), Sramka et al. (1997), Nowinski et al. (1997b), and Hardy et al. (1999); the Talairach and Tournoux atlas (1988), by Nowinski et al. (1997a), and Hardy et al. (1999); the Referentially Oriented Talairach and Tournoux atlas (1993), by Nowinski et al. (1997a); the Ono et al. (1990) atlas, by Nowinski et al. (1997b); the Afshar et al. (1978) atlas, by Niemann et al. (1999); and the Van Buren and Borke (1972) atlas, by Hardy et al. (1999). Computerized versions of printed atlases may vary substantially from a simple, direct digitization of the original material to a sophisticated, fully segmented, labeled, enhanced, and three-dimensionally extended deformable atlas.

9.2.2.3
Other Electronic Brain Atlases

Many other types of brain atlases have been developed. They include MR imaging-based atlases (Lehmann et al. 1991; Hohne et al. 1992; Kikinis et al. 1996; Schmahmann et al. 1999); cryosection-based atlases (Bohm et al. 1983; Greitz et al. 1991; Dev et al. 1992; Toga et al. 1994); multi-modal Visible Human-derived atlases (Hohne 1995; Schiemann et al. 2000); brain animations (Sundsten et al. 1994); probabilistic anatomical atlases (Evans et al. 1992; Mazziotta et al. 1995; Thompson et al. 2000); surface-based atlases (Van Essen and Drury 1997); surface-based probabilistic atlases (Van Essen et al. 2000); and probabilistic functional atlases constructed from microrecordings (Nowinski and Benabid 2002).

9.2.3
Cerefy Electronic Brain Atlas Database

The Cerefy[1] electronic brain atlas database (Nowinski et al. 1997b; Nowinski 2001a) contains electronic versions of the printed brain atlases published by Thieme:

– *Atlas for Stereotaxy of the Human Brain* (Schaltenbrand and Wahren 1977);
– *Co-Planar Stereotactic Atlas of the Human Brain* (Talairach and Tournoux 1988);
– *Atlas of the Cerebral Sulci* (Ono et al. 1990);
– *Referentially Oriented Cerebral MRI Anatomy: Atlas of Stereotaxic Anatomical Correlations for Gray and White Matter* (Talairach and Tournoux 1993).

We digitized these complementary printed atlases and then enhanced, segmented (color-coded or contoured), labeled, aligned, and organized them into atlas volumes. The atlases feature high-quality processed atlas images, and fully segmented and labeled structures. The anatomical index has about 1000 structures per hemisphere and more than 400 sulcal patterns. Their three-dimensional extensions were constructed. In addition, all two-dimensional (2D) and three-dimensional (3D) atlases were mutually coregistered.

The electronic atlas images were pre-labeled to speed up structure labeling in atlas-based applications. About 17,000 labels were placed manually for the entire Cerefy brain atlas database. Atlas pre-labeling has been used in two applications –*The Electronic Clinical Brain Atlas* (Nowinski et al. 1997a) and *Brain Atlas for Functional Imaging* (Nowinski et al. 2000a) – described in Sect. 9.3. Recent applications, the *Cerefy Neuroradiology Atlas* (Nowinski et al. 2001a) and *Cerefy Student Brain Atlas* (Nowinski et al. 2001b), featured in Sect. 9.3 use on-the-fly labeling. This allows the label of a structure to be calculated automatically at the indicated location in real time based on the color of the structure; the user can place this label interactively at any location. On-the-fly labeling works also for the warped atlas.

The *Atlas for Stereotaxy of the Human Brain* (Schaltenbrand and Wahren 1977) contains photographic plates of macroscopic and microscopic sections. The microscopic myelin-stained sections show in great detail cerebral deep structures that usually are not well visible on the scan. The original atlas axial, coronal, and sagittal microseries were digitized with high resolution. The electronic contours were derived manually from the digitized atlas and labeled. The microseries plates and contours were extended to cover both hemispheres (Fig. 9.2).

The *Co-Planar Stereotactic Atlas of the Human Brain* (Talairach and Tournoux 1988) was constructed from a single brain specimen which had been sectioned and photographed sagittally, and the

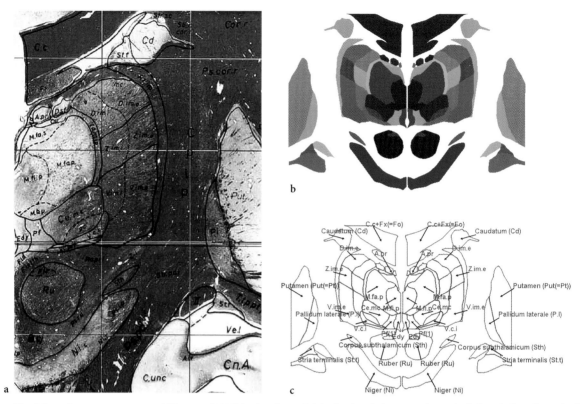

Fig. 9.2a–c. SCHALTENBRAND and WAHREN (1977) brain atlas. **a** Original printed plate covering a single hemisphere. **b** Derived corresponding color-coded image covering both hemispheres. **c** Derived corresponding contour image labeled with full and abbreviated names

coronal and axial sections were subsequently interpolated manually. To construct an electronic version, the printed plates were digitized with high resolution, and extensively preprocessed, enhanced and extended: (1) the original grids, rulers, and annotations were removed; (2) each atlas structure was assigned a unique color-coded representation, as opposed to a mixture of contour, color-coded, and texture representations in the printed atlas; (3) the left thalamic nuclei, not available in the printed atlas on the axial and coronal plates, were outlined and color-coded; (4) the right hemisphere cortex for axial orientation was added by mirroring the left hemisphere cortex; (5) Brodmann's areas and gyri, which are labeled but not segmented in the printed atlas, were constructed and color-coded for axial orientation (Fig. 9.3).

This version of the atlas is used in: *The Electronic Clinical Brain Atlas* (NOWINSKI et al. 1997a) and *Brain Atlas for Functional Imaging* (NOWINSKI et al. 2000a).

For the *Cerefy Neuroradiology Atlas* (NOWINSKI et al. 2001a) and *Cerefy Student Brain Atlas* (NOWINSKI et al. 2001b), the electronic atlas has been further processed by: (6) manual enhancing, cleaning, and smoothing of the electronic images under high magnification to facilitate generation of smooth contours and to achieve completely fully color-coded structures across all three orientations; (7) adding the lateral ventricle for the right hemisphere on several axial images; (8) adding the cortex of the right hemisphere on the coronal plates; and (9) re-coloring some structures to avoid color conflicts across all three orientations.

The TALAIRACH and TOURNOUX (1988) and SCHALTENBRAND and WAHREN (1977) atlases were constructed in color-coded image, contour, and polygonal representations (Figs. 9.2, 9.3, 9.15). The contour representation is useful when overlaying the atlas on the scan. The atlas images superimposed on the scan obscure it partially and contour representation avoids this effect (Fig. 9.11).

The *Atlas of the Cerebral Sulci* (ONO et al. 1990) studies 25 specimen brains for variations and consistencies in location, size, shape, dimensions, and relationships to the internal structures. The atlas shows the sulcal pattern variability on the cortex, such as sulcal interruptions, side branches, and connections with the surrounding sulci. The atlas contains 55 sulci and 403 patterns with their corresponding incidence rates. The original atlas was digitized, the individual patterns were separated, and each pattern was manually traced and converted into geometrical representation (a set of 2D points). In this way, the original arrows, letters, and cortical outlines were removed in the electronic atlas. Three-dimensional patterns were constructed by backprojecting the 2D patterns, placed in the Talairach space, into a cortical surface (Fig. 9.4).

The *Referentially Oriented Cerebral MRI Anatomy: Atlas of Stereotaxic Anatomical Correlations for Gray and White Matter* (TALAIRACH and TOURNOUX 1993) contains diagrams of the thalamocortical connections and commissural fibers as well as the corticofu-

gal fibers and homolateral association tracts on coronal and sagittal sections. The atlas diagrams were digitized with the same resolution as that of the TALAIRACH and TOURNOUX (1988) atlas. The original grids and annotations were removed, the stripes representing the fibers were manually cleaned up, and each tract was assigned a unique color (Fig. 9.5).

In addition, 3D extensions of the atlases were constructed (NOWINSKI et al. 1997b) (Figs. 9.4, 9.6, 9.7, 9.11, 9.15).

Each of the brain atlases included in the Cerefy database has its own strengths and their combination by mutual coregistration has several advantages. First, complementary information is merged and provided to the user, such as different parcellations. Second, the user needs to register the scan with

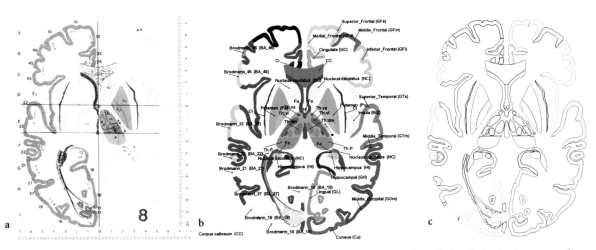

Fig. 9.3a–c. TALAIRACH and TOURNOUX (1988) brain atlas. **a** Digitized original printed axial plate. **b** Derived corresponding electronic image fully color-coded and labeled with subcortical structures, gyri, and Brodmann's areas (full and abbreviated names are used). **c** Derived corresponding color-coded contours

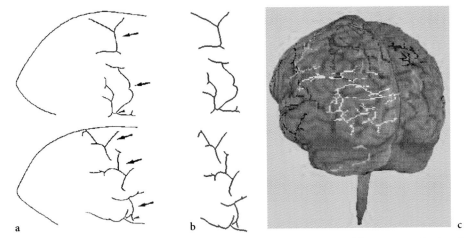

Fig. 9.4a–c. The *Atlas of the Cerebral Sulci*. **a** Original digitized patterns of the postcentral sulcus. **b** Corresponding electronic patterns composed of line segments; the arrows, letters, and cortical outlines were removed. **c** Three-dimensional patterns overlaid on an MR imaging cortical surface

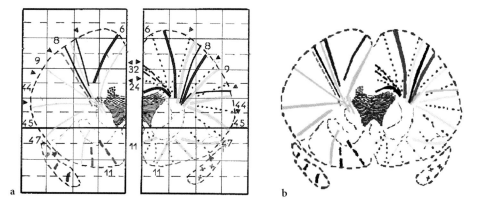

Fig. 9.5a, b. Referentially oriented TALAIRACH and TOURNOUX (1993) brain atlas. **a** Digitized original printed coronal plate with two images. **b** Derived corresponding single electronic image fully color-coded

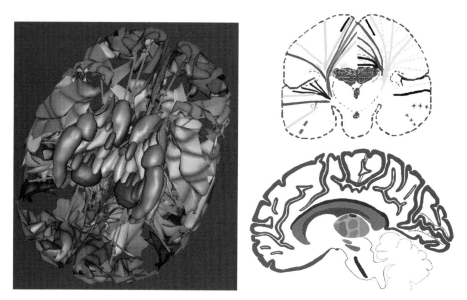

Fig. 9.6. The three-dimensional TALAIRACH and TOURNOUX atlas reconstructed from the two-dimensional TALAIRACH and TOURNOUX (1988, 1993) brain atlases

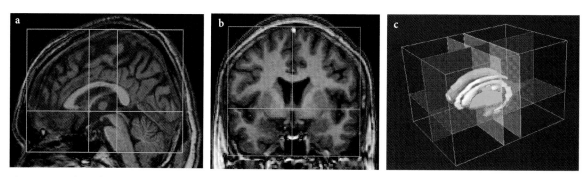

Fig. 9.7a–c. Talairach proportional grid system. **a** Sagittal orientation. **b** Coronal orientation. **c** In three dimensions

a single atlas only to have all 2D and 3D atlases in registration with this scan, as the atlas-to-atlas coregistration is scan-independent. The 2D and 3D atlases are mutually coregistered using the concept of the Talairach transformation.

9.2.4
Talairach Transformation and Landmarks

The Talairach transformation (TALAIRACH and TOURNOUX 1988) normalizes brains piecewise linearly. It is based on the Talairach landmarks: two internal landmarks lying on the midsagittal plane and six external landmarks lying on the smallest bounding box encompassing the cortex. The Talairach landmarks are: AC – the anterior commissure is the intersection of the lines passing through the superior edge and the posterior edge of the anterior commissure; PC – the posterior commissure is the intersection of the lines passing through the inferior edge and the anterior edge of the posterior commissure; L (R) – most lateral point of the parietotemporal cortex for the left (right) hemisphere; A – most anterior point of the frontal cortex; P – most posterior point of the occipital cortex; S – most superior (most dorsal) point of the parietal cortex; I – most inferior (most ventral) point of the temporal cortex.

The Talairach bounding box and the reference planes (i.e., the intercommissural plane, interhemispheric plane, and coronal planes passing through the AC and PC) divide the brain into 12 regions (Figs. 9.7, 9.9).

The Talairach transformation normalizes brain images by warping the images within each of 12 regions linearly. In this way, the volumetric image of brain is warped in three dimensions piecewise linearly. The Talairach transformation can be used to warp one atlas against another, atlas against scan, or scan against atlas.

There are several problems associated with the original Talairach landmarks. First, not all of them are available in the original atlas. Second, locations of some landmarks in the atlas contradict their definitions. Third, the cortical landmarks are not defined in a constructive way. And fourth, the intercommissural landmarks are located beyond their own structures and, despite being defined constructively, their constructions are not easily feasible on a scanner console. To overcome these problems, we have introduced a new, equivalent set of landmarks called the Talairach-Nowinski landmarks (NOWINSKI 2001b). The new landmarks are defined in a more construc-

tive way and can be more easily identified automatically. Two intercommissural lines are defined in the midsagittal plane: *central* and *tangential*. The central intercommissural line passes through the centers of the anterior and posterior commissures. The tangential intercommissural line is tangential dorso-posteriorly to the anterior commissure and ventro-anteriorly to the posterior commissure. The choice of intercommissural line is application-dependent. For neuroradiology, the tangential intercommissural line is recommended, (NOWINSKI 2001b).

9.3
Cerefy Atlas-Assisted Applications

We have developed several atlas-assisted applications based on the Cerefy brain atlas database useful in clinical practice, research, and education. Three applications are low-cost CD-ROMs: *The Electronic Clinical Brain Atlas* (NOWINSKI et al. 1997a), *Brain Atlas for Functional Imaging* (NOWINSKI et al. 2000a), and *Cerefy Student Brain Atlas* (NOWINSKI et al. 2001b). The *Cerefy Neuroradiology Atlas* is a web-enabled application (NOWINSKI et al. 2001a).

We have also developed two brain atlas add-on libraries: the *Electronic Brain Atlas Library* (NOWINSKI and THIRUNAVUUKARASUU 1998) and *Brain Atlas: Geometrical Models* (NOWINSKI 1998b). The *Electronic Brain Atlas Library* contains the atlases in image representation while the *Brain Atlas: Geometrical Models* is a library with the atlases in contour and 3D polygonal representations. These libraries are becoming the standard in stereotactic functional neurosurgery, already integrated with major image-guided surgery systems including the *StealthStation* (Medtronic/Sofamor-Danek), *Target* (BrainLAB), *SurgiPlan* (Elekta), *SNN 3 Image Guided Surgery System* (Surgical Navigation Network), and neurosurgical robot *NeuroMate* (Integrated Surgical Systems). They are also suitable for integration with scanners and radiological workstations.

The Electronic Clinical Brain Atlas (NOWINSKI et al. 1997a) contains the TALAIRACH and TOURNOUX (1988, 1993) and SCHALTENBRAND and WAHREN (1977) atlases. It provides many features not available in the original atlases, including coregistered atlases; flexible display, manipulation, and printing of atlas in multi-atlas and triplanar modes; 17,000 structures fully pre-labeled on 1,500 atlas images; and 3D animations of cerebral structures. These features along with the enclosed atlas and neuroanatomical material make it an ideal reference tool. This CD-ROM also allows the individualized atlas to be generated without loading the scan. The atlas is conformed to the scan in real time by a 2D deformation done by matching the atlas rectangular region of interest (spanned on any visible landmarks) to the corresponding region of interest defined interactively in the scan. By selecting the whole brain and placing the region of interest around it, the individualized atlas plate can easily be generated. The individualized atlas can be printed on transparent paper and overlaid on the film or this superimposition can be done off-line electronically.

The *Brain Atlas for Functional Imaging* (NOWINSKI et al. 2000a) is a tool for rapid atlas-assisted analysis of functional images. Its three major applications are: (1) interactive labeling of morphological images; (2) correlating structural and functional images enhanced by atlas-based labeling and triplanar display; (3) rapid, atlas-assisted localization analysis of functional images. This CD-ROM allows the user to load anatomical and functional datasets, correlate them by placing them in the Talairach space, identify activation loci, and label these loci automatically with Brodmann's areas, gyri, and subcortical structures by using the extended TALAIRACH and TOURNOUX (1988) atlas. The Talairach landmarks are set interactively on the anatomical images, which subsequently are normalized by the Talairach transformation. The functional images, with a known position with respect to the anatomical images, receive the identical transformation. Image warping is near real time, so exploring hundreds of images can be done on the fly. The anatomical and functional images and the atlas plates are displayed together as a single, blended dataset. Numerous tools are available for identification of activation loci, placing marks on them, and mark editing and labeling (NOWINSKI and THIRUNAVUUKARASUU 2001).

The *Brain Atlas for Functional Imaging* warps the scan against the atlas and the datasets loaded can be of various matrices provided their fields of view are the same. The *Cerefy Neuroradiology Atlas* warps the atlas against the scan and the multiple datasets loaded have to be of the same image size to be placed in register.

The *Cerefy Neuroradiology Atlas* (NOWINSKI et al. 2000c, 2001a) is a tool for rapid exploration and labeling of scans by means of the extended TALAIRACH and TOURNOUX (1988) atlas. The atlas is warped against the scan in three dimensions and displayed in all three orthogonal planes. A near real-time identification of the Talairach landmarks is semi-automatic, based on a patent-pending solution (NOWINSKI and THIRUNAVUUKARASUU 2000). The user has to spec-

ify the AC-PC plane and the Talairach landmarks are identified automatically. Computation time is less than 1 s on a standard personal computer, regardless of the number of slices. Atlas warping is near real time, so exploring and labeling hundreds of images can be done on the fly. The *Cerefy Neuroradiology Atlas* provides interactive on-the-fly labeling of the scan, triplanar navigation with all three planes warped, zoomable triplanar, data-atlas blending, reading Talairach coordinates, mensuration, addition of annotations, and drawing regions of interest. In addition, it saves the atlas-labeled and annotated scans in Dicom or XML (extensible mark-up language) files for subsequent utilization (by other clinicians such as neurosurgeons or neurologists, or for presentations). The *Cerefy Neuroradiology Atlas* is able to load multiple datasets each having its own control for scrolling and blending.

The *Cerefy Student Brain Atlas* (NOWINSKI et al. 2001b) is developed to meet, among others, requests from clinicians from developing countries and medical students for an easily affordable atlas-assisted tool for neuroanatomy. The materials and methods used for its development are based on our previous applications. The *Cerefy Student Brain Atlas* works in two modes: explore and test. In explore mode, the atlas/data are explored in triplanar mode. In test mode, the user is tested against either location or name of atlas structure. The user's testing score can be saved in an external file.

9.4
Atlas Potential

The quality and cost of interpreted scans can be considered in a 2D space over the available data and experience of person interpreting the scan (Fig. 9.8).

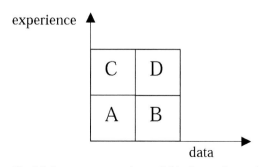

Fig. 9.8. Scan space over the available data and experience of person interpreting the scan. Scans in zone D maximize the quality while scans in zone A minimize the cost

Scan interpretation by an experienced neuroradiologist, viewing multi-modal data, is typically of the highest quality (and preferred). However, this may not be feasible technically or affordable economically. From a cost point of view, the interpretation of a unimodal scan by a radiology resident results in the lowest cost (zone A). Cases in zone D maximize the quality while cases in zone A minimize the cost. In our opinion, the potential of model-enhanced neuroradiology is that it can allow the interpreted scans to be moved from zone D towards zone A while not compromising much on their quality.

9.4.1
The Difference Made by the Cerefy Brain Atlas

We believe that the Cerefy brain atlas database is able to make a difference in neuroradiology. This will be even more evident with the use of new atlases, more powerful in terms of content, resolution, and warping abilities. We illustrate some areas where the Cerefy brain atlas makes a difference, serving as a tool for faster scan interpretation, facilitating communication of information, increasing confidence, and speeding up learning.

9.4.1.1
Atlas as a Means for Faster Scan Interpretation

The atlas can assist the neuroradiologist in speeding up scan interpretation by:
- rapid labeling of morphological and/or functional scans;
- displaying underlying anatomy for functional studies;
- facilitating multi-modal fusion;
- providing triplanar display with one plane from the scan and the other two from the atlas;
- providing higher parcellation of structures than is visible in the scan;
- displaying multiple labels for the same location in the scan corresponding to multiple, coregistered atlases;
- providing information that is not available in the scan.

Rapid and automatic labeling of scans using the *Cerefy Neuroradiology Atlas* is illustrated in Fig. 9.9. The Talairach landmarks have been calculated automatically within a fraction of second in this T1-weighted MR dataset with 112 images. The atlas is warped automatically in near real time, and the scan is interactively labeled.

An example in Fig. 9.10 illustrates display and labeling of underlying anatomy for functional images. The anatomical MR data containing 40 T1-weighted 256×256 axial images, the functional data generated for a visual experiment [functional MR blood oxygen level dependent (fMR BOLD) time series with 40 256×256 axial images], and the atlas plates are blended together as a three-into-one volume.

Multi-modal fusion using the *Brain Atlas for Functional Imaging* is illustrated in Fig. 9.10. An MR imaging dataset of 113 T1-weighted 256×256 images acquired for the whole brain with 1.5 mm slice thickness is fused with a color-coded fMR diffusion dataset of 8 512×512 images acquired in the region of tumor with 7.5 mm slice thickness. Despite having different matrices, the Talairach transformation places the anatomical and functional scans in the Talairach space such that they are in register. Then, the neuroradiologist is able to blend continuously the anatomical and

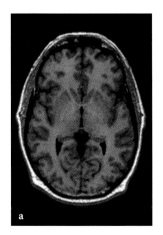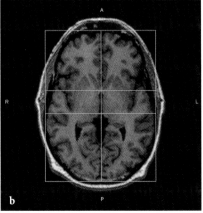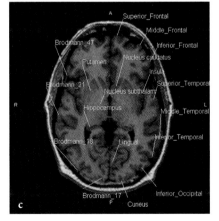

Fig. 9.9a–c. Rapid labeling of an MR scan. **a** T1-weighted image. **b** Talairach grid placed automatically on the scan. **c** Atlas-enabled interactive labeling of the scan with subcortical structures, gyri, and Brodmann's areas

functional images exploring the structure-function relationships.

Figure 9.11 shows a scan with a thalamic lesion, the problem being to identify nuclei involved in this lesion. HASSLER (1959) delimits more than 150 subdivisions of the thalamus. However, this T1-weighted MR image is almost homogeneous in the thalamic region and the identification of nuclei involved in the lesion is difficult, if not impossible. The deformable atlas, with a higher parcellation than that of the MR scan, is able to delineate invisible structures. The atlas also provides this information in all three orientations, increasing the clinician's confidence. The atlas in contour representation does not obscure the scan, as opposed to atlas plates superimposed on the scan. Moreover, the 3D display of the individualized thalamic nuclei facilitates understanding of spatial relationships.

Multiple labeling of the same location in the scan is illustrated in Fig. 9.12. By using multiple, coreg-

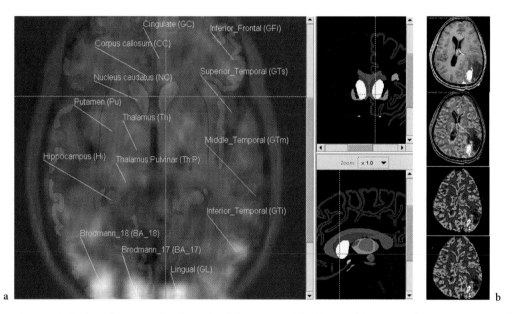

Fig. 9.10a, b. Fusion of anatomical and functional data. **a** T1-weighted MR and fMR BOLD datasets are registered and the activation loci and some cerebral structures are labeled. The data/atlas triplanar shows three-dimensional relationships. **b** Blending of the registered T1-weighted and color-coded fMR diffusion images to explore the structure-function relationships

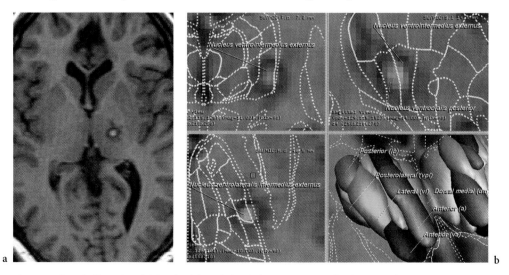

Fig. 9.11a, b. Labeling of nuclei involved in a thalamic lesion. **a** T1-weighted MR axial image. **b** Segmentation of the thalamus and labeling of the nuclei involved in the lesion simultaneously in axial, coronal, and sagittal planes by using the atlas in contour representation. The individualized 3D models of the thalamic nuclei are also labeled and displayed within the data/atlas triplanar to facilitate understanding of thalamic spatial relationships

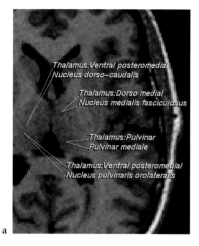
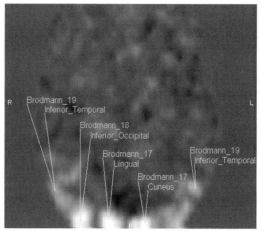

Fig. 9.12a, b. Multiple labeling of the same location in the scan by using multiple, coregistered atlases. **a** T1-weighted scan labeled by using two parcellations of the thalamus [Hassler's from the SCHALTENBRAND and WAHREN atlas (1977), and Walker's from the TALAIRACH and TOURNOUX (1988) atlas]. **b** Activation loci of an fMR BOLD scan labeled with gyri and Brodmann's

istered atlases, a scan can be labeled with various anatomical parcellations. Moreover, flipping the atlas during labeling allows the same location to be labeled simultaneously with gyri and Brodmann's areas.

Figure 9.13 shows a T1-weighted MR scan with the TALAIRACH and TOURNOUX (1993) atlas superimposed on it. Without acquiring a DWI (diffusion weighted imaging) scan, the approximate locations of the white matter tracts are traced and labeled by the atlas.

9.4.1.2
Efficient Communication of Clinical Information

The understanding of underlying anatomy in the scan is easy for a neuroradiologist; however, communicating this knowledge to others may be tedious and time-consuming. A deformable and labeled atlas is well suited for efficient transfer of this knowledge to other clinicians, such as neurosurgeons, neurologists and referring physicians, and to medical students. For instance, the *Cerefy Neuroradiology Atlas* allows the neuroradiologist to annotate the scan with text, regions of interest and measured distances, and then label the structures of interest. The annotated and labeled scan can be saved in Dicom and/or XML formats, giving the neuroradiologist the possibility of storing the atlas-enhanced scan in a PACS (picture archiving communication system) and using it in web-enabled applications. In this way, the scan interpretation done by the neuroradiologist can easily be communicated to other clinicians and medical students.

9.4.1.3
Increasing Clinical Confidence

The atlas can also increase the confidence of those radiologists who do not interpret brain scans often, or radiology residents interpreting brain scans in urgent cases when experienced neuroradiologists are not available. The atlas increases both anatomical confidence by providing detailed anatomy labeled on all three orthogonal views (as illustrated in Figs. 9.10, 9.11) and spatial confidence by showing triplanar and 3D anatomical relationships (Figs. 9.10, 9.11, 9.15).

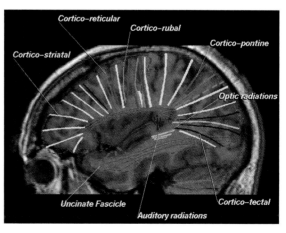

Fig. 9.13. T1-weighted MR scan with the atlas of brain connections superimposed on it marking and labeling the approximate locations of the white matter tracts

9.4.1.4
Using the Cerefy Brain Atlas as a Standard Reference

The comparison of multi-modal scans acquired in different planes is difficult. Any standardization in terms of orientation and anatomical reference would facilitate scan interpretation. The Talairach system along with the atlas offers a solution. By using the AC-PC plane as the standard (acquisition or reformatting) plane, the comparison of multi-modal studies would be greatly facilitated. The AC-PC line can easily be identified in the midsagittal plane. The TALAIRACH and TOURNOUX (1988) atlas can be used as a standard gross anatomy reference (similarly to human brain mapping where it has become the gold standard), particularly for functional studies. The use of the Talairach space and transformation facilitates multi-modal registration. Moreover, the Talairach coordinates provide a means for quantification of scans in terms of spatial positioning.

9.4.1.5
Using the Atlas in Education

Neuroeducation was one of the first applications of electronic brain atlases. A deformable, labeled atlas overlaid on radiological images greatly facilitates learning how to read and interpret real images, and is superior to the traditional use of pre-labeled cadaveric images usually static in content. In particular, the atlas can be used to interactively label data of any imaging modality, facilitating its understanding and interpretation. Figure 9.14 illustrates the educational potential of the *Cerefy Student Brain*

Atlas by using radiological images with interactive labeling.

In addition, the individualized electronic atlas along with triplanar and volumetric display of data provides spatial anatomical relationships (Fig. 9.15).

A rapid atlas warping mechanism along with interactive labeling available in the Cerefy brain atlas is useful for exploring any user dataset for educational purposes. We will be developing more educational applications by: (1) extending the atlas content by adding atlases with three-dimensional structures, blood supply regions, and cerebral vasculature; and (2) adding more modalities including T2-weighted, CT, and PET scans.

9.4.2
Atlas as an Extender

The role of the Cerefy brain atlas can also be considered as an extender. The triplanar display, where one plane is from the scan and the other two from the atlas, provides an extension of scan in three dimensions (Fig. 9.10). When segmenting and labeling the scan, the structures of which are not discernible, the atlas provides an image contrast extension (Fig. 9.11). When labeling structures not shown in the scan, the atlas provides a modality extension (Fig. 9.13). When the atlas is used as an anatomical reference, it provides knowledge extension. Fast labeling of patient-specific data by the individualized atlas is knowledge customization.

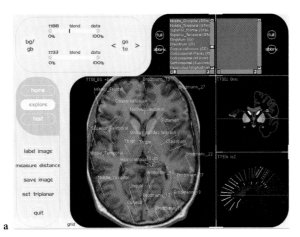
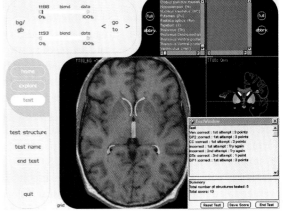

Fig. 9.14a, b. The *Cerefy Student Brain Atlas.* **a** In explore mode, the student can label interactively the radiological images. **b** In test mode, a structure is highlighted on the image and the student has to provide its name

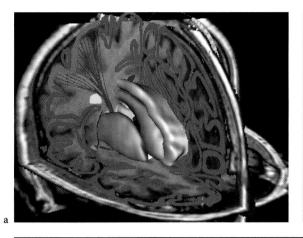
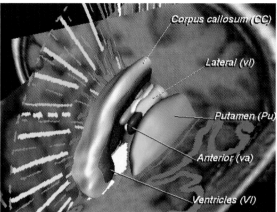

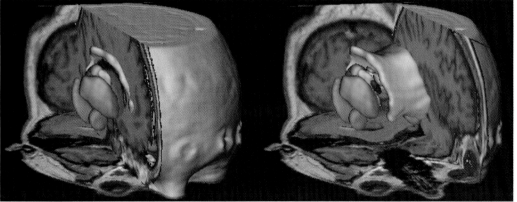

Fig. 9.15a–c. Three-dimensional polygonal atlas registered with MR volume data. **a** Data/atlas triplanar display. **b** Individualized atlas structures labeled. **c** Volumetric display

9.4.3
Atlas Limitations

Despite its increasing acceptance and use, the Cerefy brain atlas database has several limitations resulting mainly from the shortcomings inherent in the original printed material. The original TALAIRACH and TOURNOUX (1988) and SCHALTENBRAND and WAHREN (1977) atlas plates are not consistent in all three planes, so their 3D extensions are qualitative, not quantitative. Their sparseness limits the construction of accurate volumetric atlases. As a result, the scan (if not acquired in the AC-PC plane) rather than the atlases has to be reformatted when matching it to the atlas. The use of fully non-linear 3D brain warping techniques (TOGA 1998) is also limited. The electronic brain atlas database, therefore, has to be used with caution and understanding of its limitations. We have been working on the construction of the next generation brain atlas that will overcome all these problems.

9.4.4
Atlas Validation

The atlas potential discussed above has to be validated. This validation covers the accuracy, robustness, and reproducibility of the atlas. Atlas clinical utility has to be proved as measured by cost saving, time required, extent of user interaction, and ease of integration in a clinical protocol. Towards achieving this goal, we have started a trial subscription for the *Cerefy Neuroradiology Atlas* and the collected feedback will be used for validation and atlas enhancements.

9.5
Summary

The Cerefy electronic brain atlas database constructed and the applications developed from it:

– reduce time in image interpretation by providing interactive multiple labeling, triplanar display, higher parcellation than the scan itself, multimodal fusion, and display of underlying anatomy for functional images;
– facilitate communication of information about the interpreted scans from the neuroradiologist to other clinicians and medical students;
– increase the neuroradiologist's confidence in terms of anatomy and spatial relationships by providing interactive multiple labeling of the scan in the orthogonal planes and triplanar display with one plane from the scan and the other two from the atlas;
– can potentially reduce costs by providing some information from mutually coregistered atlases which otherwise has to be acquired from other modalities;
– reduces time in learning neuroanatomy and scan interpretation by providing 3D and triplanar displays and labeling of multi-modal scans.

The atlas makes a difference both for experienced neuroradiologists and for medical students. This difference will be even more prominent with the next generation of electronic brain atlases. The neuroradiologist will be able to fully benefit from this potential provided the Cerefy brain atlas is available on scanner consoles and PACS workstations, similar to the way in which it is available today to neurosurgeons in operating rooms by integrating the Cerefy atlas with key image-guided surgery systems.

The major weakness of anatomical atlases is the lack of pathology modeling. The next generation of brain atlases, the development of which will require solving problems related to atlas representation, warping, validation, and computational efficiency, should account for this by providing statistical information on relationships between the structure and the corresponding distribution of the types of lesions, and between the lesion and the corresponding distribution of structures/locations. Furthermore, the new atlases should be labeled with multiple sources of information going beyond anatomy and pathology.

Acknowledgements. The author is deeply grateful to Prof. J. Talairach and Prof. P. Tournoux for insightful discussions on their atlases. The *Electronic Clinical Brain Atlas* and *Cerefy Student Brain Atlas* was a joint development with Prof. R. N. Bryan of Johns Hopkins Hospital/Hospital of the University of Pennsylvania, USA. The *Brain Atlas for Functional Imaging* was developed in consultation with the NMR Center of Massachusetts General Hospital, USA. The key contributors to the construction of the Cerefy brain atlas database and development of the atlas-assisted applications include A. Thirunavuukarasuu, D. Belov, G.L. Yang, A. Fang, and B.T. Nguyen, among many others.

References

ADAM (1994) A.D.A.M. Animated dissection of anatomy for medicine. User's guide, ADAM Software

Afshar E, Watkins ES, Yap JC (1978) Stereotactic atlas of the human brainstem and cerebellar nuclei. Raven Press, New York

Andrew J, Watkins ES (1969) A stereotaxic atlas of the human thalamus and adjacent structures: a variability study. Williams and Wilkins, Baltimore

Bohm C, Greitz T, Eriksson L (1983) A computerized adjustable brain atlas. Eur J Nucl Med 15:687–689

DeArmond SJ, Fusco MM, Dewey MM (1989) Structure of the human brain: a photographic atlas, 3rd edn. Oxford University Press, New York

Dev P, Coppa GP, Tancred E (1992) BrainStorm: designing an interactive neuroanatomy atlas. Radiology 185:413

Duvernoy HM (1988) The human hippocampus: an atlas of applied anatomy. Bergman, Munich

Evans AC, Collins DL, Milner B (1992) An MRI-based stereotactic brain atlas from 300 young normal subjects. Proceedings of the 22nd symposium of the Society for Neuroscience, Anaheim, pp 407–408

Fix JD (1987) Atlas of the human brain and spinal cord. Aspen, Rockville

Greitz T, Bohm C, Holte S (1991) A computerized brain atlas: construction, anatomical content, and some applications. J Comput Assist Tomogr 15:26–38

Hardy TL, Deming LR, Harris-Collazo R (1999) Computerized stereotactic atlases. In: Alexander E III, Maciunas RJ (eds) Advanced neurosurgical navigation. Thieme, Stuttgart, pp 115–124

Hassler R (1959) Anatomy of the thalamus. In: Schaltenbrand G, Bailey W (eds) Introduction to stereotaxis with an atlas of the human brain. Thieme, Stuttgart

Hohne KH (1995) Voxel-Man. I. Brain and skull. Springer, Berlin Heidelberg New York

Hohne KH, Bomans M, Riemer M (1992) A 3D anatomical atlas based on a volume model. IEEE Comput Graph Appl 12:72–78

Kall BA (1992) Computer-assisted stereotactic functional neurosurgery. In: Kelly PJ, Kall BA (eds) Computers in stereotactic neurosurgery. Blackwell, Boston, pp 134–142

Kazarnovskaya MI, Borodkin SM, Shabalov VA (1991) 3-D computer model of subcortical structures of human brain. Comput Biol Med 21:451–457

Kikinis R, Shenton ME, Iosifescu DV (1996) A digital brain atlas for surgical planning, model-driven segmentation, and teaching. IEEE Trans Visualization Comput Graph 2:232–241

Kraus GE, Bailey GJ (1994) Microsurgical anatomy of the brain: a stereo atlas. Wiliams and Wilkins, Baltimore

Lehmann ED, Hawkes D, Hill D (1991) Computer-aided interpretation of SPECT images of the brain using an MRI-derived neuroanatomic atlas. Med Inform 16:151–166

Martin J (1989) Neuroanatomy. Text and atlas. Appleton and Lange, Norwalk

Mazziotta JC, Toga AW, Evans AC (1995) A probabilistic atlas of the human brain: theory and rationale for its development. Neuroimage 2:89–101

McMinn RMH, Hutchings RT, Pegington J (1993) Color atlas of human anatomy, 3rd edn. Mosby Year Book, St Louis

Netter FH (1991) The CIBA collection of medical illustrations, vol 1. Nervous system. CIBA, New Jersey

Niemann K, Naujokat C, Pohl G, Wollner C, von Keyserlingk D (1994) Verification of the Schaltenbrand and Wahren stereotactic atlas. Acta Neurochir 129:72–81

Niemann K, van den Boom R, Haeselbarth K (1999) A brainstem stereotactic atlas in a three-dimensional magnetic resonance imaging navigation system: first experiences with atlas-to-patient registration. J Neurosurg 90:891–901

Nieuwennhuys R, Voogd J, van Huijzen C (1981) The human central nervous system: a synopsis and atlas, 2nd edn. Springer, Berlin Heidelberg New York

Nowinski WL (1998a) Anatomical targeting in functional neurosurgery by the simultaneous use of multiple Schaltenbrand-Wahren brain atlas microseries. Stereotac Funct Neurosurg 71:103–116

Nowinski WL (1998b) Brain atlas: geometrical models. Thieme, New York/KRDL, Singapore (BAGM specification is available from www.cerefy.com)

Nowinski WL (2001a) Computerized brain atlases for surgery of movement disorders. Semin Neurosurg 12:183–194

Nowinski WL (2001b) Modified Talairach landmarks. Acta Neurochir 143:1045–1057

Nowinski WL, Benabid AL (2002) New directions in atlas-assisted stereotactic functional neurosurgery. Advanced techniques in image-guided brain and spine surgery. Thieme, New York

Nowinski WL, Thirunavuukarasuu A (1998) Electronic brain atlas library. Thieme, New York/KRDL, Singapore (EBAL specification is available from www.cerefy.com)

Nowinski WL, Thirunavuukarasuu A (2000) Methods and apparatus for processing medical images. Patent application PCT/SG00/00185

Nowinski WL, Thirunavuukarasuu A (2001) Atlas-assisted localization analysis of functional images. Med Image Anal 5:207–220

Nowinski WL, Bryan RN, Raghavan R (1997a) The electronic clinical brain atlas. Multiplanar navigation of the human brain. Thieme, New York, Stuttgart

Nowinski WL, Fang A, Nguyen BT (1997b) Multiple brain atlas database and atlas-based neuroimaging system. Comput Aided Surg 2:42–66

Nowinski WL, Thirunavuukarasuu A, Kennedy DN (2000a) Brain atlas for functional imaging. Clinical and research applications. Thieme, New York

Nowinski WL, Yang GL, Yeo TT (2000b) Computer-aided stereotactic functional neurosurgery enhanced by the use of the multiple brain atlas database. IEEE Trans Med Imaging 19:62–69

Nowinski WL, Thirunavuukarasuu A, Srinivasan R (2000c) Brain atlas for neuroradiology. Radiology 217 (Suppl) 217:S620

Nowinski WL, Thirunavuukarasuu A, Belov D (2001a) Web-based atlas for neuroradiology. Proceedings of the American Society of Neuroradiology 39th annual meeting, ASNR2001, 23–27 April 2001, Boston, Mass, USA, p 500 (the atlas is available from www.cerefy.com)

Nowinski WL, Bryan RN, Thirunavuukarasuu A (2001b) Cerefy student brain atlas. KRDL, Singapore

Ono M, Kubik S, Abernathey CD (1990) Atlas of the cerebral sulci. Thieme/Thieme Medical, Stuttgart

Schaltenbrand G, Bailey W (1959) Introduction to stereotaxis with an atlas of the human brain. Thieme, Stuttgart

Schaltenbrand G, Wahren W (1977) Atlas for stereotaxy of the human brain. Thieme, Stuttgart

Schiemann T, Freudenberg J, Pflesser B (2000) Exploring the visible human using the VOXEL-MAN framework. Comput Med Imaging Graph 24:127–132

Schmahmann JD, Doyon J, McDonald D (1999) Three-dimensional MRI atlas of the human cerebellum in proportional stereotaxic space. Neuroimage 10:233–260

Schnitzlein HN, Murtagh FR (1980) Imaging anatomy of the head and spine. A photographic color atlas of MRI, CT, gross, and microscopic anatomy in axial, coronal, and sagittal planes, 2nd edn. Urban and Schwarzenberg, Baltimore

Sramka M, Ruzicky E, Novotny M (1997) Computerized brain atlas in functional neurosurgery. Stereotact Funct Neurosurg 69:93–98

Sundsten JW, Brinkley JF, Eno K (1994) The digital anatomist. Interactive brain atlas. CD-ROM for the Macintosh. University of Washington, Seattle

Szikla G, Bouvier G, Hori T (1977) Angiography of the human brain cortex: atlas of vascular patterns and stereotactic localization. Springer, Berlin Heidelberg New York

Talairach J, Tournoux P (1988) Co-planar stereotactic atlas of the human brain. Thieme, Stuttgart

Talairach J, Tournoux P (1993) Referentially oriented cerebral MRI anatomy: atlas of stereotaxic anatomical correlations for gray and white matter. Thieme, Stuttgart

Talairach J, David M, Tournoux P (1957) Atlas d'anatomie stereotaxique des noyaux gris centraux. Masson, Paris

Thompson PM, Woods RP, Mega MS (2000) Mathematical/computational challenges in creating deformable and probabilistic atlases of the human brain. Hum Brain Mapp 9:81–92

Toga AW (1998) Brain warping. Academic Press, San Diego

Toga AW, Ambach KL, Schluender S (1994) High-resolution anatomy from in situ human brain. Neuroimage 1:334–344

Van Buren JM, Borke RC (1972) Variations and connections of the human thalamus. Springer, Berlin Heidelberg New York

Van Essen DC, Drury HA (1997) Structural and functional analyses of human cerebral cortex using a surface-based atlas. J Neurosci 17:7079–7102

Van Essen DC, Drury HA, Hadjikhani N (2000) A probabilistic surface-based atlas of human visual cortex. Proceedings of the human 6th brain mapping meeting, HBM 2000, June, San Antonio, Texas, USA. Neuroimage 11:S533

Yoshida M (1992) Three-dimensional maps by interpolation from the Schaltenbrand and Bailey atlas. In: Kelly PJ, Kall BA (eds) Computers in stereotactic neurosurgery. Blackwell, Boston, pp 143–152

10 Middle and Inner Ear

Emanuele Neri, Stefano Berrettini, Michela Panconi, Carla Cappelli

CONTENTS

10.1
The Middle Ear

10.1.1
Image Acquisition

As in other anatomical regions, to generate three-dimensional (3D) reconstructions of the middle ear structures, a volumetric acquisition is required. In the case of the tympanic cavity, high-resolution computed tomography (HRCT) is the imaging modality of choice; although the term "high-resolution" is traditionally applied to acquisitions performed with millimetric or sub-millimetric collimation (even with conventional CT), volumetric study is more properly used when single-slice or multislice spiral CT is used. CT is generally introduced into the diagnostic investigation of middle ear pathologies when external otoen-

E. Neri, MD, M. Panconi, MD, C. Cappelli, MD
Diagnostic and Interventional Radiology, Department of Oncology, Transplants, and Advanced Technologies in Medicine, University of Pisa, Via Roma 67, 56100 Pisa, Italy
S. Berrettini, MD
Otolaryngologic Unit, Department of Neuroscience, University of Pisa, Via Savi 10, 56126 Pisa, Italy

doscopy is unsuccessful at demonstrating the cause of the disease. Volumetric acquisitions allow the evaluation of most of the components of the tympanic cavity, such as the walls and ossicular chain, but fail to demonstrate the mucosal layer and ligaments.

Recently, the interest in the CT study of the middle ear has been renewed by detailed endoscopic studies of this region performed during interventions with dedicated devices; this technique has been called transtympanic endoscopy, since it requires the perforation of the tympanic membrane.

Our single-slice spiral CT protocol includes axial and coronal acquisitions (beam collimation, 1 mm; pitch, 1; table incremental speed, 1 mm/s; tube rotation, 1 s; tube current, 160 mA with 120 kVp; field of view, 16 cm). Axial and coronal images are obtained at a 0.5 mm reconstruction interval with a bone algorithm (Neri 2000a). If a multislice CT is used, the protocol includes axial acquisition and coronal views obtained with multiplanar reconstructions (Fujii 2000; Gotwaldt 2001).

10.1.2
3D Image Processing:
Value of Multiplanar Reconstructions

The near-isotropic imaging obtained by helical CT allows not only the accurate evaluation of anatomical details on native images but even the reconstruction of oblique planes (MPR, multiplanar reconstruction) (Ali 1993; Hermans 1995). MPR has been well known since the introduction of CT into clinical practice. Initial applications of MPR to the study of the middle ear were carried out with conventional CT (Haas and Kahle 1988; Grevers 1989), and such experiences secured for MPR an effective integrative role in CT imaging of the middle ear. With the advent of spiral CT, MPR has been made available for most users and the frequency of its application in clinical routine has increased.

An interesting application of reformatted planes in the study of the middle ear is represented by the imaging of recurrent postoperative cholesteatoma. In this case, the combined use of axial native images with coronal and sagittal reformations allows evaluation of the shape of the tissue filling the middle ear, which in the case of recurrent cholesteatoma can be identified by the prevalent scalloped limits (VEILLON 1993, 1997).

WATANABE (2000) studied MPR images of the facial nerve canal in 628 CT examinations of the temporal bone. These were created along the labyrinthine and tympanic segment, and the along the tympanic and mastoid segment of the facial nerve. Further, MPR images along the facial nerve canal and bone fracture lines were created. In all cases, the MPR images delineated the labyrinthine and tympanic segment in one image, and the tympanic and mastoid segment in another image. In two patients with traumatic facial nerve palsy, the MPR images revealed a relationship between the facial nerve canal and the bone fracture. The authors concluded that MPR of the facial nerve canal was useful in detecting facial nerve schwannoma, traumatic facial nerve palsy and congenital facial nerve palsy.

Again, the application of MPR is variable since any case that requires integration of axial images with addition planes is valuable. One example is the postoperative evaluation of cochlear implants, where the path of the electrode within the cochlear turn is not easy to assess by native images; in such cases the creation of MPR images that allow the display in a unique plane of the entire electrode permits the precise assessment of the proportion of the electrode introduced.

DIEDERICHS (1996) applied a variant of MPR, called multiplanar volume reconstruction (MPVR), to the study of the middle ear after HRCT performed with a reduced radiation dose. The aim of the study was to reduce image noise and at the same time increase the partial volume averaging to balance this effect; the technique failed to visualize the small bony structures and, for example, the stapes was not visualized.

MPR has also been proposed as an alternative to direct coronal acquisitions in order to reduce the examination time and of course the radiation dose to the patient. CALDEMEYER (1999) demonstrated that submillimetric and isotropic imaging of the middle ear can be obtained using helical CT, with 0.5 mm collimation, a single volumetric scan in the axial plane, 0.2 mm reconstruction spacing and a coronal image created with MPR. Although this approach could be questionable using a single-slice scanner, the limitation of MPR seems to be overcome by a multislice CT (FUJII 2000; GOTWALDT 2001).

10.1.3
3D Image Processing: Segmentation, Surface and Volume Rendering

During 3D image processing in the study of the middle ear, the normal subject provides optimal conditions for image segmentation and visualization, making it easy to differentiate bone from the air content of the tympanic cavity. However, the presence of abundant fluid or tissue, resulting from a pathological process, make the separation between air, bone, fluid and tissue difficult.

The reconstruction of the bone is quite simple for any image processing software, be it surface or volume rendering based. In the first case the boundary between bone and other tissues is identified at a density threshold of 160–200 HU; just below this value enhancing parenchyma after intravenous contrast can be seen (but this is quite rare in the case of the middle ear). Below this value in turn, the mucosal layer of the tympanic cavity can be found and represented if the threshold value is reduced to identify the passage between mucosa and air, as −500 HU (POZZI MUCELLI 1997). It is clear that any software working with a CT data set can reconstruct in three dimensions the morphology of the mucosal layer, but it can not represent colorimetric alterations in the course of edema, bleeding or dysplasia.

The knowledge of these segmentation values is extremely important to determine whether or not the reconstructed images correspond to reality. To this end a comparison between real anatomy and 3D reconstructed endoluminal views from seven formalin-fixed anatomical specimens was performed by our group (NERI 2000b). We found 100% agreement between the observations for endoluminal views and anatomical sections, even though in two cases the complete visualization of the middle ear cavity could not initially be obtained because of the presence of tissue remnants within the external auditory meatus. However, careful electronic removal of this tissue allowed the middle ear to be visualized, while in the case of anatomical specimens, the tissue remnants were removed manually.

Volume rendering offers an alternative approach to segmentation; although it is still dependent on thresholds, the modulation of opacity values (see Chap. 5) allows a wider range of tissue combination and display (RUBIN 1996; JOHNSON 1996). With volume rendering it is possible to visualize in the same view different tissues (that have different Hounsfield densities) or to combine the visualization of tissue and metallic components, i.e., cochlear implants (Fig. 10.1) (NERI 2001a).

One interesting feature of surface or volume rendering is the provision of a global visualization of the aerated cavities of the middle ear. The reconstruction of the air content permits estimation of the grade of pneumatization of the tympanic cavity and mastoid cells, which could change in the case of malformation and inflammation.

In contrast to the reconstruction of the air, surface and volume rendering also provide a global view of the petrous bone. Such a perspective can be useful in many situations to estimate bony alterations: the malformation of the temporal bone that occurs in hemifacial microsomia, the surgical resection of bone performed in mastoidectomies, or the presence and extent of fractures.

10.1.4
Endoluminal Views of the Middle Ear: Virtual Endoscopy (Technique)

The technical aspects of virtual endoscopy (VE) have been introduced in Chap. 6, to which the reader should refer. The application of VE to the study of the middle ear is quite simple but requires, as for other image processing methods, the availability of volumetric and high-resolution data. The optimal CT acquisition protocols are under discussion.

VE of the middle ear is obtained by creating a virtual empty space within the tympanic cavity, which is really an empty space but not accessible by direct human vision. The creation of the virtual space is generated in surface rendering by the application of binary segmentation in which a specific threshold level identifies the boundary between air and the mucosal layer of the middle ear, as discussed in the previous paragraph. In volume rendering the threshold is almost the same and the use of a high opacity level allows the mucosal surface to be enhanced. In both cases the inner wall of the tympanic cavity are displayed. The majority of commercially available software allows one to point with the computer mouse within the air space (using an axial or coronal image as reference) and generate an endoscopic view of the cavity. The virtual eye can be positioned in any space of the middle ear and directed to look towards specific structures or anatomical regions. The aim of VE of the middle ear is to obtain a 3D perspective of the tympanic cavity walls and of the ossicular chain. However, before describing the application of VE in the middle ear, we need a historical digression on the history of real endoscopy and an explanation of how real endoscopy is obtained.

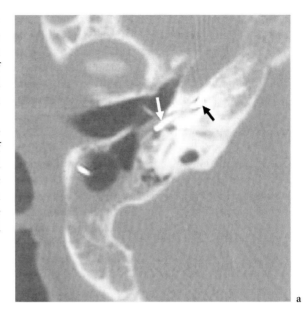

a

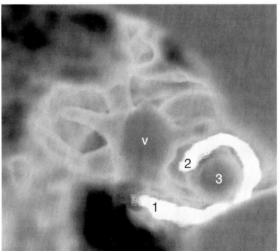

b

Fig. 10.1a, b. Spiral CT follow-up in a patient who underwent cochlear implantation of the right ear for hearing loss. **a** Axial image crossing through the basal turn of the cochlea shows the initial (*white arrow*) and final (*black arrow*) portions of the electrode. The latter reach the middle turn of the cochlea but the precise location is not measurable. **b** Volume rendering of the bone labyrinth demonstrates the entire path of the electrode within the cochlea. Electrode path from basal turn (*1*) to the middle turn (*2*) is clearly visible. The apical turn (*3*) is not reached by the electrode tip. *V* vestibule

10.1.5
Real Endoscopy: Transtympanic Endoscopy

The history of real endoscopy of the middle ear started in 1967, when Zini tried to visualize the middle ear using a system of micromirrors that allowed the exploration of the retrotympanum. This method, called indirect microtympanoscopy, is still used in clinical practice. Mer (1967) introduced a fiberoptic endoscope into the tympanic cavity through a perforation of the tympanic membrane. In 1982 the middle ear cavity was visualized with a rigid needle otoscope by Nomura (1982). Subsequently many authors started to use endoscopy for diagnosis and postsurgical follow-up.

Modern endoscopes are based on the Hopkins optical system and have a variable diameter (minimum 1 mm), length and angle depending on the region to be explored. In the majority of cases the endoscopes are based on a rigid system, but in difficult cases, such as a strong curvature of the external auditory canal, the presence of stenosis or fibrotic tissue, the use of flexible endoscopes is preferred despite their lower spatial resolution and image quality.

Transtympanic endoscopy can be used as a diagnostic tool or as a guide for otosurgical interventions. In the first case the easy access to the external auditory canal allows the visualization of the tympanic membrane, a barrier between the endoscope and the middle ear; only the presence of a pathological or surgical (myringotomy) perforation permits a limited exploration of the tympanic cavity.

The use of transtympanic endoscopy in otosurgery aims to provide real time video assistance to the surgical procedure.

10.1.6
Virtual Endoscopy (Clinical Applications): The Study of the Tympanic Cavity

In a recent study carried out by our group (Neri 2001b), a virtual endoscopic analysis of the tympanic cavity was performed by following the traditional imaging of transtympanic endoscopy. As radiologists we are confident with traditional axial or coronal imaging, but we here describe the anatomy of the tympanic cavity from the point of view of the otologist. This means that we have a further instrument to understand this complex region and that we are now closer to the surgical views than ever before.

Creating an endoscopic perspective from the external auditory canal to look toward the middle ear, the tympanic cavity can be divided into four regions on the basis of endoscopic and surgical studies: retrotympanum (posterior), epitympanum (superior), protympanum (anterior) and hypotympanum (inferior).

The anatomy of the middle ear, as displayed by VE is hereby described according to this anatomical partition. A typical VE perspective obtained from the

external auditory canal allows the accurate identification of the anatomical landmarks that define these regions (Fig. 10.2a).

The retrotympanum represents more than half of the posterior part of the tympanic cavity and includes the oval and round windows (Parlier-Cuau 1998). VE allows all the components of the retrotympanum to be displayed (Fig. 10.2b), showing eminences and depressions represented by the pyramidal and styloid eminences, pyramidal ridge, ponticulus, subiculum, and the eminence of the mastoid portion of the facial nerve (Pickett 1995; Espinoza 1989).

VE displays the pyramidal and styloid eminences as smoothed elevations of the medial wall of the tympanic cavity. The styloid or Politzer eminence, which represents the base of the styloid process, divides the retrotympanum from the hypotympanum. The pyramidal ridge is shown by VE as an elevation of the medial wall connecting the pyramidal and styloid eminences. Turning the virtual endoscope toward the stapes, the eminence of the mastoid portion of the facial nerve appears just above the oval window niche (Thomassin 1996). VE allows the recognition of two other small osseous crests, represented by the ponticulus and subiculum. On the basis of these ridges, eminences and depressions of the medial wall of the tympanic cavity, the retrotympanum can be divided into four regions: the superomedial or *posterior sinus tympani* (or *tympanic sinus of Proctor*), the inferomedial sinus or *sinus tympani*, the superolateral or *facial sinus,* and the inferolateral sinus or *fossula of Grivot* (Guerrier 1976).

At VE the posterior sinus tympani can be seen under the eminence of the facial nerve canal and posterior to the oval window. The sinus tympani appears as a parietal depression with the following landmarks: the ponticulus (superior), the subiculum (inferior-anterior), the pyramidal crest and eminence (posterior-lateral) and the promontory (anterior). Thomassin (1994) describes three types of sinus tympani on the basis of the feasibility of transtympanic endoscopy, but their morphology can be easily recognized also at VE: sinus tympani of *easy exploration*, characterized by a simple depression of the tympanic wall; sinus tympani of *difficult exploration*, represented by a depression of the wall that continues into a deep canal through the tympanic wall and opens into the retrotympanum via a small orifice; *intermediate* sinus tympani, with a deep canal and large orifice.

The promontory appears at VE as an eminence with a smooth surface that covers the round window. This opens from the tympanic cavity into the scala tympani of the cochlea.

Fig. 10.2a–c. Virtual endoscopy of the middle ear. a The endoscopic view is created positioning the virtual endoscope within the external auditory canal, looking toward the middle ear cavity. The virtual perspective allows the recognition of most of the structures composing this region: malleus head (*MH*) and handle (*HM*), long process of incus (*LPI*), sinus tympani (*ST*), promontory (*Prom*) and pharyngo-tympanic tube (*PTT*). b Detailed perspective of the *ST* and fossula of Grivot, divided by the pyramidal ridge (*PR*). At the inferior border of the *ST*, the styloid eminence (*SE*) and subiculum (*Sub*) are recognized. c Detailed perspective of the protympanum where opens the initial portion of the pharyngo-tympanic tube (*PTT*). Superiorly the epytimpanic sinus (*ES*) is visible. *M* malleus, *I* incus, *S* stapes

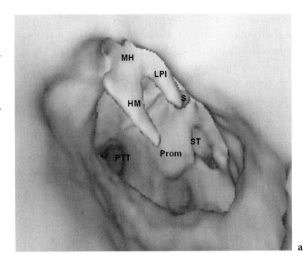

a

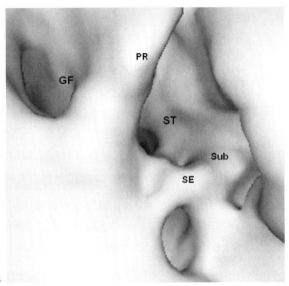

b

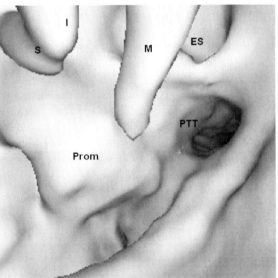

c

Other depressions of the retrotympanum are the facial sinus and the fossula of Grivot. Their visualization is obtained at VE by positioning the virtual endoscope in the retrotympanum and looking posteriorly. These depressions become important landmarks during surgical interventions with a retrofacial approach.

The protympanum represents the anterior part of the tympanic cavity that includes the pharyngo-tympanic tube. The superior border of the tube divides the protympanum from the sinus epitympani. The inferior border separates the tube from the internal carotid artery. The protympanum is easy to explore with either transtympanic endoscopy or VE (Fig. 10.2).

The hypotympanum represents the floor of the tympanic cavity, separated from the mesotympanum by a horizontal plane crossing the inferior border of the external meatus. VE display the floor, characterized by many osseous crests, the development of which is related to the dimensions of the sub-labyrinthic cells.

The epitympanum (attic or epitympanic recess) represents the superior part of the tympanic cavity. Its posterior landmark is provided by the aditus ad antrum, the anterior by the supratubal recess, the lateral by the scutum and the medial by the wall of the labyrinth at the level of the second portion of the facial nerve. The superior landmark is represented by the tegmen tympani, a thin osseous lamina 1 mm thick. By considering a sagittal plane crossing the superior ligaments of the incus and malleus, the epitympanum can be divided into a medial and lateral part. The lateral part includes Prussak's space. The superior ligament of the malleus divides the epitympanum into anterior and posterior parts. In the posterior part of the epitympanum the eminence of the lateral semicircular canal can easily be detected by either transtympanic endoscopy or VE. A significant advantage of VE in the exploration of the epitympanum is the demonstration of the entire incudo-malleolar joint obtained after the electronic removal of ligaments and soft tissues.

10.1.7
Virtual Endoscopy (Clinical Applications): The Study of the Ossicular Chain

VE allows the visualization of the entire ossicular chain, potentially from any point of view. Positioning the virtual endoscope within the external auditory canal, VE displays the long process of the incus, the stapes, and the handle of the malleus. However, the visualization of the stapes superstructure, with clear representation of the anterior and posterior crus, is difficult to obtain because of the partial volume effects of CT acquisition. From a point of view located within the epitympanum, VE can easily display the incudo-malleolar joint; this perspective is quite important in surgery of the temporal bone when mastoidectomy is performed to access the middle ear from the aditus ad antrum. The surgical field is nicely represented, and VE even allows the recognition of the eminence of the lateral semicircular canal, whose position has to be detected before drilling the bony part of the tympanic cavity (Fig. 10.3).

10.2
The Study of the Labyrinth

The labyrinth is a small organ with a complex structure. The interpretation of its anatomy by axial or coronal imaging is not difficult for experienced radiologists. However, the increased amount of information obtained by high-resolution spiral CT with single- or multislice technology, and by high-resolution MR imaging with dedicated surface coils and sequences, has changed the traditional approach. More frequently the data sets are analyzed with 3D reconstruction programs to better understand some anatomical details and clarify suspected pathological changes. The following paragraphs will review separately the application of 3D imaging to the study of the bone and membranous labyrinths.

10.2.1
Bone Labyrinth

The study of the bone labyrinth requires data sets obtained with CT. The use of spiral CT is preferred since data interpolation can increase image quality. The imaging protocol is the same as used for middle ear imaging, since the study is commonly performed for both these anatomical regions.

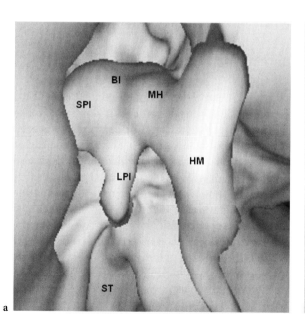 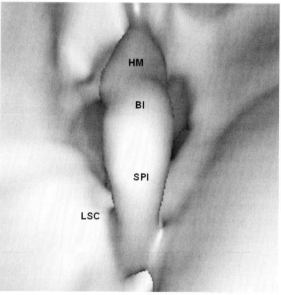

Fig. 10.3a, b. Virtual endoscopy of the ossicular chain. a Lateral view including almost the entire ossicular chain: *HM* handle of malleus, *MH* malleus head, *BI* body of incus, *SPI* short process of incus, *LPI* long process of incus, *ST* sinus tympani. b Superior view of the incudo-malleolar joint. The eminence of the lateral semicircular canal (*LSC*) represents an important surgical landmark for mastoidectomy

As in the case of the middle ear, multiplanar reconstructions can be used to study the components of the inner ear. These allow one to follow the different planes through which cochlea, semicircular canals, vestibule, first portion of the facial nerve, internal auditory canal and vestibular duct are oriented. Even if the study of the bone labyrinth includes both axial and coronal acquisitions with single-slice CT, in cooperative adult patients, this protocol is not always applicable in pediatric patients, or seems to be superfluous when the acquisition is performed with multislice CT (FUJII 2000; GOTWALDT 2001). In pediatric unsedated patients LUKER et al. (1993) showed the utility of MPR in generating coronal views that could not be obtained during image acquisition.

FRANKENTHALER (1998) used surface rendering methods to generate 3D representations of ossicles, bone labyrinth and even vessels, with excellent results, but the entire image processing framework, which required a phase of segmentation and a phase of generation of the geometric model, was extremely time-consuming. An alternative method is direct volume rendering, proposed by TOMANDL (2000). The method takes into account all the information inherent in the CT data sets and provides a semitransparent representation of the bone labyrinth. Volume rendering, performed with a powerful workstation, is done in real time and seems to be compatible with clinical routine. The selective visualization of the cochlea, vestibule and semicircular canals requires the application of different cut planes to the 3D data sets to reduce the superimposition of other bony structures, i.e., the medial wall of the tympanic cavity (Fig. 10.4). TOMANDL (2000) used a small volume of

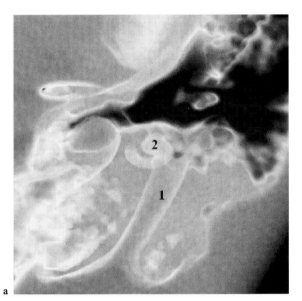

a

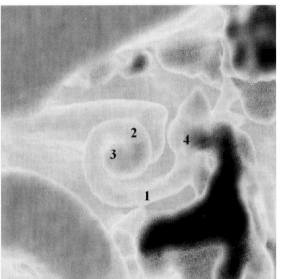

b

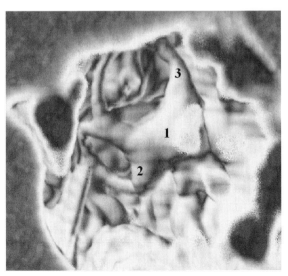

c

Fig. 10.4a–c. Volume rendering of the left labyrinth from a CT data set. a The inferior view of the labyrinth shows the bony part of the internal auditory canal (1) and the apical turn of the cochlea (2). b The lateral view from the same data set allow the visualization of the entire cochlea with basal (1), middle (2) and apical (3) turns, and of the vestibule (4). c From the medial view the vestibule (1) and ampullae of posterior (2) and superior (3) semicircular canals are displayed

interest including the labyrinthine structures; this avoided the influence of other structures and reduced rendering time.

Our group (NERI 2001a) has used CT volume rendering in the follow-up of patients who have undergone cochlear implantation. Volume rendering was helpful to display the path of the cochlear electrode and to establish the length of the portion inserted in the cochlea (Fig. 10.1b).

10.2.2
Membranous Labyrinth

The membranous labyrinth is relatively easier to represent in three dimensions than the bone labyrinth since data are directly acquired by MR imaging.

The initial method applied to MR imaging for 3D display the labyrinth was the MIP (maximum intensity projection). The final image obtained represents a projectional roadmap of the labyrinthine components. The simplicity of using MIP has made it the most widely used algorithm for 3D imaging in this case; but since MIP results from summed intensity values projected onto a bi-dimensional plane it is affected by the signal intensity of the tissue being visualized, the number of pixels of that tissue occurring along the projection, and the dynamic range of the data set. This means that small structures in a MIP may be poorly seen because they are consigned to the lower end of the display range.

A concrete solution to the limitations of MIP is volume rendering. We carried out a 3D study of the membranous labyrinth with a 1.5 T MR unit, using a 7.5 cm circular surface coil for signal reception. The imaging sequence included a 3D, T2-weighted, fast spin echo sequence in the axial plane (NERI 2000a). For 3D image processing MR data sets were processed with the software Advantage Windows 3.1 (GE Medical Systems, Milwaukee, Wis.) for generating volume renderings of the membranous labyrinth. Just as TOMANDL (2000) performed for CT data sets, a preliminary segmentation of the MR data set was carried out in order to select a volume of interest. This was done by interactive placement of cut planes through the volume, perpendicular to the plane of acquisition, in order to isolate the inner ear from the surrounding anatomical structures. Volume rendering then required the determination of the optimal signal intensity interval, including the signal of the labyrinth and the proper selection of opacity levels, for optimally displaying all its components (Fig. 10.5). In some difficult cases volume rendering failed to demonstrate the superior and lateral semicircular canals in their entirety, probably due to partial volume effects in image acquisition. KROMBACH (2000) compared MIP and volume rendering for displaying the labyrinthine components and observed that volume rendering was unique in being able to demonstrate the ampullae of the semicircular canals; in the same study the 2.5 windings of the cochlea were best depicted with MIP.

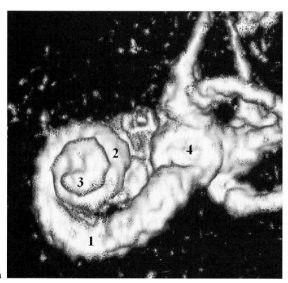
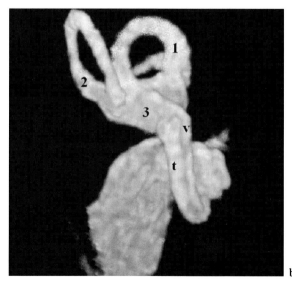

a b

Fig. 10.5a, b. Volume rendering of the left labyrinth from a high-resolution MR data set. **a** The lateral view from the same data set allows the visualization the entire cochlea with basal (*1*), middle (*2*) and apical (*3*) turns, and of the vestibule (*4*). **b** The inferior view shows with fine detail the scala tympani (*t*) and vestibuli (*v*) in the basal turn of the cochlea. (*1*) Lateral semicircular canal, (*2*) posterior semicircular canal, (*3*) vestibule

References

Ali QM (1993) Three-dimensional CT of the middle ear and adjacent structures. Neuroradiology 35:238–241

Caldemeyer KS (1999) Temporal bone: comparison of isotropic helical CT and conventional direct axial and coronal CT. AJR 172:1675–1682

Diederichs CG (1996) Spiral CT with reduced radiation dosage. Rofo Fortschr Geb Rontgenstr Neuen Bildgeb Verfahr 164:183–188

Espinoza J (1989) Surgical anatomy of the retrotympanum: on 25 temporal bones. Rev Laryngol Otol Rhinol 110:507–515

Frankenthaler RP(1998) Virtual otoscopy. Otolaryngol Clin North Am 31:383–392

Fujii N (2000) Imaging of the middle ear: high resolution multiplanar reconstruction and three-dimensional CT by 0.5 mm multislice helical CT. Radiology 217:S673

Gotwaldt TF (2001) Multidetector CT scanning of the temporal bone in patients with cholesteatoma. Eur Radiol 11 (Suppl 1):256

Grevers G (1989) Multiplanar imaging of the temporal bone: initial results. Laryngorhinootologie 68:392–395

Guerrier Y (1976) Topographic and surgical anatomy of the petrous bone. Acta Otorhinolaryngol Belg 30:22–50

Haas JP, Kahle G (1988) How best to present the radiological picture of the temporal bone today? HNO 36:89–101

Hermans R (1995) Spiral CT of the temporal bone: value of imaging reconstruction at submillimetric table increments. Neuroradiology 37:150–154

Johnson PT (1996) Three-dimensional CT: real-time interactive volume rendering. AJR 167:581–583

Krombach GA (2000) MRI of the inner ear: comparison of axial T2-weighted, three-dimensional turbo spin-echo images, maximum-intensity projections, and volume rendering. Invest Radiol 35:337–342

Luker GD, Lee BC, Erickson KK (1993) Spiral CT of the temporal bone in unsedated pediatric patients. AJNR Am J Neuroradiol 14:1145–1150

Mer SB (1967) Fiberoptic endoscope for examining the middle ear. Arch Otolaryngol 85:387–393

Neri E (2000a) Virtual endoscopy of the middle and inner ear with spiral computed tomography. Am J Otol 21:799–803

Neri E (2000b) High-resolution magnetic resonance and volume rendering of the labyrinth. Eur Radiol 10:114–118

Neri E (2001a) Outcome of cochlear implantation: assessment by volume rendered spiral CT. Eur Radiol 11 (Suppl 1):256

Neri E (2001b) Virtual endoscopy of the middle ear. Eur Radiol 11:41–49

Nomura YA (1982) Needle otoscope (an instrument of oto-endoscopy of the middle ear). Acta Otolaryngol (Stockh) 93:73–79

Parlier-Cuau C (1998) High-resolution computed tomographic study of the retrotympanum: anatomic correlations. Surg Radiol Anat 20:215–220

Pickett BP (1995) Sinus tympani: anatomic considerations, computed tomography, and a discussion of the retrofacial approach for removal of disease. Am J Otol 16: 741–750

Pozzi Mucelli RS (1997) Virtual endoscopy of the middle ear with computed tomography. Radiol Med 94:440–446

Rubin GD (1996) Perspective volume rendering of CT and MR images: applications for endoscopic imaging. Radiology 199:321–330

Thomassin JM (1994) La chirurgie sous guidage endoscopique des cavitée de l'oreille moyenne. Springer, Berlin Heidelberg New York

Thomassin JM (1996) Surgery under oto-endoscopic control. Rev Laryngol Otol Rhinol 117:409–415

Tomandl BF (2000) Virtual labyrinthoscopy: visualization of the inner ear with interactive direct volume rendering. Radiographics 20:547–558

Veillon F (1993) CT and MR imaging versus surgery of recurrent cholesteatoma in the post-operative middle ear: a 72 case study. Radiology 185:p248

Veillon F (1997) Imaging of recurrent postoperative cholesteatoma. International congress of head and neck radiology. Strasbourg, France, p 170

Watanabe Y (2000) High-resolution computed tomography using multiplanar reconstruction for the facial nerve canal. Acta Otolaryngol 542:44–48

Zini C (1967) La microtympanoscopie indirecte. Rev Laryngol Otol Rhinol 88: 736–738

11 Virtual Endoscopy of Paranasal Sinuses

JOACHIM KETTENBACH, WERNER BACKFRIEDER, MARTIN CITARDI, RAMIN SHAHIDI,
HELMUT RINGL, MONIKA CARTELLIERI, WOLFGANG BIRKFELLNER

CONTENTS

J. KETTENBACH, MD
Department of Diagnostic Radiology, University Hospital of
Vienna, Waehringer Guertel 18–20, 1090 Vienna, Austria
W. BACKFRIEDER, MS, PhD
Department of Biomedical Engineering and Physics, Univer-
sity of Vienna, General Hospital Vienna, Waehringer Guertel
18–20, 1090 Vienna, Austria
M. CITARDI, MD
Department Ear Nose and Throat, Cleveland Clinic Founda-
tion, 9500 Euclid Avenue, Cleveland, OH 44195, USA
R. SHAHIDI, PhD
Image Guidance Laboratories, Stanford University, Stanford
University Medical Center, Department of Neurosurgery, 300
Pasteur Drive, Room S-006, Stanford, CA 94305-5327, USA
H. RINGL, MD
Department of Diagnostic Radiology, University Hospital of
Vienna, Waehringer Guertel 18–20, 1090 Vienna, Austria
M. CARTELLIERI, MD
Department of Otolaryngology, University Hospital of Vienna,
Waehringer Guertel 18–20, 1090 Vienna, Austria
W. BIRKFELLNER, MS, PhD
Department of Biomedical Engineering and Physics, Univer-
sity of Vienna, General Hospital Vienna, Waehringer Guertel
18–20, 1090 Vienna, Austria

11.1
Introduction

Minimally invasive surgery for the nasal sinuses has became an important area of surgical intervention. Even with careful diagnostic endoscopic assessment the majority of abnormalities within the paranasal sinuses are not evident. To identify such abnormalities or anatomic variants that may compromise the ventilation prior to surgery is important for both the surgeon and the patient. To demonstrate areas of diseased mucosa CT is now considered the modality of choice. The surgeon, however, must combine high-quality axial CT imaging sets and reformat them mentally, which requires extensive experience. Thus, transformation of the perspective-free CT images into a perspective view of the endoscope is necessary, which has led to the development of virtual endoscopy of the paranasal sinuses. To date, studies have confirmed a good correlation of virtual endoscopy with intraoperative endoscopy, but intensive training is necessary for successful sinus surgery. Therefore, noninvasive virtual endoscopy has become an important part of surgical education and of planning individual sinus surgery procedures. When the endoscopic view is compromised either intraoperative image guidance or navigational imaging tools may provide image guidance during a procedure and may complement the surgeon's view.

The concept of functional endoscopic sinus surgery, developed by MESSERKLINGER in the early 1970s, revolutionized and radically altered the techniques used for diagnosis and treatment of patients with sinus disease (MESSERKLINGER 1978, 1994; STAMBERGER and POSAWETZ 1990). MESSERKLINGER's initial work, however, was conducted with information derived from conventional tomograms. This technique has now been replaced by CT, considered an essential component of the diagnostic investigation of patients presenting with symptoms suggestive of benign disease of the paranasal sinuses. CT identifies anatomic variants that may compromise the ventilation of the sinuses and can demonstrate areas of diseased mucosa that are responsible for recurrent disease. The CT scan further provides valuable information about the presence of potential hazards such as septations of the frontal or sphenoid sinuses, and the proximity of the orbit, internal carotid artery and optic nerve to areas of disease. Furthermore, CT is the ideal method for the demonstration of delicate bone structures of the ethmoid labyrinth. Even with careful diagnostic endoscopic assessment, the majority of these latter abnormalities may not be evident. The ability to identify radiologically prior to surgery those abnormalities that may increase surgical morbidity is important for both the surgeon and the patient. The surgeon, however, must combine high-quality axial imaging sets and has to reformat them mentally, which requires extensive experience. Therefore, a transformation of the perspective-free CT images into a perspective view of the endoscope is necessary for successful surgical exploration.

Advances in computer technology have led to the development of hardware and software imaging techniques that have been successfully utilized by the entertainment industry. These techniques have been adopted by the medical field, which has resulted in numerous imaging advances (GILANI et al. 1997). This has led to even more robust three-dimensional imaging, allowing newer generation display techniques (FISHMAN et al. 1987; KELLER et al. 1989; RUBIN et al. 1993). While advances in CT and MR technologies have resulted in greater resolution of small structures, initial applications for virtual endoscopy (VE) were introduced by VINING et al. (1994a, b). To date, studies have confirmed a good correlation of VE with intraoperative endoscopy (GILANI et al. 1997; ROGALLA et al. 1998; HOPPER et al. 1999; YAMASHITA et al. 1999; NAKASATO et al. 2000). The endoscopic view, however, can be decreased during surgery by blood and humidity covering the surface of the lens. To overcome this obstacle, either intraoperative image guidance (FRIED et al. 1998a) or navigational imaging tools may provide image guidance during a procedure and may complement the surgeon's view (SHAHIDI et al. 1998a; NAKASATO et al. 2000; GREIML and BACKFRIEDER 2000). Although not widely used currently, in the near future these tools may support the surgeon in approaching sinonasal disease.

11.2
Image Acquisition and Postprocessing

11.2.1
Computed Tomography

Preoperative coronal CT of the paranasal sinuses is now a standard imaging procedure (CHAKERES 1985; SOM 1985; CHOW and MAFEE 1989; BEUS et al. 1995), although some authors prefer axial image acquisition and coronal reconstruction (HOSEMANN 1996). Using axial CT acquisition is advantageous for the patient, since extended positioning of the patient's head during image acquisition in the coronal plane can be avoided. The disadvantage, however, is more limited spatial resolution. However, spiral CT and multi-row detector computed tomography (MRDCT) techniques overcome this limitation by using thin collimation and overlapping reconstruction algorithms (SUOJANEN and REGAN 1995; ROGALLA et al. 1998). Thus reconstructed axial images obtained from diagnostic scans can be used to generate high-quality virtual endoscopic reconstructions. For multiplanar visualization, sagittal and coronal MPR (multiplanar reconstruction) images can be obtained with a 0.5 mm slice thickness and a 2–3 mm interval. Typical helical CT data acquisition parameters for paranasal sinuses are given in Table 11.1.

The bone reconstruction algorithm is routinely used in CT scanners and heightens the depiction of edges. In addition, an increased kernel hardness provides greater edge sharpness. Nonionic contrast media can be applied to differentiate between vascular and less vascular structures.

11.2.2
Magnetic Resonance Imaging

There are several advantages of MR imaging over CT. Of particular note is the minimal artefact caused by dental fillings and the capability of multiplanar imaging. For the paranasal and nasopharyngeal area 4 or 5 mm slices are used. For the detailed analysis of smaller areas such as the cribriform plate, thinner (≤3 mm) slices are preferable (Table 11.2). Newer sequences such as FLASH (fast low angle shot sequence) and FISP (fast imaging with steady state processing) may provide improved detail with thin 1 mm adjacent sections or with a three-dimensional (3D) volume. T1-weighted 3D volumetric gradient-echo sequences provide isotropic voxels, which are suitable for 3D rendering. For vessel visualization,

Table 11.1. Typical helical CT and MRDCT acquisition parameters for paranasal sinuses

	Coronal acquisition (helical CT)	Axial acquisition (helical CT)	Axial acquisition (MRDCT)
	120–140 kV, 140 mAs	120–140 kV, 50–130 mAs	140 kV, 150 mAs
Scan time	1.0 rev/s	0.75–1.0 rev/s	0.75 rev/s
Collimation	3.0 mm	1.5–3.0 mm	4×1 mm
Table feed	1.5–3.0 mm/s	1.5–3.0 mm/s	5 mm/s
Pitch	1	1–2	
Patient position	Supine or prone; head hyperextended	Supine	
Gantry orientation	Tilted to approximate a plane perpendicular to the orbitomeatal line	Parallel to hard palate	
Imaging range:	Nose to sphenoid sinus	Maxillary alveolar ridge to the superior aspect of the frontal sinus	
Contrast	Optional; 100 ml nonionic contrast i.v. (2 ml/s, delay 50 s)		
Threshold range	–520 to –200 HU		
Reconstruction algorithm	Bone; sharp to extrasharp edges		
Reconstruction kernel	Sharp to extrasharp edges		
Reconstruction thickness	2–3 mm	1–1.5 mm	

Table 11.2. Advantages of CT and MR imaging of sinusal region

Advantages of MR	Advantages of CT
No radiation	Superior bone detail
Superior detail of soft tissues and brain	Availability
	Lower cost to patient
Multiple pulse sequences	
No bone-hardening artifact	
Dental artifacts localized	
Multiplanar capability	
No intravenous contrast needed	
Intrinsic sensitivity to blood flow	

3D time-of-flight (TOF) MR angiography (MRA) is preferred over phase contrast angiography because of the better delineation of vessel walls. The actual pulse sequence for T1- and T2-weighted images depends on the magnetic field strength. For a 1.0 T scanner, a 256×256 matrix and spin echo sequences with a TR (repetition time) of 0.6 s and a TE (echo time) of 17 ms are used for mild T1-weighted images. Sequential images are separated by 1 mm spacing and 4 acquisitions are used for thin (3 mm) sections to improve the signal-to-noise ratio, whereas two acquisitions are sufficient for thicker sections. For T2-weighted sequences, a TR of 3.0 s with a TE of 45/90 ms can be used. A head coil is commonly used; however, the best detail is obtained with specially designed surface coils. The preferred orientation of the imaging plane is axial and coronal, except in special circumstances when a sagittal plane may be preferable (VALVASSORI et al. 1998).

11.2.3
Postprocessing

Several research groups have developed visualization techniques for medical imaging data. An overview of the computational tasks and diversities of technologies which support the different applications in the field of medical imaging can be found in EZQUERRA et al. (1999).

In particular three techniques are commonly used for displaying volumetric data regardless of the modality used to obtain them (GILANI et al. 1997). The first is a "flat" depiction of the data set that shows the 3D set by highlighting selected threshold limits, also called maximum intensity projection (MIP).

The second technique, surface rendering, is a more realistic 3D depiction in which the data set is manipulated so that structures of the surfaces are shown, further highlighted by shading techniques, and called shaded surface display (SSD). For SSD threshold ranges from about –520 to –200 HU are recommended to eliminate voxels denser than –500 HU.

Surface rendering techniques use an intermediate step, called segmentation, to transform the volume data into a mesh of polygons (LORENSEN and CLINE 1987). Due to the large quantity of voxels to be processed and the complexity of the presentation, most segmentation techniques are semiautomatic. Manual segmentation is time-consuming and may contain operation errors; fully automatic procedures are not generally applicable. The resulting mesh of polygons can be rendered using the standard graphics hardware support. The drawback is often a time-consuming preparation phase and reduced accuracy, since information about the inner parts of the objects is lost (GEIGER and KIKINIS 1995; HONG et al. 1997; BARTZ and SKALEJ 1999).

The third technique, volume rendering, provides dimensional views generated by casting rays from an observation point either outside the imaging volume or from inside through the remaining part of the volume. Volume rendering can show a greater spectrum of 3D information by concentrating not only on chosen "surface" features, but also by displaying structures as though they were partially transparent (LEVOY 1987; SHAHIDI et al. 1996; DARABI et al. 1997; BRADY et al. 1998; MEISSNER et al. 1998). When a perspective view, chosen by the operator, is added, this mode is called perspective volume rendering (PVR), a refinement of volume rendering (RUSINEK et al. 1989; MAGNUSSON et al. 1991). There is no loss of information but volume rendering is limited in its visualization of small, complicated internal structures within a large data set (PFISTER et al. 1999). Once imaging data is generated, it is transferred to a dedicated workstation equipped with high-performance graphic cards and reconstruction software. It is recommended that the data set be reduced according to reconstruction needs. For example, since bony detail is less important than mucosal surface visualization the upper 4 bits of the 12 bit data set contains much unnecessary bone information that can be discarded (GILANI et al. 1997). Processing will then take place with the 8 bit range, which contains all information relevant to the examination and speeds up information processing and manipulation. Depending on the rendering technique (surface rendering or volume rendering) either pixels or voxels are segmented to represent the mucosal surface. Pixels and voxels can be assigned colors and opacities. By altering the surface reflectivity, lighting direction and lighting coordinates, the surface appearance of the imaged tissues can be manipulated to achieve the appearance of mucosal membranes.

11.2.4
Path Generation

The following techniques can be used to guide a virtual camera through the virtual endoscopy models.

11.2.4.1
Manual Camera Movement

Using a mouse, the camera position, the field of view of the camera and focal point are interactively changed. User controls can rotate the camera about its origin or its focal point. The software may provide a collision detection of camera and anatomic surface, thus applying a force model to keep the camera inside the sinonasal structures.

11.2.4.2
Keyframing

Keyframing is a computer animation technique that interpolates between user-selected essential points. Cubic splines are used to calculate intermediate parameter values at any desired resolution (KOCHANEK and BARTELS 1984). Key frames can be used easily to generate motion through open interior and exterior environments. An operator selects "key" locations in the patient's sinuses that must be viewed and the order in which these designated "key" images are viewed. For camera location and orientation manual camera movement is used. Each key image has an unique spatial coordinate, a directional coordinate defining viewer placement in space, and a field of view defining how wide a perspective is included in the view. For most of the images, a 60–80° field of view is appropriate to simulate the endoscopic perspective. ROGALLA et al. (1998) used a viewing angle of 120° to create an overlap of 30° on all four sides with adjacent views. The computer then connects these key views (around 150 for the sinuses) as an interpolated continuous film along a desired route. This route is also known as a flight path. This interconnecting technique is also known as a spline path, generated at a rate of 25–30 frames/s. Using this technique RUBIN et al. (1993) reported that several person-hours were required to generate an elaborate flight path. For path definition through each of the nasal passages ROGALLA et al. (1998) required a mean time for path definition and movie calculation of 8 (±2) min and 3 (±1) min, respectively (GILANI et al. 1997; ROGALLA et al. 1998; SHAHIDI et al. 1998b).

11.2.4.3
Automatic Path Planning

Most of the tubular organs in the sinuses present a challenge for both manual camera movement and key-framing. To guide a virtual endoscope, a robot path-planning algorithm can be adapted (LENGYEL et al. 1990). The camera is treated as a point robot and the walls of the organs as obstacles. These obstacles are identified as ranges of threshold values or tissue labels. The path planner labels all voxels within the 3D data set with a specified distance to a particular goal, normally defined as the terminus of the organ to be explored. Then, given a starting point, the path-planning algorithm finds the shortest path to the goal. The voxel coordinates for each point in the path are recorded and the path smoothed using the found points as key points. Then a flight path can be choreographed by exploring the nostrils and then the internal surfaces of the paranasal sinuses on both sides, entering them through their native ostia. Entering the maxillary sinus through the hiatus semilunaris, all aspects of the sinus can be explored and a mucosal web can be easily identi-fied. The same can be done by entering the frontal sinuses through the frontal recess. A nasopharyngeal reconnaissance with the camera panning around the nasopharynx may be included as well. In addition, the variables can be changed to make the soft tissue become transparent, so that the underlying bony anat-omy becomes visible. Therefore, variations in the optic chiasm or the carotid siphon can be viewed while still demonstrating the partially transparent nasopharyn-geal margin. Using variations in opacity, structures the surgeon either may wish to avoid or may want to target for an minimally invasive procedure (i.e., biopsy, drain-age) can be discriminated and selectively visualized. Showing the back side of the nasal septum and conchae, the turbinates and nares are viewed in much greater detail and with a larger field of view than is allowed with indirect mirror examination. Another advantage is that structures not accessible by conventional endoscopy can be entered or views can be obtained that are not easily achievable with conventional techniques (Table 11.3). Unusual perspectives can be examined to visual-ize precise areas of pathology from multiple perspec-tives. This may allow a more thorough evaluation of even small lesions. However, manual path definition is needed if mucosal swelling precludes entering a sinus. In this case coronal MPR is valuable to control the path definition. To date, path definition through the nose must be done manually. Automated path definition is desirable but appears to be more difficult due to the complex anatomy.

Table 11.3. Advantages of virtual endoscopy of paranasal sinuses

Highly interactive, remarkably sharp and detailed pictures of the nasal and paranasal sinuses

Visualization of complex anatomic relationships obscured by bone and soft tissue

Unusual perspectives can be examined (back side of the nasal septum and conchae)

Turbinates and nares are viewed in much greater detail and with a larger field of view than allowed with indirect mirror examination

Data set obtained as part of a routine diagnostic examination

No additional morbidity beyond that of a routine CT or MR examination

Complementary visualization in anatomically difficult or impossible to reach regions or in the case of overlap of pathologic processes

With the field of view decreased during sinus surgery, a navigational system allow the localization of anatomic landmarks

Noninvasive teaching element for students and trainees

11.3
Endoscopic Sinus Surgery Training

Endonasal sinus surgery requires extensive training before it can be performed adequately. The near-field endoscopic anatomy is very different from the typical anatomic presentation seen in cross-sectional images or in an anatomy atlas. Even the experienced endos-copist can easily become disoriented or even lost due to the complex and variable anatomy and the proxim-ity of important structures (MAY et al. 1994; HOSE-MANN 1996; WEBER et al. 1998). Therefore intensive training is necessary to avoid severe complications, and this is even more important given the fact that endoscopic surgery remains the major reason for lawsuits against physicians in the United States (ANON et al. 1994).

ECKE et al. (1998) combined computer graphics and virtual reality techniques to create an interactive nasal endoscopy simulator (NES) for nasal endos-copy and endonasal sinus surgery. The system con-sisted of a graphics workstation, a tracking system for measuring the position of the endoscope and sur-gical instruments in space, a head model, image data sets of the nasal cavity and paranasal sinus area, and complementary software. The current NES is com-prised of a visual and auditory virtual reality system that provides both educational and planning options for sinus surgery. However, the usual resistance when touching relevant anatomic structures is not provided by this release. Thus, a "force feedback system" was implemented that allows for such a response (RUDMAN et al. 1998). The use of VE for training can familiarize the operator with endoscopic anatomic appearance and provide anatomic landmarks to assist with orientation. The information gained from such training can provide confidence, and preoperative VE may lead to more effective and safer endoscopic procedures. In the near future virtual reality simulation will become an important part of surgical education and planning for individual sinus surgery procedures. The continuing development such devices will lead to an improved educational environment for residents in training and practitioners (WIET et al. 1997).

11.4
Clinical Applications

Recently developed rendering techniques, including a perspective mode, result in highly interactive, remarkably sharp and detailed pictures of the nasal and paranasal sinuses. These images including VE are easy to reconstruct using a widely available workstation equipped with advanced software. DE NICOLA et al. (1997) evaluated the ability to perform CT-based VE of the paranasal sinuses using surface rendering. However, the authors used a 3 mm slice thickness and no reconstruction overlap. The reconstruction algorithm and surface rendering yielded low-quality images. The primary limitation of surface rendering is that structures may have a density value more or less value than the chosen threshold value. This caused a discontinuity or continuity of the rebuilt nasal-sinus surfaces that did not always correspond to reality. In addition, overlap of different structures such as mucosa-purulent secretions were visualized only as shape modification. HOPPER et al. (1999) theorized from their work that volume rendering provides a tremendous advantage because of its ability to

make mucosal surfaces transparent and therefore to reveal underlying structures or pathology. ROGALLA et al. (1998) evaluated the applicability of VE in the sinonasal region based on volume-rendered spiral CT data in 45 patients. Using low-dose spiral CT of the sinuses the imaging data were transferred to a workstation running software for volume rendering (EasyVision, Philips Medical Systems, Eindhoven, The Netherlands). Six orthogonal views of the maxillary sinuses and the nasopharynx and a fly through movie of the nose were obtained. Coronal reconstructions and VE with respect to detectability of pathology were compared, while in 30 patients who underwent subsequent endoscopic surgery, surgeons were asked to rank the degree of assistance of the preoperative VE. Overall, anatomic details were depicted more often with coronal reconstructions than with VE; however, a high degree of similarity between VE and the intraoperative impression was reported by the surgeons. The authors concluded that VE of the nose and paranasal sinuses may develop into a standard means to guide surgeons during endoscopic interventions (ROGALLA et al. 1998) (Figs. 11.1–11.3).

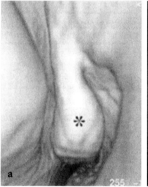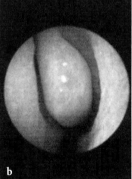

Fig. 11.1. a Left infundibulum (*asterisk*) on virtual endoscopy. **b** The endoscopic view of the infundibulum prior to resection. Note the almost identical anatomic structure. (Courtesy of ROGALLA et al. 1998)

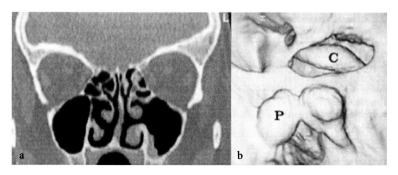

Fig. 11.2. a Coronal reconstruction of axial CT slices. Recurrent sinusitis can be seen in the base of the left maxillary sinus after functional sinus surgery. **b** Corresponding virtual endoscopy of the left maxillary sinus demonstrating the polypoid character of the mucosal swelling (*P*). The medial concha (*C*) can be seen through an osseous defect in the medial wand. (Courtesy of ROGALLA et al. 1998)

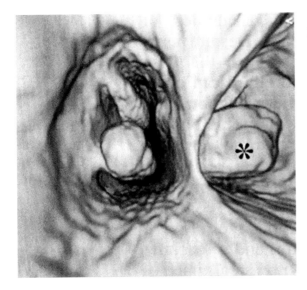

Fig. 11.3. View from the nasopharynx through the conchae nasales. Polypoid swelling of the dorsal aspect of the inferior right conchae (*asterisk*). The swelling is less prominent on the left side. (Courtesy of Rogalla et al. 1998)

Hopper et al. (1999) evaluated the feasibility of highlighting surgical sites using CT-based virtual reality of the paranasal sinuses before sinus surgery in 25 patients with significant paranasal sinus disease. For all 25 planned surgeries, the virtual images showed the entire surgical site marked on the 2D coronal images as well as the orientation of the planned surgical site to adjacent normal anatomy. For surgery of the maxillary sinuses, tagging and electronic removal of the middle turbinate and uncinate processes mimicked the actual surgery and allowed complete visualization of the infundibulum and the planned surgical site. Therefore, planned endoscopic paranasal sinus surgical sites could be easily and reliably highlighted using CT virtual reality techniques with respect to the patient's normal endoscopic anatomy. This is particularly true in complex surgical accesses to the frontal and sphenoid sinuses. Displaying the superficial anatomy with the planned surgical window highlighted and with the actual surgical window opened, which demonstrating the bony depth, proved to be very useful (Figs. 11.4, 11.5).

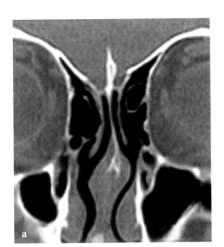
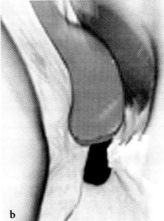
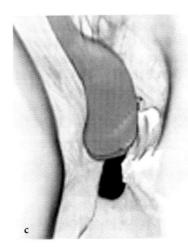

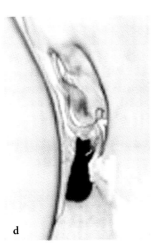

Fig. 11.4a–d. With the use of volumetric rendering a simple and rapid process to tag structures and pathologic processes can be performed. In this normal subject the middle turbinate and uncinate processes have been tagged in *green* and *red*, respectively (**a,b**). Once tagged, a simple click-on command removes the tagged structures. Sequentially, the uncinate process (**c**) and the middle turbinate (**d**) have been removed, allowing full exposure of the infundibulum. The whitish areas represent cut-away bone. (Courtesy of Hopper et al. 1999)

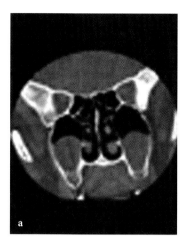
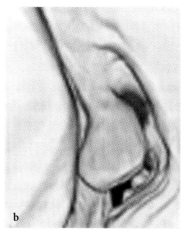
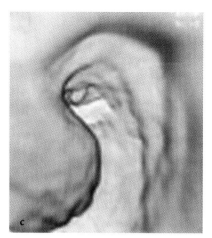

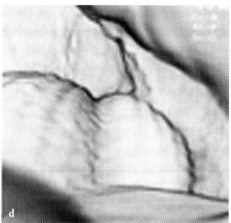

Fig. 11.5a–d. Maxillary sinus exposure. This patient with large bilateral retention cysts (**a**) first had the uncinate processes tagged, (**b**) segmented (*red*) and removed (**c**), allowing direct visualization of the infundibulum. Once the maxillary sinus ostia were easily visible and traversed, the cysts could be viewed directly (**d**). (Courtesy of HOPPER et al. 1999)

To specify a safe surgical entrance point for paranasal mucoceles the value of MPR and virtual CT sinuscopy was evaluated and compared with results confirmed by surgical endoscopy (NAKASATO et al. 2000). The combination of the two techniques was important in depicting safe puncture sites through an endonasal approach to treat simple mucoceles. Virtual endoscopic images revealed the interface between air and soft tissue. Since it was difficult to approach deeper lesions, VE was applicable only to the most superficial lesions. These authors concluded that a navigational system might overcome this limitation.

If mucosal swelling causes occlusion of natural ostia VE cannot access the sinus and manual path definition might be necessary, provided the access can be defined on coronal reconstructions. VE is advantageous for viewing the entry site of the tuba auditiva, a region not well depicted on coronal reconstructions. On the other hand, septal deviations are easier to define on coronal slices; decisions about the septum can be impossible using VE because slight curves in general escape detection due to the per-

spective distortion of the images. Further, normal bone variations can be imaged only on cross-sectional slices if they are hidden behind the surface structure.

Correlation with cross-sectional images is still advantageous since these images provide precise localization and definition of structures behind a surface. This is particularly true if a sinus is completely blocked or closed and VE is impossible.

11.5
Image-Guided Sinus Surgery

When the endoscope tip gently touches the mucosa, the view is easily obstructed by blood, mucus or pus. Continuing surgery with an obstructed view is dangerous. The endoscope must be withdrawn to wash the tip and it will take time to reach the area of interest again. Therefore, it is vitally important to keep the endoscope tip away from inner walls to maintain a good endoscope view. This principle will also avoid damage to fragile tissues that can occur when they are struck by the endoscope.

However, disorientation may occur for several reasons:

- The position of the endoscope tip inside the patient is not directly visible and therefore surgeons usually guess at the location on the basis of the inserted length, orientation and monitor screen view.
- The viewing direction varies from 0° (straight forward) to 120° (backward viewing) and may rotate on its axis. Thus when the viewing direction exceeds 0° disorientation may occur.
- The endoscopic view is limited to the mucosal surface and landmarks used to position the endoscope within the patient may become indistinguishable because of damage by disease or injuries from previous surgery.

To provide spatial orientation and therefore to increase safety and effectiveness of sinus surgery the use image guidance has been proposed by several groups (KLIMEK et al. 1996; FRIED et al. 1997, 1998b; YAMASHITA et al. 1999).

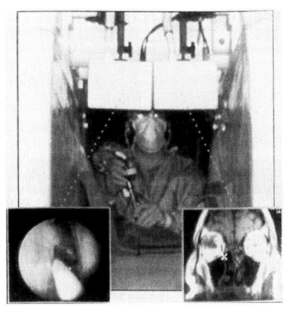

Fig. 11.6. The surgeon operates standing in the vertical open space at the interventional MR unit. During functional endoscopic sinus surgery (FESS) the surgeon views the display from the two head-high screens that show the video camera image from the endoscope (*lower left*) and the MR image (*lower right*), with crosshairs to identify the position of the pointer tip. The image scan plane is defined by the location of the pointer. (Courtesy of FRIED et al. 1998a)

11.5.1
Image-Guided Sinus Surgery Using MR Imaging

The first image-guided endoscopic surgeries using intraoperative MR imaging were reported by FRIED et al. (1998b). The procedures were experimental and intended to test the unusual working environment of a unique new "open-configuration" MR unit for head and neck surgery using near real-time image guidance. Twelve patients underwent endoscopic sinus surgery while under general anesthesia in a new open MR unit that provides the surgeon with access to the patient while imaging is being performed. Eleven patients had chronic sinusitis (eight of them had bilateral disease) and one had a right nasoethmoid and antral tumor. All 12 surgeries were performed without complications and both the endoscopic view and the MR scans were available at the surgical field. The image plane was surgeon-controlled, and the MR scanner updated images in as little as 14 s. The MR scanner provided adequate visualization of both the disease and the related anatomy and allowed the surgeon to navigate during the procedure (Fig. 11.6).

Intraoperative MR imaging has several advantages over CT-based guidance systems. MR imaging provides a multiplanar capability and has better soft tissue differentiation than CT. The intraoperative data reflect tissue changes during surgery and provide optimum feedback for surgical guidance. Apparently intraoperative MR imaging has a role in the treatment of head and neck disorders and warrants further study (HSU et al. 1998). The operating environment, however, poses some challenges; in particular, all instruments, including the endoscope, must be made from MR-compatible materials.

11.5.2
Image-Guided Sinus Surgery Using a Navigational System

A navigational system should support the surgeon to prevent complications during surgery, by means of probes to localize landmarks or critical structures such as the optical nerve. The following image-guided surgical navigation systems currently commercially available were used for functional endoscopic sinus surgery (FESS): the Viewing Wand (ISG Technologies, Mississauga, Ontario, Canada) using a six-degree-of-freedom (DOF) mechanical-arm probe (ANON et al. 1994); a system with the mechanical arm replaced by an optical tracker (KLIMEK et al. 1996); the InstaTrak system (Visualization Technology, Woburn, Mass.) with a six DOF electromagnetic sensor attached to an aspirator, working as a probe (FRIED et al. 1997); and the ARTMA Virtual Patient system (ARTMA Biomedical, Vienna, Austria), an electromagnetic tracking device developed by TRUPPE et al. (1996).

FREYSINGER et al. (1997) compared the ISG Viewing Wand with the ARTMA Virtual Patient system for generating an endoscopic 3D navigation for ear nose and throat (ENT) surgery by using augmented reality techniques. Initial experiences were very promising, and the two systems achieved a comparable intraoperative accuracy. However, interference of magnetizable objects with the sensor technology may cause localization errors using the ARTMA system. With the Viewing Wand there were mechanical limitations as well as the weight imposed by the arm. The Insta-Trak System was reviewed in a multicenter clinical study (n=55) that assessed the system's capability for localizing structures in critical surgical sites (FRIED et al. 1997, 1998a). Several new advances including an automated registration technique that eliminates the redundant CT scan, compensation for head movement, and the ability to use interchangeable instruments were described. However, some regions such as the ethmoid roof and frontal sinus could not be accessed with a straight rigid probe. In addition no information about the viewing direction of the endoscopes is available.

To overcome these limitations a 3D-model-based navigation system for endoscopic sinus surgery was developed (YAMASHITA et al. 1999). To prevent disorientation during surgery and to optimize training, this system aided navigation by showing a single perspective view of the patient and the endoscope models. This virtual endoscope had a viewing cone with a simulated light to indicate the viewing direction and visual field in real time. The system's three clipping planes automatically followed the endoscope and helped to keep the surgeon aware of the endoscope's actual position. Compared with conventional navigation using a triplanar display, the perspective view was referenced more frequently. The triplanar display was almost completely ignored, apparently because it was too difficult to interpret during surgery. A significant refinement was introduced by the research team at the Stanford University Department of Neurosurgery Image Guidance Laboratory. This group developed a surgical set-up

based on modern frameless stereotactic techniques. It enabled surgeons to explore the underlying layers of the patient's anatomy through a surgical endoscope with the endoscope display overlaid in real time with volumetrically reconstructed images of the patient's 3D data. This represents a marked improvement over conventional image guidance systems, which display only 2D reconstructed images based on a single point in the surgical volume (SHAHIDI et al. 1996, 1998b). CBYON software (CBYON Suite's Image Enhanced Endoscopy Module) was used to review the preoperative sinus CT. During this review, it was noted that the sphenoid sinus had pneumatized around the left optic nerve. A 3D model of the intrasinus portion of the nerve was made through virtual patient reconstruction. Subsequently, the anatomic relationships among the optic nerve and adjacent sinus pneumatization were reviewed by adjusting the transparency/opacity of the bone and soft tissue. The CBYON system was auto-registered with the ENT head frame. The endoscopic video image and the perspective volume rendered endoscopic image were registered for image-enhanced endoscopy (IEE). During IEE, the perspective volume rendering (PVR) image and the corresponding standard endoscopic image were displayed; the system updated both images simultaneously. The 3D model could easily be seen on the PVR image without direct entry into the sphenoid sinus. IEE provided a means for visualization of structures that could not be seen during standard endoscopy, by making visible surfaces transparent (Fig. 11.7).

It has been shown through IRB (institutional review board) approved surgical procedures that the combination of two technologies – real and virtual endoscopy – will provide the means for minimally invasive surgical interventions while maintaining maximum exposure and orientation (SHAHIDI et al. 1996, 1998b).

11.5.3
Developing an Interactive Navigational System

A display system for navigation in ENT surgery to be used for intraoperative navigation has been proposed (GREIML and BACKFRIEDER 2000). An off-line mode (disabled connection to the tracking system) is provided for training purposes.

First, the visual information is generated by using all available imaging modalities such as CT, MR imaging, single photon emission computed tomography (SPECT) and positron emission tomography

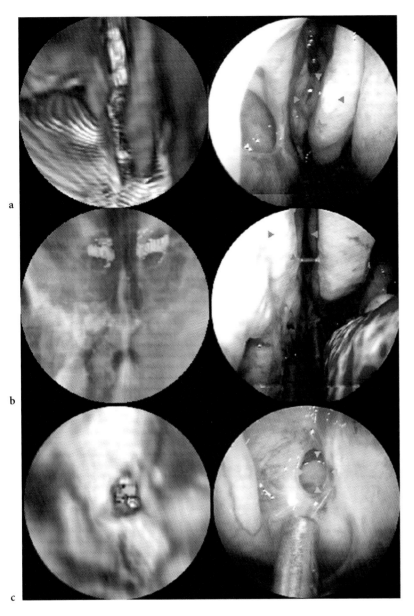

a

b

c

Fig. 11.7a–c. A 3D model of the intra-sinus portion of the nerve was made through virtual patient reconstruction. The endoscopic video image and the perspective volume rendered endo-scopic image were autoregistered for image-enhanced endoscopy using the CBYON system. During FESS, the per-spective volume rendered image and the corresponding standard endoscopic image were displayed; the system updated both images simultaneously

(PET). By virtue of their specific properties these imaging modalities can provide complementary information: CT may be used for osseous structures, MR imaging for depicting soft tissues and tumor, and SPECT and PET to analyze the metabolic state of tissues. The information from these different modalities, visualized within different frames of references, can be integrated into one standardized frame. This process involves fusion of volume data sets resulting from the registration of respective anatomic structures within the data sets. Before image registration, anatomic and pathologic structures must be selected (segmented). The segmentation of the structures is completed semi-automatically using algorithms that fit the image modality, e.g., region growing, morphologic procedures, thresholding operations. Image registration is then performed by minimizing the distance between the surfaces of respective segmented structures, accomplished by "chamfer matching" (BORGE-FORS 1988). The volume data set is then rendered according to the position of the endoscope. The 3D view of the anatomic structures is calculated and displayed using the intrinsic imaging properties of the endoscopic optics. In addition to this view, the current position of the endoscope's tip is visualized on a 3D view and on three corresponding orthogonal slices. An optical tracking system (FlashPoint,

Image Guided Technologies, USA) can be used for monitoring the position of the endoscope relative to the patient, which can be located near the endoscope's operator.

A drawback of VE systems is that they do not simulate the distorted optical model of a real endoscope. By wrapping the image plane around a sphere a camera model can be used to simulate the real endoscope. This effect has been calibrated and verified by EISENKOLB and BACKFRIEDER (1999) (Figs. 11.8, 11.9). The user interface shows a simple layout for easy handling to meet the needs in the FESS. Complementary information to the real endoscope view can be supplied as demonstrated in Fig. 11.10. The selection of the current slices (transverse, coronal, sagittal) is performed either by user input or automatically by the tracking system using the endoscope's tip as reference point. The 3D view is generated using a transparent volume rendering algorithm (LEVOY 1987). The endoscope is modeled as an object within the volume data set. To improve the rendering

performance an image-based method is used with the position of the endoscope calculated first. If the endoscope appears inside a subvolume, the corner of that volume is mapped to the image plane and those pixels defined that are affected by the positional change of the endoscope. Therefore, only a small proportion of the rays need to be recalculated during the rendering process, which allows interactive display speed. It is possible to zoom in and out as well as to rotate the viewpoint to allow a view of the volume data from different angles and to enlarge areas of interest. It is also possible to generate stereoscopic images of the volume data, which can be displayed in the 3D overview window. When using the appropriate hardware (double buffering monitor, shutterglasses etc.) the operator perceives a 3D impression of the anatomic structures and the position of the endoscope. The endoscopic rendering at the display system uses the algorithm described by EISENKOLB and BACKFRIEDER (1999). The "preview" mode is used for fast image generation with less

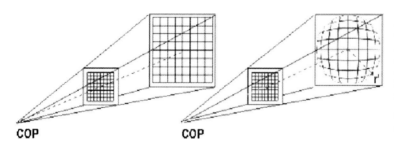

Fig. 11.8. Camera model for virtual endoscopy: simple perspective model (*left*); perspective camera model with endoscopic distortion (*right*). The left figure shows a perspective camera model used in computer graphics, the right section shows the fish-eye distortion of a real endoscope as used for endoscopic volume rendering

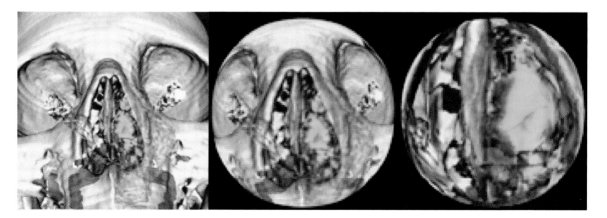

Fig. 11.9. Three-dimensional and virtual endoscopy reconstruction: an overview of the 3D reconstruction of a patient with nasopharyngeal tumor (*left*); plane rendering of virtual endoscopy (*middle*); perspective rendering to simulate the endoscopist's view (*right*)

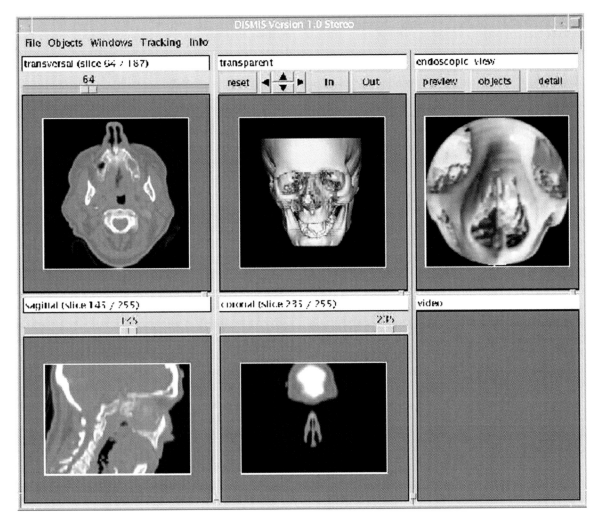

Fig. 11.10. User interface of the prototype navigational system. Orthogonal slices are displayed in the *upper left, lower left* and *lower middle* windows; transparent rendering (*upper middle window*); endoscopic rendering (*upper right window*)

accuracy; the "detail" version takes more time but produces a more precise output. The "object" mode includes the colors and opacities from the object map.

11.5.3.1
Tracking System

The optical tracking system used in this setting (FlashPoint 3D Localizer, Image Guided Technologies, USA) consists of a static optical sensor assembly with three high-resolution linear digital cameras and a tracking sensor attached to the endoscope. Placing at least three light-emitting diodes (LEDs) at well-defined positions on an instrument, enables that instrument to be tracked (Fig. 11.10). The tracking system sends a reference point to the display process during the registration step, which allows the calculation of the endoscope position relative to the volume data set. During tracking the distance and rotational parameters of the endoscope in relation to the reference point are sent to the display process, which in turn calculates the position of the endoscope tip inside the volume data set. The tracking system provides 6 degrees of freedom for tracking the endoscope's movements. The process of communication between tracking and the display process is based on the computation time needed for the transparent rendering. To prevent an overflow of the display process, the tracking process sends approximately two new positions per second to the display process. This is within the interactive speed range determined to be necessary for clinical use.

11.5.3.2
Results

The most time-consuming task is the 3D rendering algorithm. It takes about 2 s to render the 256×256 pixels image shown in Fig. 11.11, whereas the volume consists of 320×320×216 voxels using an 8 bit resolution. Rendering can be improved by applying a rendering mask and entering only selected voxels when tracking the endoscope. The amount of time saved depends on the position of the endoscope (parallel or orthogonal to the viewing direction). The average speed-up is around 3.5 times, which leads to approximately 2 frames per second. Unfortunately, when selecting a new viewpoint this advantage is lost. A precomputation of the 3D view from different selected viewpoints (keyframes) was deemed not practical. Hardware would be available that uses parallel perspective rendering (PFISTER et al. 1999). This may provide interactive frame rates; under certain conditions, however, colorization of voxels may fail. Also planned is the implementation of stereoscopic rendering for the 3D view window.

11.6
Conclusion

VE and PVR allow evaluation of the nasal cavity, nasopharynx and paranasal sinuses obtained from CT or MR imaging with no additional morbidity. Despite the fact that all anatomic information is provided on axial slices, VE will not show new informa-

tion. However, VE displays relevant structures in a manner that can also be visualized by the surgeon. Anatomic and pathologic details can be visualized using unconventional angles, perspectives and locations not conventionally accessible, and complex 3D anatomic relationships obscured by bone and soft tissue can be visualized. However, a manual segmentation tool might be useful to compensate for uncertain reconstructions in regions subject to artifacts. To date VE of the paranasal sinuses has found only limited clinical applications; however, VE may be more commonly used with high-resolution imaging data obtained with MRDCT. An operator could then use a virtual endoscopic reconstruction rather than large numbers of single images to review a clinical case. Currently VE of the paranasal sinuses is more a preoperative tool for assisting surgeons than for diagnostic purposes. Another potential of VE is in education and training. Highly developed visualization software might even allow virtual surgery based on CT data for training purposes. To take advantages of both CT (detailed delineation of bony anatomy) and MR imaging (superior soft tissue detail), multimodal image fusion algorithms and integration into real-time navigational or image-guidance systems will improve visualization.

In the case of a decreased field of view during FESS a navigational system may aid in determining a safe surgical entrance point or in allowing the localization of anatomic landmarks. Intraoperative imaging based on MR guidance is helpful but still in a very early phase of development. CT guidance for procedures in regular operating rooms is more applicable for most procedures. Although routine surgeries may

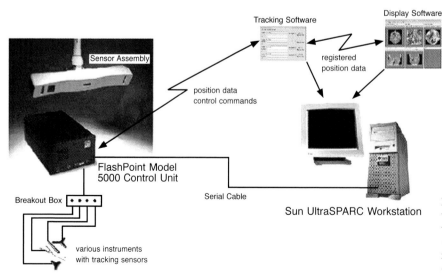

Fig. 11.11. System architecture for surgical navigation: tracking system hardware (FlashPoint 5000) and tracking application workstation (Sun UltraSparc)

not benefit from MR guidance, applications for real-time guidance will develop, particularly in cases of tumor resection, complex cases such as skull base surgery, and in access for hypophysectomy and orbital nerve compression. Real-time guidance is also helpful for biopsies, thermal ablations and revisions. In the very near future clinical applications will be available using VE, PVR and 3D-positioning tracking of a real endoscope to complement the endoscopist's view during surgery.

Acknowledgements. Software development was supported by Project P12463-MED of the Austrian Science Fund and by the Ludwig-Boltzmann Institute for Clinical and Experimental Radiology, Vienna. The authors are grateful to Monika Eisenkolb, MS, for providing the endoscopic view functions and to Fritz Vorbeck, MD, of the Department of Radiology, Vienna University Hospital, for providing MR and CT data.

References

Anon JB, Lipman SP, Oppenheim D (1994) Computer-assisted endoscopic sinus surgery. Laryngoscope 104:901–905

Bartz D, Skalej M (1999) VIVDENI – virtual ventricle endoscopy. In: Data visualization. Springer, Berlin Heidelberg New York, pp 155–166

Beus J, Kauczor HU, Schwikkert HC (1995) Coronal paranasal sinus CT: using the spiral technique. Aktuelle Radiol 5:189–191

Borgefors G (1988) Hierarchical chamfer matching: a parametric edge matching algorithm. IEEE Trans Pattern Anal Machine Intell 10:849–865

Brady LM, Jung KK, Nguyen HT (1998) Interactive volume navigation. IEEE Trans Visual Comput Graph 4:243–255

Chakeres DW (1985) Computed tomography of the ethmoid sinuses. Otolaryngol Clin North Am 18:29–42

Chow JM, Mafee MF (1989) Radiologic assessment preoperative to endoscopic sinus surgery. Otolaryngol Clin North Am 22:691–701

Darabi K, Resch KDM, Weinert J (1997) Real and simulated endoscopy of neurosurgical approaches in an anatomical model. Lectures Notes Comput Sci 1205:323–326

De Nicola M, Salvolini L, Salvolini U (1997) Virtual endoscopy of nasal cavity and paranasal sinuses. Eur J Radiol 24:175–180

Ecke U, Klimek L, Muller W (1998) Virtual reality: preparation and execution of sinus surgery. Comput Aided Surg 3:45–50

Eisenkolb M, Backfrieder W (1999) Virtual endoscopy of multi-modal data in ORL-surgery. Phys Media 15:28

Ezquerra N, Navazo I, Morris TI (1999) Graphics, vision, and visualization in medical imaging: a state of the art report. Eurographics '99, pp 21–80

Fishman EK, Drebin B, Magdid D (1987) Volumetric rendering techniques: applications for three-dimensional imaging of the hip. Radiology 163:737–738

Freysinger W, Gunkel AR, Thumfart WF (1997) Image-guided endoscopic ENT surgery. Eur Arch Otorhinolaryngol 254:343–346

Fried MP, Kleefield J, Gopal H (1997) Image-guided endoscopic surgery: results of accuracy and performance in a multicenter clinical study using an electromagnetic tracking system. Laryngoscope 107:594–601

Fried MP, Kleefield J, Taylor R (1998a) New armless image-guidance system for endoscopic sinus surgery. Otolaryngol Head Neck Surg 119:528–532

Fried MP, Topulos G, Hsu L (1998b) Endoscopic sinus surgery with magnetic resonance imaging guidance: initial patient experience. Otolaryngol Head Neck Surg 119:374–380

Geiger B, Kikinis R (1995) Simulation of endoscopy. In: Ayache N (ed) Lecture notes in computer science. Computer vision, virtual reality and robotics in medicine. Springer, Berlin Heidelberg New York, pp 276–282

Gilani S, Norbash AM, Ringl H (1997) Virtual endoscopy of the paranasal sinuses using perspective volume rendered helical sinus computed tomography. Laryngoscope 107:25–29

Greiml W, Backfrieder W (2000) A display system for surgical navigation. ORL surgery. Proc 4th Centr Eur Semin Comput Graph 1:207–216

Hong L, Muraki S, Kaufmann A (1997) Virtual voyage: interactive navigation in the human colon. SIGGRAPH 97 conference proceedings, ACM SIGGRAPH. Addison Wesley, Reading, Mass, pp 27–34

Hopper KD, Iyriboz AT, Wise SW (1999) The feasibility of surgical site tagging with CT virtual reality of the paranasal sinuses. J Comput Assist Tomogr 23:529–533

Hosemann W (1996) Endonasal surgery of the paranasal sinuses: concepts, techniques, results, complications and revision interventions. Eur Arch Otorhinolaryngol S1:155–269

Hsu L, Fried MP, Jolesz FA (1998) MR-guided endoscopic sinus surgery. AJNR Am J Neuroradiol 19:1235–1240

Keller PJ, Drayer BP, Fram EK (1989) MR angiography with two-dimensional acquisition and three-dimensional display. Radiology 173:527–532

Klimek L, Moesges R, Schloendorff G (1996) Longterm experience with different types of localization systems in skull-base surgery. In: Taylor RH, Lavallee S, Burdea C, Mosges R (eds) Computer-integrated surgery. MIT Press, Cambridge Mass, pp 6735–6738

Kochanek DH, Bartels RH (1984) Interpolating splines with local tension, continuity, and bias control. Comput Graph 18:33–41

Lengyel J, Reichert M, Donald BR (1990) Real-time robot motion planning using rasterizing. Comput Graph 24:327–335

Levoy M (1987) Display of surfaces from volume data. IEEE Comput Graph Appl 8:29–37

Lorensen WE, Cline HE (1987) Marching cubes: a high resolution 3D surface construction system. Comput Graph 21:163–169

Magnusson M, Lenz R, Danielsson PE (1991) Evaluation of methods for shaded surface display of CT volumes. Comput Med Imaging Graph 15:247–256

May M, Levine HL, Mester SJ (1994) Complications of endoscopic sinus surgery: analysis of 2108 patients-incidence and prevention. Laryngoscope 104:1080–1083

Meissner M, Kanus K, Strasser W (1998) VIZARD II, a PCI-card for real-time volume rendering. Eurographics/ Siggraph workshop on graphics hardware, pp 61–67

Messerklinger W (1978) Endoscopy of the nose. Urban and Schwartzenberg, Baltimore

Messerklinger W (1994) Background and evolution of endoscopic sinus surgery. Ear Nose Throat J 73:449–450

Nakasato T, Katoh K, Ehara S (2000) Virtual CT endoscopy in determining safe surgical entrance points for paranasal mucoceles. J Comput Assist Tomogr 24:486–492

Pfister H, Hardenbergh J, Knittel J (1999) The volume pro real-time ray-casting system. SIGGRAPH 99, computer graphics proceedings, annual conferences series, pp 251–260

Rogalla P, Nischwitz A, Gottschalk S (1998) Virtual endoscopy of the nose and paranasal sinuses. Eur Radiol 8:946–950

Rubin GD, Dake MD, Napel SA (1993) Abdominal spiral CT angiography: initial clinical experience. Radiology 186:147–152

Rudman DT, Stredney D, Sessanna D (1998) Functional endoscopic sinus surgery training simulator. Laryngoscope 108:1643–1647

Rusinek H, Mourino MR, Firooznia H (1989) Volumetric rendering of MR images. Radiology 171:269–272

Shahidi R, Argiro V, Napel S (1996) Assessment of several virtual endoscopy techniques using computed tomography and perspective volume rendering. Lect Notes Comput Sci 1131:521–526

Shahidi R, Tombropoulos R, Grzeszczuk R (1998a) Clinical applications of three-dimensional rendering of medical data-sets. Proc IEEE 86:555–568, http://neurosurgery.stanford.edu/igl/image/movies/ent-2.mpg, http://neuro-surgery.stanford.edu/igl/image/movies/nose-2.mpg

Shahidi R, Wang B, Epitaux M (1998b) Volumetric image guidance via a stereotactic endoscope. Proceedings MICCAI '98. Springer, Berlin Heidelberg New York

Som PM (1985) CT of the paranasal sinuses. Neuroradiology 27:189–201

Stammberger H, Posawetz W (1990) Functional endoscopic sinus surgery: concept, indications and results of the Messerklinger technique. Eur Arch Otorhinolaryngol 247:63–76

Suojanen JN, Regan F (1995) Spiral CT of the paranasal sinuses. AJNR Am J Neuroradiol 16:787–789

Truppe MJ, Freysinger W, Gunkel AR (1996) Remote-guided surgical navigation in ENT surgery. Stud Health Technol Inform 29:280–282

Valvassori GE, Buckingham RA, Carter BL (1998) Head and neck imaging. Thieme Medical, New York, pp 187–190

Vining DJ, Shifrin RY, Haponik EF (1994a) Virtual bronchoscopy. Radiology 193:261

Vining DJ, Winston-Salem MD, Shifrin RY (1994b) Virtual reality imaging of the airways. Radiology 193:446

Weber R, Keerl R, Hosemann W (1998) Complications with permanent damage in endonasal paranasal sinus operations – more frequent in experienced surgeons? Laryngorhinootologie 77:398–401

Wiet GJ, Yagel R, Stredney D (1997) A volumetric approach to virtual simulation of functional endoscopic sinus surgery. Stud Health Technol Inform 39:167–179

Yamashita J, Yamauchi Y, Mochimaru M (1999) Real-time 3-D model-based navigation system for endoscopic paranasal sinus surgery. IEEE Trans Biomed Eng 46:107–116

12 Virtual Laryngoscopy

Joachim Kettenbach, Mike E. Leventon, Marvin P. Fried, Vik M. Moharir, Wolfgang Birkfellner, Rudolf Hanel, William E. Lorensen, Ron Kikinis, Ferenc A. Jolesz

12.1
Introduction

Two-dimensional CT or MR imaging data converted to virtual endoscopy enables computer-generated three-dimensional (3D) visualization of a cavity. To date, this technique has been used experimentally to study the colon, bronchi, ear and other organs, and recently has been used for clinical applications.

J. Kettenbach, MD
Department of Diagnostic Radiology, University Hospital of Vienna, Waehringer Guertel 18–20, 1090 Vienna, Austria
M.E. Leventon, MS, PhD, M.P. Fried, MD, V.M. Moharir, MD
Surgical Planning Laboratory, Department of Radiology, Brigham and Women's Hospital Boston, 75 Francis Street, Boston, MA 02115, USA
W. Birkfellner, MS, PhD, R. Hanel, MS
Department of Biomedical Engineering and Physics, University of Vienna, General Hospital Vienna, Waehringer Guertel 18–20, 1090 Vienna, Austria
W.E. Lorensen
GE Corporate Research and Development, Building KW Room C215, 1 Research Circle, Niskayuna, NY 12309, USA
R. Kikinis, MD
Surgical Planning Laboratory, Department of Radiology, Brigham and Women's Hospital Boston, 75 Francis Street, Boston, MA 02115, USA
F.A. Jolesz, MD
Director of MR Division and Image Guided Therapy Program, Department of Radiology, Brigham and Women's Hospital Boston, 75 Francis Street, Boston, MA 02115, USA

As demonstrated by several authors virtual laryngoscopy (VL) was created from the cross-sectional image data of CT and MR images. Since VL is based on the individual patient's anatomy this allows navigation through the computer-generated 3D visualization, simulating a traditional endoscopic technique. Therefore, the individual laryngeal anatomy similar or equivalent to that produced with standard endoscopic procedures can be explored noninvasively. VL may therefore overcome the drawbacks of conventional laryngoscopy and may add the ability to assess the transmural extent of disease and the view of the airway distal to areas of luminal compromise. Combined with positional sensor techniques, image fusion of actual endoscopy and virtual endoscopy (VE) may provide guidance for correct placement of biopsy needles and minimally invasive surgical tools. This technology may well provide clinical benefit in preoperative planning, staging and intraprocedural guidance for head and neck disease and merits further study. VL complements the findings of actual endoscopy, or in some applications might replace these findings, thus reducing the costs of hospital admission and the risks inherent in this procedure.

Conventional endoscopy is currently the gold standard for evaluating the upper airways such as the larynx or the tracheal lumen. Rigid endoscopes, however, require general anesthesia, which may limit clinical application in high-risk patients, whereas flexible endoscopy depends on a cooperative patient and on a very experienced endoscopist. Furthermore, congenital anomalies or acquired stenoses may inhibit passage of the endoscope. In addition, viewing is limited strictly to the lumen, which limits the transmural evaluation of lesions. There is also the potential risk of perforation in procedures such as esophagoscopy.

Cross-sectional imaging using spiral CT or MR imaging and postprocessing of imaging data sets may offer an additional evaluation tool for those difficult clinical situations (and provide additional information about the larynx) that cannot be obtained with laryngoscopy. Multiplanar reconstruction (MPR), shaded surface display (SSD) or 3D reconstructions have been researched for otolaryngology head and neck surgery (Marsh and Vannier 1983; Cline et al. 1987; Wiengand et al. 1993; Altobelli et al. 1993; Eisele et al. 1994; Korves and Klimek 1995; Girod et al. 1995; Vannier and Marsh 1996; Schubert et al. 1996). Thus, the radiologist can point out pathologic findings to the clinician using several essential images without having to demonstrate all axial slices. However, MPR, SSD and color-coded reconstructions may reduce the original data, containing less diagnostic information than the CT or MR volume data set. Therefore a diagnosis should always be based on the original axial images (Table 12.1).

From advances in imaging technology and improvements in computer technology, a new 3D display and visualization tool has emerged: VE (Rosenberg et al. 1994; Valvassori 1994; Schenck et al. 1995; Lorensen et al. 1995; Fried et al. 1996; Vining et al. 1996; Jolesz et al. 1997; Frankenthaler et al. 1998). VL describes a new method of diagnosis, using computer processing of imaging data sets such as from spiral CT, multi-row detector CT (MRDCT) scans or MR imaging. This provides simulated visualization techniques of the individual laryngeal anatomy similar or equivalent to those produced with standard endoscopic procedures (Robb 2000; Satava 2000). So far, the colon, bronchi, ear and other organs (Jolesz et al. 1997; Frankenthaler et al. 1998; Aquino and Vining 1999; Assimos and Vining 2001) have been evaluated in the initial assessment of VE.

When the progression of the endoscope is limited, as in the case of a difficult airway (stenosis), VL is advantageous. This is particularly true in high-risk patients with non-passable stenoses or in postoperative examinations if no biopsies are required (Table 12.2). Furthermore, VL should be particularly helpful during assessment of the difficult airway when neoplasm, infection, inflammation or congenital defects compromise the lumen.

The benefit of VL can be even greater if a 3D reconstruction of a patient's anatomy based on the individual's CT and MR data is generated. This will allow navigation through the reconstruction, simulating a traditional endoscopic technique. A concomitant display of the global view and a view of the related CT or MR slice may provide information beyond traditional endoscopy in localizing and analyzing tissue.

12.2
Image Acquisition

Any CT or MR techniques that provide high-resolution cross-sectional images or volumetric data acquisition can be postprocessed to obtain 3D reconstructions and VL (Table 12.3).

12.2.1
Computed Tomography

In early studies, a CT dataset with a 3 mm collimation and a pitch of 1:1 or larger was commonly used to cover larger imaging volumes, such as the entire tracheobronchial tree (Ferretti et al. 1996; Greess et al. 2000). This protocol limited the delineation of structures smaller than the slice thickness. To overcome this limitation, spiral CT is now standard for imaging the larynx.

With spiral CT, although slice thickness is set before scan acquisition, the volumetric data set can be manipulated to "shift" slices by any distance up to that of the original slice thickness. This overlapping of image reconstruction ensures that the X-ray beam will pass through the center of any lesion and that the true density of the lesion will be displayed. To provide a sufficiently high spatial resolution for VL computation, a rather thin slice thickness of image acquisition is desirable. This, however, limits the total length of the imaging volume within a single breath-hold. The greatest disadvantage of spiral CT thus far is the limited number of milliamperes that can be delivered. Consequently, spiral CT often produces a grainier image than does conventional CT. However, this disadvantage is becoming negligible as manufacturers improve the detector efficiency and heat capacity of the X-ray tubes.

Using "conventional" spiral CT, reasonable longitudinal coverage of the anatomic structures can be obtained with a collimation of 3 mm, a pitch of 1.5 and an overlapping reconstruction increment (2–3 mm). This allows a good correlation between VE and the anatomic findings (Baum et al. 2000) (Table 12.4).

To improve the diagnostic value a short additional spiral parallel to the corpus of the mandible may reduce artefacts behind the dental arches in a patient with dental fillings. For optimal tissue contrast, a volume of 150 ml contrast medium, a flow rate of 2.5 ml/s and a start delay of 70–80 s are necessary. To visualize the carotid artery, a start delay of 20 s is recommended. Dynamic enhanced CT is only necessary

Table 12.1. Specific advantages of multiplanar reconstruction, shaded surface display and color-coded 3D reconstructions

Multiplanar reconstruction (MPR)	Delineates structures that may be overlooked with axial slices (often due to partial volume effects)
	Coronal MPRs ideal to show whether a tumor is crossing the midline
Shaded surface display (SSD)	Especially suited for visualizing dense tissue such as bones or bone transplants, but not for soft tissue or tumors of the hypopharynx or larynx
	Helpful if there is extensive bony destruction of the skull, spine, hyoid or laryn skeleton
Color-coded 3D reconstructions	Good depiction of the spatial relationship between extensive tumors and great vessels, bone, lymph nodes, etc.
	Advantageous in extensive tumors invading surrounding structures (very useful for developing a cooperative surgical strategy or treatment plan

Table 12.2. Specific features of conventional and virtual laryngoscopy

Conventional laryngoscopy	Virtual laryngoscopy
No assessment beyond passage of endoscope if lumen compromised	Assessment of regions inaccessible with standard endoscopic procedures especially in high-risk patients or non-passable stenoses
Invasive, requires sedation, risk of perforation	Noninvasive, does not require sedation. Can be repeated as often as needed
High-resolution visualization strictly limited to the laryngeal lumen and mucous surface	Three-dimensional (3D) information on anatomic structures and pathologic processes beyond the mucosal surface demonstrates the extent of disease, and involvement of surrounding vessels
Interactive	Provides more degrees of freedom regarding motion than conventional endoscope (e.g., backward views)
Enables intervention (biopsy, lavage)	Image guided intervention if combined with a tracking system
	VE most accurate in evaluation of subglottic and nasopharyngeal anatomy

Table 12.3. Specific advantages of imaging modalities

Computed tomography	Magnetic resonance tomography
Short examination time and fast imaging data acquisition enables breath-hold mode and functional imaging (Valsalva, "i" phonation, etc.)	3D volume acquisition of tumor pathology
Excellent delineation of air and bone. Preferable to estimate the degree to which the airway is compromised	Excellent soft tissue contrast and depiction of paraglottic and pre-epiglottic space invasion or involvement of laryngeal cartilage by cancer
Tends to underestimate neoplastic cartilage invasion and may lead to inadequate treatment	More sensitive but less specific in detection of neoplastic cartilage
Availability	No ionizing radiation

Table 12.4. Recommended parameters for virtual endoscopy using a spiral CT scanner

Collimation (mm)	Pitch	Reconstruction index (mm)	Tube current (mAs)	Effective mAs (mAs/pitch)
3	4–5	2	80	<20
2	4	1	120	30
1	3	0.8	200	67

in certain special cases such as when a glomus tumor is suspected.

Patients are advised not to swallow, followed by slight hyperventilation and continuous shallow expiration to keep the vocal cords in an expiratory position. Additional functional CT imaging during phonation of the vowel "i" and/or a Valsalva maneuver are of great importance to confirm vocal cord mobility. Therefore, imaging during "i" phonation is an essential part of every thorough examination of the hypopharynx and larynx region.

Other investigators recommend imaging data acquisition during a single breath-hold, which reduces motion artefacts caused by swallowing or respiration. In addition, the intensity of vascular enhancement is significantly heightened during breath-hold, which improves lymph node detection and reduces the amount of contrast medium required (CURTIN 1996).

Shorter acquisition times reduce motion artefacts (especially in the Z direction) even further, as in the new multislice detector CT (BERLAND and SMITH 1998; BODE et al. 2001). These volumetric data sets consist of stacked slices, the number of which can be chosen even retrospectively to match the resolution requirements of the task at hand (usually around 1 mm or less).

To cover the entire larynx within a single breath-hold the following protocol could be used on a MRDCT scanner: 4×1 mm collimation, 120 kV, 200 mAs, and a 0.5 s rotation (BRUNING et al. 1999). MRDCT allows near-isotropic imaging of the larynx and the image quality is as good as direct coronal scanning with no risk of amalgam artefacts (BAUM et al. 2000). Thin structures (the base of the skull, the orbital floor and the hard palate) as well as the floor of the mouth can be evaluated sufficiently with MPR.

The selected threshold CT values can be –600 HU to –100 HU for the mucous membranes, and +250 HU for bone. Under these conditions almost all structures remain distinct and scanning of the larynx provides an excellent contrast between air-containing spaces, such as the larynx, and soft tissue surfaces (SAKAKURA et al. 1998). CHOI et al. (2000) concluded that the airways can be reconstructed even from low-dose spiral CT (tube current 50 mA) without appreciable loss of image quality.

12.2.2
Magnetic Resonance Tomography

Generally, MR seems to be the optimal method of examination in cooperative patients, especially for

evaluation of the larynx before an attempted partial laryngectomy. MR is more sensitive than CT in the detection of neoplastic cartilage invasion, but seems to have a somewhat lower specificity, particularly if there is thyroid cartilage involvement (CASTELIJNS et al. 1998). For MR imaging, T1-weighted 3D volumetric gradient echo sequences are advantageous since they provide a good delineation of tumor tissue, vessels and other soft tissue structures.

The choice between the CT and MR imaging is determined by the clinician's experience with these modalities. Both are highly sensitive for the detection of neoplastic invasion of the pre-epiglottic and paraglottic space, subglottic region and cartilage. The high negative predictive value of both CT and MR imaging allows exclusion of neoplastic cartilage invasion quite reliably. Because of reactive inflammation, MR imaging tends to overestimate neoplastic cartilage invasion, which may possibly result in overtreatment, while CT tends to underestimate neoplastic cartilage invasion, which could lead to inadequate therapeutic decisions (ZBAREN et al. 1997a; BECKER 2000).

The specificity of both CT and MR imaging is, however, limited and both methods may therefore overestimate the extent of tumor spread (BECKER 1998). However, the overall accuracy of CT and MR imaging in detecting neoplastic invasion of cartilage is 80% versus 82% (ZBAREN et al. 1996) and the two techniques show equal staging accuracy (ZBAREN et al. 1997a, b). CT and MR imaging show tissue volume beyond the lumen and usually do not require sedation. The problem with these noninvasive techniques is that they present information in a cross-sectional, 2D format, which the physician must mentally reconstruct into a 3D picture. This can be difficult at times in areas of intricate anatomy, such as that of the head and neck (JOLESZ et al. 1997). Thus, a 3D imaging technique to visualize the larynx could combine the benefits of endoscopic and radiologic imaging.

12.3
Postprocessing

CT and MR images are usually transferred to computer workstations using internal network communication. Depending on computer hardware, images may undergo filtering for reduction of unwanted signal (GERIG et al. 1992; FRANKENTHALER et al. 1998). The next step, so-called segmentation, consists of a manual or automatic technique for isolating and outlining anatomic structures stacked into individual 3D objects.

Several approaches have been published in the recent literature on medical image segmentation. Although each technique may be used separately, multiple techniques are often used in conjunction to solve different segmentation problems (PHAM et al. 2000). In some techniques, interactive exploration of the data sets is provided in near real time; earlier techniques of postprocessing required predefined landmarks or visualization paths (Table 12.5).

Table 12.5. Software and hardware used for virtual endoscopy

Software (vendor)	Hardware (vendor)
Iris Explorer (Silicon Graphics)	Indigo2 Maximum IMPACT (Silicon Graphics)
Navigator (GE Medical Systems)	Sparc-10 workstation (Sun Microsystems)
Vitrea and Voxel View (Vital Images)	O2 (Silicon Graphics)

Most commonly surface rendering (LORENSEN et al. 1995) or volume rendering (RUBIN et al. 1996) was used to generate a VE. Segmented entities may include only the mucous surfaces, but some authors have used bone, cartilage and air-containing structures as well. Finally, a special computer program combines all the 3D objects into a complete model, which is used for VL.

Depending on the technique applied, manual postprocessing may take between 15 min (RODENWALDT et al. 1996) and several hours. Virtual camera elements and free-defined virtual light, as well as variable viewing angles, are valuable features of user interfaces for VE. The camera and global views can be enlarged or reduced, rotated 360° in any axis, and translocated in the vertical or horizontal plane. The camera lens may face any direction and provide a viewing angle from 1° to 180°.

Reconstructed 3D images contain no more information than do the corresponding series of axial single scans. However, there is consensus that the viewer can better appreciate spatial relationships in a 3D display than in a series of single scans (REMY-JARDIN et al. 1998). By eliminating redundant details, the information can be reduced to its essentials. Advanced interfaces provide a display of multiple images: a camera view; a global or external view; and a view of the related CT or MR slice.

12.4
Clinical Applications

The larynx can easily be approached by conventional endoscopy. There are, however, indications where a VL may be advantageous, with encouraging clinical results (SILVERMAN et al. 1995; ASCHOFF et al. 1998). Using fast volumetric imaging techniques and advanced postprocessing techniques, a VE of the larynx can be generated with high quality at the time of scanning or retrospectively.

In a pilot study the feasibility and clinical value of high-resolution VL based on spiral CT data sets was investigated (ASCHOFF et al. 1998). Twelve patients with laryngeal pathology (three with tumors of the vocal cords, two with laryngeal carcinomas, one with invasion of the larynx by thyroid carcinoma, and six with subglottic stenoses) underwent examination by helical CT (collimation 1 mm). Imaging data were processed using a workstation with standard visualization software and VL was then compared with the findings of conventional endoscopy. Because of swallowing artefacts, reconstruction failed in two of the 12 patients. VL provided the correct diagnosis in eight of 12 cases (laryngeal tumors, subglottic stenoses) and was capable of simulating the visual findings of endoscopy in cases of laryngeal tumors and subglottic stenoses. Small tumors of the vocal cords, however, were not adequately visualized and none of the carcinomas of the vocal cords was recognized at VL or in cross-sectional CT images. The major problem that affected the results was motion artefacts resulting from involuntary swallowing.

ASCHOFF et al. (1998) concluded that VE may play an important role in evaluating the larynx while searching for tumors. However, the lack of detailed information about the mucous surface or motion artefacts limit the value of VE and prevent the detection of tumors within the mucous surface or the vocal cords.

FRIED et al. developed a VE of the larynx using 2D CT or MR data (FRIED et al. 1998a; MOHARIR et al. 1998). Patients representing a normal airway, a posterior glottic stenosis and a squamous cell carcinoma of the glottic fold were included and 2D CT and MR images of the patients were subject to postprocessing for 3D reconstruction. The resulting models included extraluminal anatomy that is not typical of current virtual endoscopic techniques and were imported into an experimental VE program for airway lumen generation and interactive viewing.

Their VE program allowed for display of multiple images: a camera view; a global or external view;

and a view of the related CT or MR data as orthogonal display (Figs. 12.1, 12.3). The camera and global views could be enlarged or reduced, rotated 360° in any axis, and translocated in the vertical or horizontal plane. The camera lens could face any direction and provide a viewing angle from 1° to 180°. Any anatomic structure could be added or deleted, individual anatomic components could be rendered transparent, and color and light intensity could be controlled.

In a patient suffering from a recent onset of inhalation stridor following a motor vehicle accident a laryngeal videostroboscopic examination was done demonstrating an interarytenoid web which limited the lateral excursion of the vocal cord. Subglottic structures could not be visualized on the laryngeal videostroboscopic examination, and therefore it was difficult to evaluate the extent of stenosis. Using a spiral CT scan (collimation 2 mm), a VL and 3D color-coded reconstruction of the larynx were generated. Since VE allows great flexibility in viewing control (the virtual camera can have a viewing angle of 1° to 180°) the area of stenosis could be visualized in both the camera and global views. The retroverted view from the trachea provided another perspective on the laryngeal structures. Using VL it could be seen that the stenosis did not extend into the subglottic area (Fig. 12.2).

Using the 3D color-coded view, the segmented structure was made transparent and the transmural extent of disease was visualized. A posterior global view, with the web removed, demonstrated a noncompromised airway distal to the stenosis (Fig. 12.3).

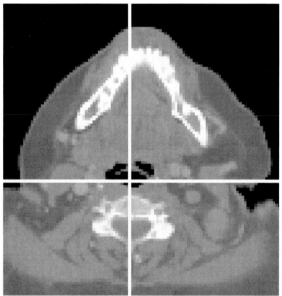

a

Fig. 12.1a, b. A 56-year-old woman with no laryngeal or airway pathology. **a** The related 2D CT slice. The cross-hairs indicate the camera location, which faces inferiorly to show the camera view on the right. The related CT slices scroll along during the virtual endoscopy to continuously update the camera location. **b** The *left* side shows the 3D color-coded posterior global view during virtual endoscopy. The left and right arytenoid cartilages are colored in *white*. The lumen has been rendered partially transparent to show the thyroid cartilage (*purple*). The epiglottis is in *red*, along with the aryepiglottic fold and the cuneiform tubercle. The vocal folds are rendered *orange*. The *green* line indicates the camera position during virtual endoscopy. The camera faces inferiorly to give the view on the *right*, showing the vocal folds, arytenoid cartilages, the edge of the cuneiform tubercle, and thyroid cartilage. The vocal folds are orange, the arytenoid cartilages in *white*, and the epiglottis, located along the superior and right perimeter, is in *red*. The lumen has been rendered partially transparent to expose the thyroid cartilage, in *purple*

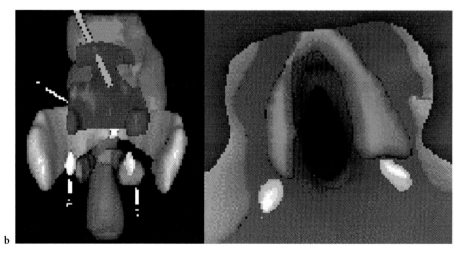

b

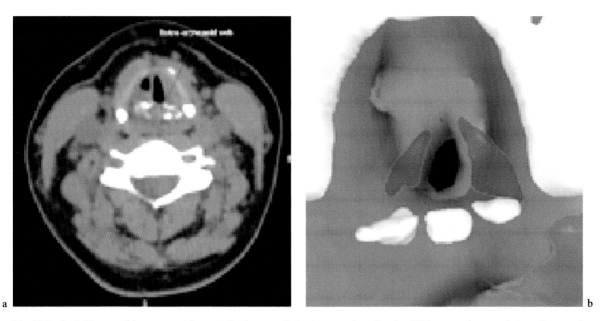

Fig. 12.2a, b. A 39-year-old woman with posterior laryngeal glottic stenosis. **a** On the CT image, a laryngeal stenosis caused by the interarytenoid web can be seen. **b** The virtual camera moves below the vocal folds. The area of stenosis (segmented in *yellow*) does not extend into the subglottic area

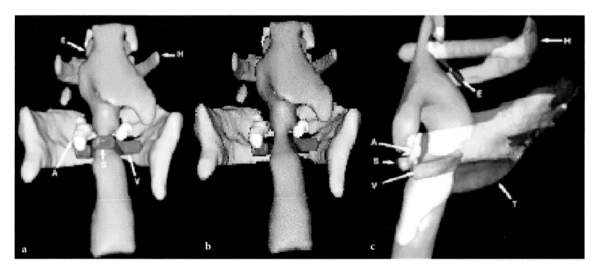

Fig. 12.3a–c. Patient with posterior laryngeal glottic stenosis. **a** A posterior global view of a 3D model reconstructed for virtual laryngoscopy. The airway lumen is in *peach* and the thyroid cartilage is rendered *green*. *A* left arytenoid cartilage, *S* stenotic intra-arytenoid web, *V* right vocal fold, *H* hyoid bone, *E* epiglottis. **b** Posterior global view with the intra-arytenoid web rendered invisible. The airway lumen narrowing between the arytenoid cartilages (*white*) and vocal folds (*red*) is evident. Below the vocal folds, the diameter of the airway lumen expands, showing no further evidence of stenosis. **c** A lateral global view of the virtual endoscopy. The airway lumen, in *orange*, runs superior to inferior. The hyoid bone (*H*) and thyroid cartilage (*T*) have been rendered transparent

GALLIVAN et al. (1999) evaluated the use of CT and VE in 21 patients with head and neck tumors distributed throughout the upper aerodigestive tract. Video-recorded images and operative records were compared with each other. Patients underwent complete head and neck examination, flexible laryngoscopy, axial CT with contrast, CTVE (computed tomography virtual endoscopy) and, in most cases, operative endoscopy. VL accurately demonstrated abnormalities caused by intraluminal tumor, but with appositions of normal tissue against tumor, inaccurate depictions of surface contour occurred. Contour resolution was limited, and mucosal irregularity could not be defined. There was very good overall correlation between virtual images, flexible laryngoscopic findings, rigid endoscopy, and operative evaluation in cases where oncologic resections were performed. VL appeared to be most accurate in the evaluation of subglottic and nasopharyngeal anatomy in this series of patients. However, the image quality was limited in situations where there was apposition of tissue folds.

GIOVANNI et al. (1998) described VE of the larynx and trachea of infants constructed from CT images, to establish the relevant pretreatment measurements (length, diameter and degree of narrowing) based on a mathematical model. A preliminary study carried out in eight infants, in parallel with their clinical treatment, showed immediate and precise measurements that could not have been achieved with conventional laryngoscopic techniques. Three-dimensional presentations and graduation of encroachment of the external stenoses was feasible.

In their survey, RODENWALDT et al. (1997) used a spiral CT data set to reconstruct the inner surface of the upper airway facilitating VL in over 80 patients, and compared the results with conventional endoscopy. VL allowed exact identification of the anatomic structures and suspected pathologic endoluminal findings, such as tracheal stenoses. When compared with conventional endoscopic examinations, the noninvasive VL technique offered additional indications in high-risk patients or in patients with non-passable stenoses. Another advantage of VE might be in the follow-up of patients who have had prolonged intubation (DROSNES and ZWILLENBERG 1990). Therefore, it might be worthwhile to follow those patients using a noninvasive method such as CT and VE to confirm the formation of laryngeal granuloma or other postintubation laryngeal lesions.

12.5
Multimodality Information Integration

In many minimally invasive procedures, the physician has a limited view of the operating field and cannot visualize structures beyond the exposed surfaces. Particularly during endoscopic procedures, the endoscopist is confronted with difficult hand-eye coordination problems since he or she is looking at a camera's view of the surgical field with a totally different reference frame. In other cases, endoscopies are complicated by the similarity in visual appearance of different tissues

(such as tumor and healthy tissue), although such tissues have high contrast in some medical images.

The best examples of this are breast cancer and brain glioma, which can be difficult to distinguish from normal tissue. Better use of 3D imaging can improve visualization and help the physician overcome the limitations of existing procedures. In particular, enhanced reality visualization, in which the physician's field of view is augmented with additional structural information, can provide useful guidance in planning and executing a minimally invasive procedure.

To date, current methods of VE are limited in their 3D display of extraluminal anatomy. For example, during virtual bronchoscopy, blood vessels and the lung parenchyma are often not seen. The lack of a global context and physical clues during viewing may lead to confusion of the patient's anatomy (SUMMERS 1997).

Three-dimensional anatomic reconstruction has been reported to complement understanding of laryngeal anatomy, especially in the subglottic area, which cannot be seen clearly by endoscopy or conventional axial CT. In particular this was advantageous in the detection of subglottic cancers, or the invasion of glottic or supraglottic cancers into the subglottic area (SAKAKURA et al. 1998).

GREESS et al. (2000) demonstrated that in all regions of the head and neck, MPRs were useful as additional planes. SSDs were valuable when there was extensive bony destruction (skull, spine, skeleton and larynx). Color-coded 3D reformations might be done for extensive tumors and before multi-specialty surgery. Although perspective volume rendering has been touted as a new and promising method for the future, it seems that MPRs or SSDs are more useful for visualizing pathologic findings in their topographic relation to anatomic structures (GREESS et al. 2000).

Different imaging modalities and image fusion techniques may further enhance visualization. Information about blood vessels may be used from angiograms, about soft tissue structures from MR imaging, about bones from CT, or about metabolic activity from SPECT (single photon emission computed tomography) or PET (positron emission tomography). Therefore, various tissue types and different physiologic functions can be highlighted.

This problem was addressed by incorporating a method of 3D anatomic reconstruction into a virtual endoscopic technique that can use merged CT and MR images (FRIED et al. 1997). Using this technique, the transparent airway lumen and the global view allowed for appreciation of the transmural extent of the tumor and patency of blood vessels (Figs. 12.4–12.6).

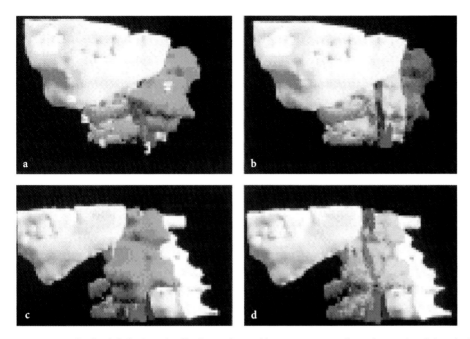

Fig. 12.4. Multiple global views (**a–d**) of a patient with a squamous cell carcinoma involving the left area of the vocal fold reconstructed from CT (5 mm thick consecutive axial images) and MR imaging (acquired with 1.5 cm thick axial spoiled gradient recalled images). The patent carotid artery (in *red*) and the compressed jugular vein (*blue*) can be seen.

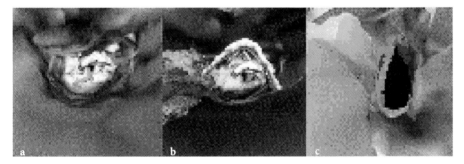

Fig. 12.5a–c. The virtual laryngoscopy begins in the oropharynx. The camera looks down toward the epiglottis, beyond which the tumor protrudes into the larynx. The (**a**) image displays the airway with the walls opaque. The epiglottis is in *off-white* and the tumor in *green*. The (**b**) figure shows the walls transparent. The transmural extent of the tumor and its relationship to surrounding structures is seen. The (**c**) image displays the virtual camera view further down the airway with the walls made partially transparent. The vocal cords (*red*) and tumor are visualized

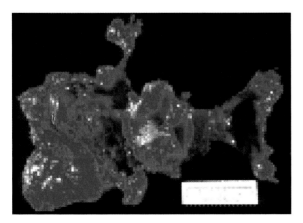

Fig. 12.6. Gross pathology, posterior view. The larynx and the contents of the dissected right and left sides of the neck are shown. The resected gross pathology specimen confirmed the virtual laryngoscopy findings of extension beyond the limits of the larynx and occlusion of the jugular vein

To overcome the limitation of anatomic details, anatomic rendition of even the smallest of structures, such as the vocal folds and arytenoid cartilages, proved to be valuable (MOHARIR et al. 1998) (Fig. 12.3). Combined use of MR and CT data to generate a VE combined with a 3D anatomic reconstruction allows for visualization of soft tissue, cartilage and bone. This should be particularly helpful when evaluating tumors and their surrounding viscera, such as the jugular veins, carotid arteries, and others. A simultaneous display of the global view and related CT or MR slice further improves the understanding of the location of the virtual camera in relation to its extraluminal spatial context.

12.6
Instrument Tracking

Correct localization and orientation relative to the surrounding anatomy is an important feature of VE. Complementing actual endoscopy with virtual images, however, requires knowledge of the endoscope's location within the patient. Various tracking devices or sensors (mechanical, optical or electromagnetic) can be attached to rigid endoscopes or smaller sensors can be introduced into the working channels of flexible endoscopes (BIRKFELLNER et al. 1998a). By tracking the 3D position of the instruments, their position can be shown/overlaid on scans of the patient, such as MR or CT scans (FRIED et al. 1997).

Several technologies are available to achieve this goal. The most widely used technology currently is optical tracking (KHADEM et al. 2000). Optical tracking systems determine the position of several optical beacons in space, providing excellent technical accuracy of typically less than 1 mm (also referred to as fiducial localization error, FLE). These systems carry a severe drawback for applications in surgical navigation in ENT (ear nose and throat) surgery: the system cannot operate when the line-of-sight between beacon and camera is obstructed (FITZPATRICK et al. 1998). Therefore, the beacons must be mounted outside the patient, which makes the use of an optical tracker together with a flexible endoscope impossible.

Electromagnetic tracking is another approach designed to track the position of a flexible endoscope. In these systems, the position of a small sensor to measure magnetic flux or magnetic induction is determined relative to a reference field emitter. The electromagnetic field passes without significant distortion through body tissue; thus, it is possible to attach a small sensor to the tip of a flexible instrument such as a catheter (SOLOMON et al. 1999). Tracking of electromagnetic trackers can be severely distorted when conductive or ferromagnetic materials (such as instruments made of surgical steel) are within the vicinity of the field emitter or the sensor (BIRKFELLNER et al. 1998b). Therefore, electromagnetic digitizers are not as widespread as optical trackers in the field of surgical navigation, in general.

In an experimental case study, JOLESZ et al. (1997) used an electromagnetic tracking system [Magelan, Biosense, NY; now called Biosense CARTO Nonfluoroscopic Mapping and Navigation System (CARTO System)] to combine VL with conventional laryngoscopy. This setting was used during an image-guided intubation of a 55-year-old male patient with a large endolaryngeal bulging of a retropharyngeal tumor. Since the tumor compromised the larynx, the augmented endoscopy-guided intubation was performed just before the patient underwent surgery (Fig. 12.7).

A VL was created from prior (2 days earlier) cross-sectional MR imaging data of the patient, designed to simulate an intubation. A miniature electromagnetic sensor (1.2 mm diameter) of the tracking system was then integrated within a catheter-like sensor probe. The patient's position was then registered on the MR scan by choosing five landmarks on the patient's MR scan and pointing the probe to the corresponding landmarks on the patient. The flexible endoscope and the probe were both introduced into the endotracheal tube. Thus, the endoscope's position was registered in real time on the imaging data set and visualized on a split screen display, presenting five views simultaneously. These views were updated at about 1–2 frames per second, demonstrating the progress of the endotracheal intubation, which was completed successfully with no complications.

This experiment demonstrated that an augmented endoscopy of the larynx is feasible and safe, with the added benefits of the ability to assess the transmural extent of disease and view the airway distal to areas of luminal compromise.

The most promising technologies for flexible instrument tracking are either combined magneto-optical tracking systems, which allow for reducing errors from the environment in electromagnetic trackers (BIRKFELLNER et al. 1998a), or flexible optical fibers that measure torsion and bend. Such systems are, however, not yet available on the market.

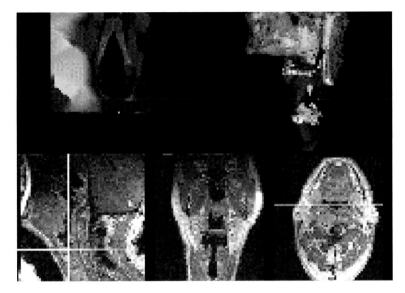

Fig. 12.7. *Upper left:* the rendered image represented the virtual view corresponding to the endoscope's position and orientation. *Upper right:* the exterior global virtual view with a yellow marker demonstrates the actual position of the endoscope's tip. *Bottom left to right:* three orthogonal slices of the MR scan are shown with cross-hairs highlighting the position of the endoscope and the positional sensor within the tube during intubation

12.7
Other Applications

OSSOFF and REINISCH (1994) envisioned the surgeon positioned at a computer workstation to perform laryngologic, otologic and rhinologic surgery. The only contact he or she will have with the patient is through robotic "hands" on the end of thin rods. These hands thread through the laryngoscope and hold tissue with no tremor. Force- or tension-feedback systems may further enhance robotic applications in ENT surgery. A virtual endoscopic view could be registered on the real endoscopic view.

Endoscopic procedures within the larynx have also been performed within open interventional MR imaging systems. In this setting, the position of the endoscope was registered with an optical tracking system to define the location of three orthogonal MR imaging planes. The MR images are displayed simultaneously on two adjacent monitors or in a multi-window format display. This combination of endoscopy and cross-sectional imaging can also be achieved with virtual endoscopic presentation, which is based on previously acquired images. These images can be updated with real time MR imaging obtained intraoperatively (FRIED et al. 1996, 1998b; HSU et al. 1998).

12.8
Conclusion

The developments of spiral CT and multidetector array technology have opened new possibilities, sub-stantially improved speed and isotropic spatial resolution. With current imaging techniques, exophytic lesions, tumors and stenoses of the larynx even a few millimeters in size can be detected easily. MRDCT in the near future will increase the temporal and spatial resolution of VL. Swallowing artefacts may then be less likely even in uncooperative or severely ill patients who may not be candidates for conventional endoscopy.

In general, there is a very good overall correlation between virtual images, flexible laryngoscopic findings, rigid endoscopy, and operative evaluation in cases where oncologic resections were performed.

For precise assessment of location, length and severity of an airway stenosis additional MPRs, simultaneously displayed with an interactive VE, allow real-time interpretation. Dedicated software could then allow interactive treatment planning. However, current imaging modalities do not allow the identification of mucous membrane alterations, such as distinct thickening (as long as the thickness itself can be segmented by specially designed algorithms). The lack of detailed information about the mucous surface, the small size, movement during expiration, and artefacts caused by swallowing may prevent the detection of small tumors. Therefore, the value of VL, at least for T1-stage tumors within the mucous surface or the vocal cord, is limited and it remains to be seen whether surface-flattening algorithms (HAKER et al. 2000) can overcome this challenge.

Clinical acceptance of VL will increase when information can be generated from diagnostic scan data without the necessity to repeat the scan with a modified protocol. However, reconstruction of VL is still time-consuming, and it may take several hours for completion of a single VE endoscopy, not including the steep learning curve that still exists.

As a supportive diagnostic procedure, VL offers a valuable overview of extension and localization of laryngeal or tracheal stenoses with regard to possible therapeutic management. Functional imaging with the vocal cords in "i" phonation can be applied to allow detection of small lesions, and VL techniques may be adapted to pass the almost closed, vibrating cords during a breath-hold maneuver.

Though VL cannot be used for biopsy, it carries the potential for improving preoperative planning, staging and intraprocedural guidance for head and neck pathology. Combined with positional sensor techniques, actual endoscopy and VL may well provide clinical benefit to guide the correct placement of biopsy needles or laparoscopes and mote cutting tools, which is problematic if these tools are outside the visual field. This could allow the margins of lesions to be biopsied, improving delineation of the extent of pathology.

VL seems to be advantageous in subglottic stenoses as an additional visualization tool, but is less useful for primary diagnosis. Compared with the conventional endoscopic examination, the noninvasive VL technique offers additional applications, especially in high-risk patients or in patients with non-passable stenoses. Particularly in the subglottic area, which cannot be seen clearly by endoscopy or conventional axial CT, the VE and 3D reconstructions provide a good representation of the laryngeal and neck anatomy that is quite helpful in understanding laryngeal anatomy.

Some challenges still must be overcome: the handling of huge data sets; the selection of a variety of user-selectable parameters; and the fact that 3D anatomic rendering is only as good as the 2D CT and MR images from which it is reconstructed. Luminal views are inferior in detail to their endoscopic counterparts.

VL may well provide clinical benefit in preoperative planning, staging and intraprocedural guidance for head and neck disease and merits further study. VL complements the findings of actual endoscopy, or in some applications might replace these findings, thus reducing the costs of hospital admission and the risks inherent in this procedure.

However, prior to expanded implementation, time and cost issues must be addressed. The cost of incorporating 3D reconstruction into VE is currently prohibitive and needs to be reduced in the future.

Acknowledgements. For their support during the software development at the Surgical Planning Laboratory, Brigham and Women's Hospital, we are grateful to Hiroshi Shinmoto, Abdalmajeid M. Alyassin, Liangge Hsu, H. Atsumi, S. Nakajima, M. Prokop, H. Shinmoto, P. van Kipshagen. For proofreading the manuscript, we are grateful to Mary McAllister, Department of Radiology and Radiological Science at the Johns Hopkins University Hospital, Baltimore, Md. This work was supported by the Ludwig Boltzmann Institute for Clinical and Experimental Radiology (Director: Prof. Christian Herold), Vienna, Austria.

References

Altobelli DE, Kikinis R, Mulliken JB (1993) Computer assisted three-dimensional planning in craniofacial surgery. Plast Reconstr Surg 92:576–585

Aquino SL, Vining DJ (1999) Virtual bronchoscopy. Clin Chest Med 20:725–730

Aschoff AJ, Seifarth H, Fleiter T (1998) High-resolution virtual laryngoscopy based on spiral CT data. Radiologe 38:810–815

Assimos DG, Vining DJ (2001) Virtual endoscopy. J Endourol 15:47–51

Baum U, Greess H, Lell M (2000) Imaging of head and neck tumors–methods: CT, spiral-CT, multislice-spiral-CT. Eur J Radiol 33:153–160

Becker M (1998) Diagnosis and staging of laryngeal tumors with CT and MRI. Radiologe 38:93–100

Becker M (2000) Neoplastic invasion of laryngeal cartilage: radiologic diagnosis and therapeutic implications. Eur J Radiol 33:216–229

Berland LL, Smith JK (1998) Multidetector-array CT: once again, technology creates new opportunities. Radiology 209:327–329

Birkfellner W, Watzinger F, Wanschitz F (1998a) Calibration of tracking systems in a surgical environment. IEEE Trans Med Imaging 17:737–742

Birkfellner W, Watzinger F, Wanschitz F (1998b) Systematic distortions in magnetic position digitizers. Med Phys 25:2242–2248

Bode A, Dammann F, Pelikan EH (2001) Analysis of artefacts by virtual endoscopy visualization of spiral CT data. Rofo Fortschr Geb Rontgenstr Neuen Bildgeb Verfahr 173:245–252

Bruning R, Sturm C, Hong C (1999) The diagnosis of stages T1 and T2 in laryngeal carcinoma with multislice spiral CT. Radiologe 39:939–942

Castelijns JA, Hermans R, van den Brekel MW (1998) Imaging of laryngeal cancer. Semin Ultrasound CT MR 19:492–504

Choi Y, McAdmans HP, Jeon SC (2000) Low-dose spiral CT: application to three-dimensional imaging of central airways. Radiology 217:385

Cline HE, Dumoulin CL, Hart HR Jr (1987) 3D reconstruction

of the brain from magnetic resonance images using a connectivity algorithm. Magn Reson Imaging 5:345–352

Curtin HD (1996) Larynx. In: Som PM, Curtin HD (eds) Head and neck imaging, 3rd edn. Mosby Year Book, St Louis, pp 612–710

Drosnes DL, Zwillenberg DA (1990) Laryngeal granulomatous polyp after short-term intubation of a child. Ann Otol Rhinol Laryngol 99:183–186

Eisele DW, Richtsmeier WJ, Graybeal JC (1994) Three-dimensional models for head and neck tumor treatment planning. Laryngoscope 104:433–439

Ferretti GR, Vining DJ, Knoplioch J (1996)Tracheobronchial tree: three-dimensional spiral CT with bronchoscopic perspective. J Comput Assist Tomogr 20:777–781

Fitzpatrick JM, West JB, Maurer CR Jr (1998) Predicting error in rigid-body point-based registration. IEEE Trans Med Imaging 17:694–702

Frankenthaler RP, Moharir V, Kikinis R (1998) Virtual otoscopy. Otolaryngol Clin North Am 31:383–392

Fried MP, Hsu L, Topulos G (1996) Image-guided surgery in a new magnetic resonance suite: preclinical considerations. Laryngoscope 106:411–417

Fried MP, Kleefield J, Gopal H (1997) Image-guided endoscopic surgery: results of accuracy and performance in a multicenter clinical study using an electromagnetic tracking system. Laryngoscope 107:594–601

Fried MP, Moharir VM, Shinmoto H (1998a) Virtual laryngoscopy. Ann Otol Rhinol Laryngol 108:221–226

Fried MP, Topulos G, Hsu L (1998b) Endoscopic sinus surgery with magnetic resonance imaging guidance: initial patient experience. Otolaryngol Head Neck Surg 119:374–380

Gallivan RP, Nguyen TH, Armstrong WB (1999) Head and neck computed tomography virtual endoscopy: evaluation of a new imaging technique. Laryngoscope 109:1570–1579

Gerig G, Kubler O, Kikinis R (1992) Nonlinear anisotropic filtering of MRI data. IEEE Trans Med Imaging 11:221–232

Giovanni A, Nazarian B, Sudre-Levillain I (1998) Geometric modeling and virtual endoscopy of the laryngo-tracheal lumen from computerized tomography images: initial applications to laryngo-tracheal pathology in the child. Rev Laryngol Otol Rhinol 119:341–346

Girod S, Keeve E, Girod B (1995) Advanced in interactive craniofacial surgery planning by 3D simulation and visualization. Int J Oral Maxillofac Surg 24:120–125

Greess H, Nomayr A, Tomandl B (2000) 2D and 3D visualisation of head and neck tumours from spiral-CT data. Eur J Radiol 33:170–177

Haker S, Angenent S, Tannenbaum A (2000) Nondistorting flattening maps and the 3-D visualization of colon CT images. IEEE Trans Med Imaging 19:665–670

Hsu L, Fried MP, Jolesz FA (1998) MR-guided endoscopic sinus surgery. AJNR Am J Neuroradiol 19:1235–1240

Jolesz FA, Lorensen WE, Shinmoto H (1997) Interactive virtual endoscopy. AJR 169:1229–1235

Khadem R, Yeh CC, Sadeghi-Tehrani M (2000) Comparative tracking error analysis of five different optical tracking systems. Comput Aided Surg 5:98–107

Korves S, Klimek L (1995) Image- and model-based surgical planning in otolaryngology. J Otolaryngol 24:265–270

Lorensen WE, Jolesz FA, Kikinis R (1995) The exploration of cross-sectional data with a virtual endoscope. In: Satava RM, Morgan K, Sieberg et al (eds) Interactive technology

and the new paradigm for health-care: medicine meets virtual reality III proceedings. IOS Press, Amsterdam, pp 221–230

Marsh JL, Vannier MW (1983) The "Third" dimension in craniofacial surgery. Plast Reconstr Surg 71:759–767

Moharir VM, Fried MP, Vernick DM (1998) Computer-assisted three-dimensional reconstruction of head and neck tumors. Laryngoscope 108:1592–1598

Ossoff RH, Reinisch L (1994) Computer-assisted surgical techniques: a vision for the future of otolaryngology-head and neck surgery. J Otolaryngol 23:354–359

Pham DL, Xu C, Prince JL (2000) Current methods in medical image segmentation. Annu Rev Biomed Eng 2:315–337

Remy-Jardin M, Remy J, Artaud D (1998) Volume rendering of the tracheobronchial tree: clinical evaluation of bronchographic images. Radiology 208:761–770

Robb RA (2000) Virtual endoscopy: development and evaluation using the visible human datasets. Comput Med Imaging Graph 24:133–151

Rodenwaldt J, Kopka L, Roedel R (1996) Three-dimensional surface imaging of the larynx and trachea by spiral CT: virtual endoscopy. Rofo Fortschr Geb Rontgenstr Neuen Bildgeb Verfahr 165:80–83

Rodenwaldt J, Kopka L, Roedel R (1997) 3D virtual endoscopy of the upper airway: optimization of the scan parameters in a cadaver phantom and clinical assessment. J Comput Assist Tomogr 21:405–411

Rosenberg SI, Silverstein H, Willcox TO (1994) Endoscopy in otology and neurootology. Am J Otol 15:168–172

Rubin GD, Beaulieu CF, Argiro V (1996) Perspective volume rendering of CT and MR images: applications for endoscopic imaging. Radiology 199:321–330

Sakakura A, Yamamoto Y, Uesugi Y (1998) Three-dimensional imaging of laryngeal cancers using high-speed helical CT scanning. J Otorhinolaryngol Rel Spec 60:103–107

Satava RM (2000) New imaging strategies for laparoscopic management of cancer. Semin Laparosc Surg 7:87–92

Schenck JF, Jolesz FA, Roemer PB (1995) Superconduction open-configuration MR imaging system for image-guided therapy. Radiology 195:805–814

Schubert O, Sartor K, Forsting M (1996) Three-dimensional computed display of otosurgical operation sites by spiral CT. Neuroradiology 38:663–668

Silverman PM, Zeiberg AS, Sessions RB (1995) Helical CT of the upper airway: normal and abnormal findings on three-dimensional reconstructed images. AJR 165:541–546

Solomon SB, Magee C, Acker DE (1999) TIPS placement in swine, guided by electromagnetic real-time needle tip localization displayed on previously acquired 3-D CT. Cardiovasc Intervent Radiol 22:411–414

Summers RM (1997) Navigational aids for real-time virtual bronchoscopy. AJR 168:1165–1170

Valvassori GE (1994) Update of computed tomography and magnetic resonance in otology. Am J Otol 15:203–206

Vannier MW, Marsh JL (1996) Three-dimensional imaging, surgical planning, and image-guided therapy. Radiol Clin North Am 34:545–563

Vining DJ, Liu K, Choplin RH (1996) Virtual bronchoscopy: relationships of virtual reality endobronchial simulations to actual bronchoscopic findings. Chest 109:549–553

Wiegand DA, Page RB, Channin DS (1993) The surgical work-station: surgical planning using generic software. Otolaryngol Head Neck Surg 109:434–440

Zbaren P, Becker M, Lang H (1996) Pretherapeutic staging of laryngeal carcinoma: clinical findings, computed tomography, and magnetic resonance imaging compared with histopathology. Cancer 77:1263–1273

Zbaren P, Becker M, Lang H (1997a) Staging of laryngeal cancer: endoscopy, computed tomography and magnetic resonance versus histopathology. Eur Arch Otorhinolaryngol Suppl 1:S117–S122

Zbaren P, Becker M, Lang H (1997b) Pretherapeutic staging of hypopharyngeal carcinoma: clinical findings, computed tomography, and magnetic resonance imaging compared with histopathologic evaluation. Arch Otolaryngol Head Neck Surg 123:908–913

13 Tracheobronchial Tree

Luca Salvolini and Elisabetta Bichi Secchi

13.1
Introduction

CT is universally established as the imaging modality of choice in depicting airways diseases, and is clearly complementary to fibreoptic bronchoscopy in patient evaluation (NAIDICH and HARKIN 1995). Before the introduction of volumetric scanning, the display of the tracheobronchial tree relied on axial CT sections alone, as pioneering two- and three-dimensional (2D and 3D) reconstruction attempts were disappointing due to data misregistration and dose and time required for redundant scanning, while poor proton content and very low spatial resolution limited the application of intrinsically 3D MR imaging in the evaluation of the central airways and lungs. Although transverse slices have already been established as powerful diagnostic tools, by spiral scanning it is now possible to develop the diagnostic power of CT even further, and to obtain additional rendered images of the trachea and bronchi of otherwise unachievable quality, thanks to lack of scaling and respiratory misregistration, reduction of motion artefacts, and retrospective reconstruction of overlapping slices (STORTO et al. 1995; NAIDICH et al. 1997; MAROM et

L. SALVOLINI, MD, E. BICHI SECCHI, MD
Department of Radiology, University Hospital "Umberto I", Via Conca, 60020 Torrette di Ancona, Ancona, Italy

al. 2001a, b). Since spatial resolution is maximal in the transverse plane, in most cases additional reformations are not required for diagnosis, although in selected cases they may increase diagnostic confidence by improved perception of image data, and aid patient management by simplifying communication with referring physicians (REMY et al. 1997). Due to their redundant nature and time limitations in everyday practice, it is essential to define precisely the selected clinical settings in which 2D and 3D rendering could be useful for solving specific problems in the diagnostic evaluation of the tracheobronchial tree.

13.2
Technical Considerations

13.2.1
Image Acquisition

Close attention to the correct technical parameters for data acquisition (HOPPER et al. 1998a, b) and retrospective reconstruction of an adequate series of transverse images are mandatory to achieve the best results from 2D and 3D reconstructions. It is in fact impossible to "ameliorate" original data by means of additional rendering, as every step introduces biases and segmentation, thus decreasing the amount of information compared with the raw data. Thin (2–3 mm) collimation and tailored reconstruction field of view are the main factors influencing spatial resolution in the XY plane, and are both essential for accurate evaluation of the trachea and bronchi. Breathholding is crucial to avoid motion artefacts. Pitch should then be adjusted to the required collimation and longitudinal extension and patient capabilities, and can be brought up to 2:1 without loss of relevant diagnostic information (SARTONI GALLONI et al. 1999). The body volume of interest must be covered in a single volumetric scan; in the thorax, the mA and kV settings can be significantly reduced, while maintaining thin collimation, in order to allow splitting of the spiral acquisition into two shorter subvolumes to avoid tube overheating. In order to optimize rendered image quality, no more than three and no fewer than two transverse images per rotation should be reconstructed for rendering (BRINK 1995). A standard kernel should be used in the reconstruction of such sections for rendering, in order to minimize possible bias. Finally, given the redundancy of possible postprocessing options and their continuous evolution, the most appropriate technique for each case must be selected from among the range of possibilities that we are now going to summarize and briefly discuss.

13.2.2
Rendering Techniques

Two-dimensional multiplanar reconstruction (MPR) is in most cases sufficient to reinforce diagnostic confidence when needed, in conjunction with axial images, and/or to solve questions unanswered by reviewing transverse sections of central airways pathology (QUINT et al. 1995; PERHOMAA et al. 1997; LEE et al. 1997). These can be performed by real-time interaction, effectively supporting axial images in displaying tracheobronchial anatomy without extensive editing and time requirements. Double obliquity of the reconstructed section is very useful in bronchial segments developing in non-orthogonal planes, but not all software allows for this possibility. Curved planar reconstruction (CPR) should be avoided, although useful in displaying tortuous bronchi, because of inherent anatomical distortion and possible measurement errors. Multiplanar volume reconstruction (MPVR), formerly known as "sliding thin slabs" (REMY-JARDIN et al. 1996a; BHALLA et al. 1996), is very useful in depicting bronchial diseases and reinforcing the evidence of nodular patterns by better anatomical display of vessels, by maintaining the interactivity and detail of MPR while displaying the whole structure of interest in one single, thicker section. Care must be taken when highlighting maximum or minimum intensity voxels within the reconstructed MPVR image not to overestimate bronchial wall thickness or to overlook thickened segments, respectively.

Three-dimensional projection techniques (minimum intensity projection, MinIP) applied to the entire volume may lead to loss of spatial information and imprecise assessment of the severity of bronchial stenoses, due to partial volume effects and extensive

data editing (REMY-JARDIN et al. 1996b). Shaded surface display (SSD) applications are limited to panoramic display of complex anatomical and/or pathological situations affecting the central airways (LACROSSE et al. 1995), as massive preliminary editing for removing surrounding chest structures and the thresholding process required for 3D surface segmentation may introduce biases, hamper real-time interactivity, and lead to loss of information such as density values (ADACHI et al. 1993; KAUZCOR et al. 1996; LO CICERO et al. 1996). Volume rendering applications to airways studies, thanks to the increased computational speed of 3D workstations, appear promising. Because both spatial and density information are maintained, multiple structures and tissues can be displayed, and a gradual rather than abrupt transition of interface voxels permits the representation of the tracheobronchial linings as close to reality as possible (REMY-JARDIN et al. 1998a).

Finally, either by SSD or volume rendering, simply by changing our point of view (Fig. 13.1) we can appreciate the inner surface of central airways, thus performing so-called virtual bronchoscopy (VB) (VINING et al. 1996; RUBIN et al. 1996b; FERRETTI et al. 1996; ROGALLA 2001). As CT and endoscopy are clearly complementary tools in the diagnostic evaluation of pathological processes affecting the airways, the tracheobronchial tree has been one of the first and more extensively studied possible applications of virtual endoscopy. VB allows perspective rendering of the trachea and bronchi in real time, with no need to remove overlapping anatomy.

As with "classical" 3D techniques, however, there is not a single threshold value that allows correct display of the whole airway from the trachea down to more peripheral bronchi (NEUMANN et al. 1999). Moreover, the diagnostic power of VB in the periphery of bronchial system, if a single slice spiral-scanner is used, is limited by the spatial resolution that can be employed when a consistent longitudinal extension of the CT study is needed to display structures, such as the tracheobronchial tree, that develop in space in the craniocaudal direction. Whichever technique is used, it should be emphasized that axial CT usually already provides all relevant information for correct diagnostic routine evaluation of the airways (NAIDICH 1996). That is why additional rendering must be used only in selected cases, starting from the simpler techniques, in defined clinical settings, for solving specific questions, with a particular benefit in mind (GRENIER and BEIGELMAN 1996; SCHAEFER-PROKOP and PROKOP 1996; RUBIN et al. 1996a; PADHANI 1998).

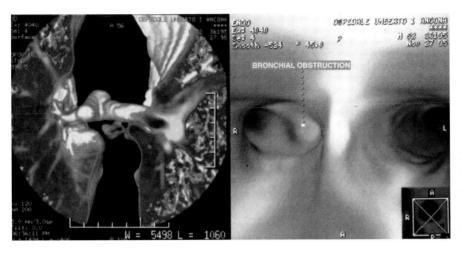

Fig. 13.1. Neoplastic occlusion of an intermediary bronchus, as seen from below, by external 3D SSD (*left*), and from inside the lumen of the trachea, by VB (*right*)

13.3
Clinical Applications

13.3.1
General Principles and Guidelines

If the tracheobronchial tree is to be studied by state-of-the-art technique, that is with single-slice spiral scanning using thin collimation, then we have to deal with a large number of reconstructed transverse sections, from which it may sometimes be difficult to extrapolate a mental representation of the airways. Their complex anatomy makes it difficult at times to figure out precise relationships of pathological processes and surrounding anatomy in three dimensions. In such selected cases, in which additional features besides maximal spatial resolution (that is found in the *XY* plane) could be of help in diagnostic evaluation, additional rendering may find effective application (SALVOLINI et al. 2000). The clinical value of 2D and 3D reconstructions lies in their ability to improve perception of image features that could be more effectively displayed than in axial slices, due to the large number of images to evaluate, poor representation of oblique structures lying in non-orthogonal planes, difficult appraisal of interfaces parallel to the transverse plane, and the poor synthetic representation of extended and complex pathological processes and anatomical structures developing in space in different directions. Constant reference to transverse CT sections is always necessary, so as not to lose orientation and for recognizing otherwise misleading artefacts.

Due to continuous technical evolution, it is essential to return the discussion about 3D rendering to the clinical environment. From several studies performed worldwide, it is possible to define a series of a few effective applications of selected techniques, in specific situations that are encountered in everyday practice, in which they could really help in the understanding of complex situations, or allow better integrated multidisciplinary patient management. In whichever clinical situation we are willing to use additional rendering, we should attain one of the following goals: easier identification of information relevant to diagnosis; better diagnostic confidence leading to more effective decision-making; a change in patient management by choice of one procedure, examination or treatment rather than another; or better patient outcome, thanks to more accurate planning and closer guidance, or simplified follow-up, of subsequent procedures (FERRETTI and COULOMB 2000).

13.3.2
Central Airways

When dealing with tracheobronchial stenoses it is not always easy to appreciate slight variations in the transverse section of the airways in a redundant series of axial slices. Reduction of the vertical diameter of bronchi and the precise craniocaudal extent of stenosed segments may be difficult to assess by review of transverse sections alone. A limited longitudinal extent could hamper detection of focal stenoses such as post-intubation webs or anastomotic strictures. In such cases, MPR/MPVR are usually sufficient as an adjunct to complete diagnostic evaluation (REMY-JARDIN et al. 1996b). They have been demonstrated to maintain the same diagnostic accuracy as original CT sections but, as additional benefit is not statistically relevant, their use might be restricted to selected cases of actual need. Additional gain in diagnostic confidence is difficult to demonstrate, even though not negligible. Three-dimensional SSD models are more impressive but not more accurate, and they find application only as a road-mapping for reconstructing lesion-oriented, double-obliquity MPR sections directly on the 3D airways cast. Also, for the evaluation of very asymmetric central stenoses, congenital strictures and malformations, and post-surgical remodelling, even though the understanding of the overall complex tracheobronchial morphology could be made easier by looking at 3D reconstructions than by performing multiple MPR sections at different angles, time and information loss, lack of interactivity, thresholding artefacts, and cumbersome segmentation as we proceed to the peripheral bronchi limit the extensive application of "conventional" 3D techniques in this field. External volume rendering perspectives are very interesting, thanks to increased computational speed and to the combination of 3D anatomical display, as in SSD, and retained density information, as for MPR, which make it possible to display tracheobronchial walls and surrounding structures simultaneously. The MinIP technique has no role, due to the possibility of overlooking small lesions as a result of the dominant negative density of air column, loss of data regarding the walls of the airways, and incorrect grading of severe stenoses, as in SSD. Virtual endoscopy can be performed in a time comparable to 2D reconstructions, with no need to edit surrounding structures. Slight parietal alterations are detected with increased confidence by a bronchoscopic perspective (McAdams et al. 1998b), but without real advantages over simpler planar images (Ferretti et al. 1997; Rapp-Bernhardt et al. 2000). In particular with SSD-based VB, motion and beam-hardening artefacts, scanning and reconstruction and display settings, and mucus plugs can dramatically modify virtual images. Because of incorrect segmentation and partial volume effects, differential diagnosis between occlusions and tight stenoses requires constant referral to 2D transverse and MPR images. This dependence upon thresholding is claimed to be reduced by volume rendered VB, but computational effort and thus the time required is increased. It is not recommended to perform measures directly on VB perspective images, due to perceptual distortion: it is better to use planar sections for this purpose.

When evaluating the locoregional extent of central lung cancer, MPR/MPVR is the method of choice, because preserving tissue information, and thus voxel density values, is essential when looking for neoplastic encasement of surrounding structures. By multiplanar display it is possible to better depict the relationships between pathological tissue and bronchovascular interfaces, revealing even slight signs of infiltration (Fig. 13.2), and to achieve more accurate staging thanks to more precise evaluation of subcarinal and aortopulmonary window lymph node stations (Padhani et al. 1995; Touliopoulos and Costello 1995). There is currently no real indication for the application of more complex rendering in this field: the actual role of volume rendering, although useful in displaying hilar vascular encasement and mediastinal involvement, is yet to be defined.

The integration of CT and bronchoscopy is essential for correct patient management. Endoscopy and CT are complementary examinations in the diagnostic routine investigation of tracheobronchial lesions, and it is still a matter of debate as to which technique should be performed first, depending on the clinical presentation (Henschke et al. 1987). The role of conventional CT as a road map for bronchoscopy and diagnostic accuracy is well established. Helical CT has gone one step further owing to increased scanning speed and abolition of respiratory misregistration. In specific applications, the use of additional rendering may increase the synergy of CT with fibreoptic endoscopy, promoting information exchange by sharing the same perspective and overcoming the perceptual limitations of axial scanning.

It is obvious that VB aroused great initial interest: nevertheless, it is essential to define its few genuine clinical applications – which are in fact not all of those initially claimed (Vining 1996). Much emphasis has been put on the possibility of "bypassing" impassable stenoses by VB (Adachi et al. 1993; Kauzcor et al. 1996; Fleiter et al. 1997): this is true, but even the review of basic transverse sections, supplemented by planar reconstructions if needed, already allows for the demonstration of airway patency distal to segmental stenoses and occlusions that is mandatory for unblocking endobronchial obstructions by laser therapy. If stenting is needed, measurements can be performed faster and better on planar images: external and internal perspective rendering are only of use to orientate exactly the orthogonal longitudinal reformats and cross-sections on such 3D models of the affected airway. Retained secretions are difficult to differentiate from pathology on VB images alone. Mucosal detail is largely lost: volume rendered VB could partially overcome this limitation (Hopper et al. 2000), but no virtual technique could ever substitute for visual appraisal, palpation attempts and

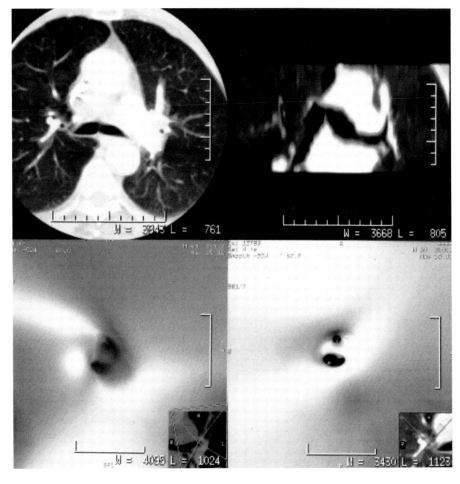

Fig. 13.2. Neoplastic stenosis of the apicodorsal segmental branch of the left
upper lobe bronchus. Cor-
onal MPVR (*top right*)
and VB (*bottom left*) allow
much more confident
diagnosis of the slight
reduction in bronchial
diameter, which is difficult
to detect on CT axial
sections alone (*top left*).
The normal appearance of
normal right upper lobe
apical bronchus on VB in
the same patient, with the
origins of subsegmental
branches (*bottom right*), is
shown for comparison

tissue sampling. In a very few cases VB can demonstrate pathological findings overlooked by bronchoscopy (Fig. 13.2), but only in anecdotal reports has the
correct diagnosis been missed on review of the CT
axial images. In fact, the diagnostic accuracy of VB
in lesion detection is almost totally inherent in volumetric thin collimation CT scanning, and not, or
only in very small part, dependent on an endoscopic
perspective. In some cases, 3D reconstructions may
better depict additional details that may be important in planning endobronchial procedures. Reproducing the course of an endoscope towards a lesion
from central to peripheral airways can assign a new
value to the bronchus sign. It could also be possible
to reduce by preliminary 3D/VB review the examination time in subsequent bronchoscopic examinations
in patient at risk of complications (GILKESON et al.
2001), or in children (KONEN et al. 1998; WAI-MAN
LAM et al. 2000), and to reduce the number of unnecessary procedures, and of endoscopies performed
in the follow-up after surgery and endobronchial
unblocking techniques (MCADAMS et al. 1998b).

In short, even if most reports, including ours (SAL-
VOLINI et al. 1997), agree about the good correlation
between real and virtual bronchoscopy, we think
that claiming that "VB will substitute for real examinations" is definitely not correct (LIEWALD 1998;
GLUECKER et al. 2001). The main role for VB is to
increase the synergy of CT with bronchoscopy, not
to compete with actual endoscopy for diagnosis. In
clinical practice, apart from targeted examinations,
we must suspend our virtual exploration not far from
the point where the fibreoptic endoscope also has to
stop: displaying by endoscopic perspective what axial
CT already shows and cannot be appreciated by the
endoscopist for correlation makes little sense. On the
whole, investigating the clinical impact of 3D rendering by estimating its diagnostic accuracy may not
be the correct way of evaluating a technique whose
effect is mainly to increase diagnostic confidence:
with a few exceptions this is not a diagnostic tool but
rather an invaluable communication device in complex cases or situations, such as endoscopic procedure planning, requiring the integration of different

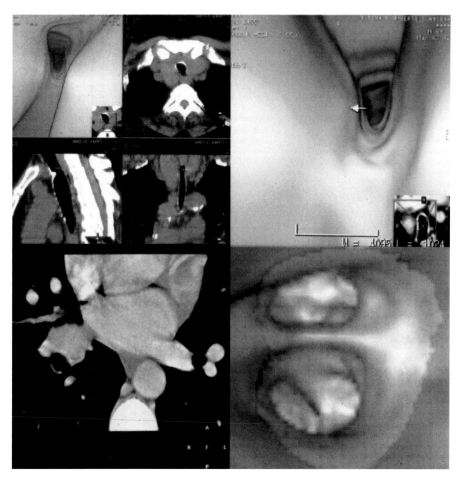

Fig. 13.3. Transbronchial needle aspiration (TBNA) planning by VB. By correlating the SSD and VB endoluminal perspective and MPR reference sections showing extraluminal structures (*top left*), it is possible to display the ideal puncture site (*top right*) to approach during TBNA, for right paratracheal adenopathy, in a patient whose trachea is compressed by a large goitre. By volume rendered VB (*bottom right*) it is possible to show directly through the semitransparent bronchial walls the "target" right hilar lymph node to be sampled, displayed by previous CT (*bottom left*)

competences and languages. Clinicians seem to be the most enthusiastic supporters of such techniques (FERRETTI et al. 2000). We think that it is possible, by displaying the whole range of possibilities available, to compensate the pitfalls of one technique with the advantages of the other, thus working together to obtain better results by the integration of two procedures such as CT and endoscopy that are routinely performed in every diagnostic investigation of bronchogenic lesions.

Perhaps the most intriguing application in this field is the possibility of displaying by VB the position of mediastinal lesions in relation to endoscopic landmarks before transbronchial needle aspiration (TBNA) (Fig. 13.3). By SSD-based VB, the position of the virtual endoscope tip is displayed in real-time interaction on axial and orthogonal MPR, showing the location of the target lymph node lying outside bronchial wall in relation to the endoscopic findings (FERRETTI et al. 1997; SALVOLINI et al. 2000). The ideal entry portal and puncture direction and depth for tissue sampling can be shown by the VB view

and will correspond to the instantly correlated position and direction of the tip of the virtual endoscope on planar reference images. Thanks to volume rendered VB software, it is possible to modulate the opacity of the walls of the reconstructed airways, thus simultaneously displaying directly on VB images pathological structures, such as lymph nodes, through a semitransparent tracheobronchial surface or by means of a windowing function (VINING et al. 1997; MCADAMS et al. 1998a). These tools could assist the clinician, who is usually forced to reproduce the same process during TBNA with the help solely of his imagination, after review of the CT sections. This can be useful in centres without extensive experience, where TBNA is affected by low diagnostic yield: preliminary VB review could save time and reduce the number of samples required for diagnosis. It is not yet clear, in the absence of large, prospective studies evaluating cost/benefit ratios and patient outcome, whether VB rendering in this situation could have a role in centres with more experience, or in spreading the application of a still largely underused diagnostic technique (HARKIN and WANG 1997; WANG 1998).

Peribronchial air collections in transplant recipients and after resection/anastomosis have been shown to be detected with increased confidence, as have other kinds of fistulas, by MPR/MPVR sections (COSTELLO 1994). Elastic recoil of bronchial branches can hamper their display on axial images alone. Minimum intensity MPVR can reinforce the evidence of extraluminal air, but care must be taken not to erase bronchial wall features. Correlating the VB and bronchoscopy findings could facilitate the detection of fistulas or leaks that could be difficult to appreciate without knowing their location relative to endoscopic landmarks. Volume rendered images can impressively depict fistulous paths that may be not so evident on axial sections (REMY-JARDIN et al. 1998a).

Three-dimensional conformational radiotherapy (CRT) aims to concentrate external beam irradiation on a neoplastic target, sparing the surrounding vital structures, by spatially modulating the isodose conformation in three dimensions, thanks to dose distribution algorithms based on axial CT sections and MPR orthogonal reconstructions (FISHMAN et al. 1991). Precise distinction between pathological and normal tissue needs CT density values to be retained, which is why only 2D reconstructed MPR images are used. Volume rendering could play an important role in the future, by combining 3D information and tissue classification. In intraluminal brachytherapy the isodoses must be calculated on exactly orthogonal reconstructed cross-sections and MPR perpendicular section pairs. Three-dimensional models are useful for obtaining such lesion-oriented 2D reconstructions; occasionally they may display some additional features that could be relevant for treatment planning, but they currently have no elective indications. Volume rendered VB may assist in calculating the effects of planned intraluminal dose distribution on surrounding structures: software evolution, stereotactic data registration, real-time interaction and multimodality image matching could allow, in the near future, CRT planning and execution in a virtual environment reconstructed by cross-sectional imaging data (REMY et al. 1997).

Finally, dynamic and functional studies, such as dynamic appraisal of bronchial reactivity and airways collapse and correlations with pulmonary function tests, could benefit from MPVR or 3D rendering to speed up data analysis, and allow better estimates of airways diameters and the volume of the whole tracheobronchial tree and lungs (GOLDIN and ABERLE 1997).

13.3.3
Peripheral Airways

As we proceed to the periphery, correct segmentation of the more distal airways becomes increasingly difficult; the threshold has to be adjusted individually and according to the order of the bronchial segment that has to be displayed, in order to minimize partial volume effects. Additionally, bronchial wall features that are essential for correctly diagnosing small airways diseases are largely lost and/or manipulated in data editing and segmentation, when minimum or maximum intensity projection or 3D techniques are applied. The dominant negative density of air contained in the lumen can hamper the detection of slight parietal lesions when using MinIP MPVR, and the conspicuity of the walls of small bronchi, which is of importance in looking for bronchiectasis and inflammatory changes, may appear to be artificially increased by the maximum intensity projection (MIP) thin slabs technique. Multidetector, subsecond technology allowing high-resolution scanning of extended segments, closer segmentation techniques, and the evolution of faster and really interactive volume rendering software retaining tissue information and navigational aids will extend 3D VB and volume rendering applications to the peripheral bronchi.

To date, only 2D MPVR sections, and especially axial/para-axial reconstructions of targeted "volumetric high-resolution computed tomography (HRCT)" slabs, are able to effectively supplement conventional HRCT scans for the depiction of pathology in the smaller bronchi (GAVELLI et al. 1998). By taking the possibilities of focused thin collimation spiral scanning and retrospective raw data reconstruction to the limit, it has been experimentally demonstrated that it is possible to obtain isotropic voxels, thus attaining the same degree of spatial resolution in all three dimensions (KALENDER 1995). This is obtained by means of a slightly summated axial MPVR display of thin (1–2 mm) axial reconstructed overlapping sections, reconstructed at a minimum (0.5 mm) interval. In searching for bronchiectasis, it is possible to display on a sole MPVR oblique reformat the entire extent of the affected segment. Virtual reality bronchographic-like images may overcome some of the limitations of transverse sections in the detection of mild degrees of bronchial dilation (REMY-JARDIN et al. 1998b). Bronchiolar pathology is detected with increased confidence on MIP MPVR focused slabs (REMY-JARDIN et al. 1996a; BHALLA et al. 1996). Small nodular lesions can be well appreciated by better anatomical depiction of vascular bundles on slightly

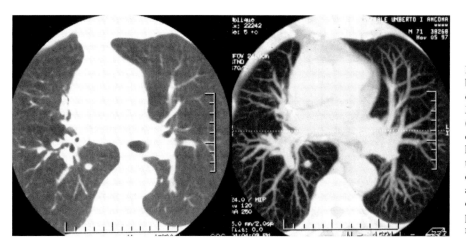

Fig. 13.4. Thanks to better anatomical display of vascular markings, MIP MPVR rendering (*right*) can improve the detection of a small right lower lobe lung nodule, that may have been misclassified as a section of a vessel perpendicularly crossing the transverse plane on the CT axial native axial section (*left*)

summated, thicker MIP planar slices (Fig. 13.4). Precise knowledge of the relations between peripheral bronchi and lung nodules can influence the choice of a transbronchial versus percutaneous approach for needle biopsy, or the selection of different tissue sampling devices. MinIP and MIP display of thin slabs allows areas of reduced density such as bronchiectasis and increased reticular markings, respectively, to be better displayed.

Whatever the clinical situation, it has yet to be demonstrated that thin collimation volumetric scanning can substitute for conventional HRCT, even if some of the multidetector scanners on the market no longer permit single-slice thin collimation acquisition (MEHNERT et al. 2000). All the techniques described here are thus to be considered as an adjunct to HRCT evaluation, to be performed after conventional studies, on target areas of interest (ENGELER et al. 1994). Multislice, subsecond acquisition now allows the thin collimation exploration of the whole tracheobronchial tree in a single breath-hold: the usefulness of this approach and its impact on switching from hard copy towards monitor reporting must be carefully evaluated. Increased patient radiation dose and ways of reducing it are becoming one of the most important focal points in multislice CT imaging: by reconstructing thicker axial or multiplanar sections it is possible, by summing the data on single images, to keep image noise, and thus dose requirements, low (PROKOP 2001). Increased redundancy of reconstructed images while using multislice thin collimation CT leads to increased demand for more efficient ways of analysing data and transferring diagnostically relevant information. Alternative rendering methods could help to solve this problem (KLINGEN-BECK-REGN et al. 1999; RYDBERG et al. 2000; UFFMANN and PROKOP 2001). It is left to the clinician's judgement to match dose, costs, time requirements, and possible benefits of introducing additional rendering techniques in routine diagnostic investigation, in the gamut of different situations that can be encountered in everyday practice (REMY et al. 2000).

13.4
Conclusions

Diagnostic analysis is still firmly based on the review of CT axial sections, even though we are increasingly moving towards monitor cine viewing instead of looking at hard copies: improvements in speed, automated processing for rendering, and more user-friendly interfaces will be needed before alternative rendering techniques can really compete with transverse section assessment (KIRKGEORG and PROKOP 1998; EIBEL et al. 2001; RUBIN 2000). Earlier studies have not shown that 3D rendering can significantly increase the diagnostic capabilities of CT (SCHOEPF et al. 1998; RAPP-BERNHARDT et al. 2000; FERRETTI et al. 2000). In selected clinical situations, however, the improved perception of image features due to additional rendering may allow the radiologist to better perceive and classify a lesion, or the clinician to more easily appreciate pathological findings and surrounding structures for endoscopic diagnostic and therapeutic procedure guidance or surgical planning. Because of time requirements and additional costs, however, we must seek real clinical settings in which the appropriate application of specific postprocessing imaging techniques, in selected cases, after meticulous data acquisition and analysis, may actually improve clinical care, not simply provide beautiful pictures, by applying the most appropriate technique to solve a specific problem in a particular patient in that well-defined clinical situation: and that must be done in conjunction with the referring physician, in everyday clinical practice. Time and prospective studies will finally tell whether advanced rendering techniques truly contribute to more effective decision-making in the clinical investigation of tracheobronchial diseases, as in other fields.

Endoscopy as the gold standard and CT are both indispensable in routine evaluation of airway pathology: the goal is to increase their synergy, making the most of standard examinations that would have been performed anyway in standard patient evaluation, and not performing dedicated examinations for 3D rendering. Technical evolution might take us one step further than endoscopy in the peripheral airways, but, of course, even endoscopic hardware technology will evolve (Tanaka et al. 1994); in a few years time it might even be possible to direct a robotic device or an endoscope, or the hand of a surgeon, towards a lesion in a virtual environment, by matching imaging data and actual anatomy: this is not a competition, however, but a team challenge (Bricault et al. 1998; Vannier and Haller 1999). Technological evolution is not a goal in itself, but only a faster and better way to get what we need. Our clinical role is to define what we need, how to obtain it better and faster, and when. We are not wanting to substitute for endoscopists, but are trying to make an effort to have a dialogue with clinicians by sharing a common language (Aberle 1998; Ravin 1998; Haponik et al. 1999). If we are not able to keep track of the clinical and critical application of imaging and rendering techniques, and to communicate efficiently to referring colleagues the information they need, the clinicians, with the help of technicians skilled in data processing, will fulfil their own needs on clinician-directed workstations designed for specific applications fields.

References

Aberle DR (1998) Future directions of research in thoracic imaging. Radiology 206:11–13

Adachi S, Kono M, Takemura T (1993) Evaluation of 3D spiral CT bronchoscopy in patients with lung cancer. Radiology 189:264–265

Bhalla M, Naidich DP, McGuinness G (1996) Diffuse lung disease: assessment with helical CT – preliminary observations of the role of maximum and minimum intensity projection images. Radiology 200:341–347

Bricault I, Ferretti G, Cinquin P (1998) Registration of real and CT-derived virtual bronchoscopic images to assist transbronchial biopsy. IEEE Trans Med Imaging 17:703–714

Brink JA (1995) Technical aspects of helical CT. Radiol Clin North Am 33:825–841

Costello P (1994) Spiral CT of the thorax. Semin Ultrasound CT MR 15:90–106

Eibel R, Tturk T, Kulinna C (2001) Value of multiplanar reformations (MPR) in multislice spiral CT of the lung. Rofo Fortschr Geb Rontgenstr Nuklearmed 173:57–64

Engeler CE, Tashjian JH, Engeler CM (1994) Volumetric high-resolution CT in the diagnosis of interstitial lung disease and bronchiectasis: diagnostic accuracy and radiation dose. AJR 163:31–35

Ferretti G, Coulomb M (2000) 3D virtual imaging of the upper airways. Rev Pneumol Clin 56:132–139

Ferretti G, Vining DJ, Knoplioch J (1996) Tracheobronchial tree: three-dimensional spiral CT with bronchoscopic perspective. J Comput Tomogr 20:777–781

Ferretti G, Knoplioch J, Bricault I (1997) Central airway stenoses: preliminary results of spiral-CT-generated virtual bronchoscopy simulations in 29 patients. Eur Radiol 7:854–859

Ferretti GR, Thony F, Bosson JL (2000) Benign abnormalities and carcinoid tumors of the central airway: impact of CT bronchography. AJR 174:1307–1313

Fishman KE, Magid D, Ney DR (1991) Three-dimensional imaging. Radiology 181:321–337

Fleiter T, Merkle EM, Aschoff AJ (1997) Comparison of real-time virtual and fiberoptic bronchoscopy in patients with bronchial carcinoma: opportunities and limitations. AJR 169:1591–1595

Gavelli G, Giampalma E, Cenni M (1998) High-resolution volumetric computerized tomography of the lung: optimization of technique and image quality as function of its clinical diagnostic use and dose to the patient. Radiol Med 95:322–328

Gilkeson RC, Ciancibello LM, Hejal RB (2001) Tracheobronchomalacia: dynamic airway evaluation with multidetector CT. AJR 176:205–210

Gluecker T, Lang E, Bessler S (2001) 2D and 3D CT imaging correlated to rigid endoscopy in complex laryngo-tracheal stenoses. Eur Radiol 11:50–54

Goldin JG, Aberle DR (1997) Functional imaging of the airways. J Thorac Imaging 12:29–37

Grenier P, Beigelman C (1996) Spiral CT of the bronchial tree. In: Remy-Jardin M, Remy J (eds) Spiral CT of the chest. Springer, Berlin Heidelberg New York, pp 185–200

Haponik EF, Aquino SL, Vining DJ (1999) Virtual bronchoscopy. Clin Chest Med 20:201–217

Harkin TJ, Wang KP (1997) Bronchoscopic needle aspiration of mediastinal and hilar lymph nodes. J Bronchol 4:238–249

Henschke CI, Davis SD, Auh Y (1987) Detection of bronchial abnormalities. Comparison of CT and bronchoscopy. J Comput Tomogr 11:432–439

Hopper KD, Iyriboz TA, Mahraj RPM (1998a) CT bronchoscopy: optimization of imaging parameters. Radiology 209:872–877

Hopper KD, Kasales CJ, Wise SW (1998b) The optimization of helical thoracic CT. J Comput Tomogr 22:418–424

Hopper KD, Iyriboz AT, Wise SW (2000) Mucosal detail at CT virtual reality: surface versus volume rendering. Radiology 214:517–522

Kalender WA (1995) Thin-section three-dimensional spiral CT: is isotropic imaging possible? Radiology 197:578–580

Kauzcor HU, Wolcke B, Fischer B (1996) Three-dimensional helical CT of the tracheobronchial tree: evaluation of imaging protocols and assessment of suspected stenoses with bronchoscopic correlation. AJR 167:419–424

Kirkgeorg MA, Prokop M (1998) Increasing spiral CT benefits with postprocessing applications. Eur J Radiol 28:39–54

Klingenbeck-Regn K, Schaller S, Flohr T (1999) Subsecond multi-slice computed tomography: basics and applications. Eur J Radiol 31:110–124

Konen E, Katz M, Rozenman J (1998) Virtual bronchoscopy in children: early clinical experience. AJR 1699–1702

Lacrosse M, Trigaux JP, Van Beers BE (1995) 3D spiral CT of the tracheobronchial tree. J Comput Tomogr 19:341–347

Lee KS, Yoon JH, Kim TK (1997) Evaluation of tracheobronchial disease with helical CT with multiplanar and three-dimensional reconstruction: correlation with bronchoscopy. Radiographics 17:555–557

Liewald F (1998) Comparison of virtual and fiberoptic bronchoscopy. Thorac Cardiovasc Surg 46:361–366

Lo Cicero JL III, Costello P, Campos CT (1996) Spiral CT with multiplanar and three-dimensional reconstructions accurately predicts tracheobronchial pathology. Ann Thorac Surg 62:811–817

Marom EM, Goodman PC, McAdams HP (2001a) Focal abnormalities of the trachea and main bronchi. AJR 176:707–711

Marom EM, Goodman PC, McAdams HP (2001b) Diffuse abnormalities of the trachea and main bronchi. AJR 176:713–717

McAdams HP, Goodman PC, Kussin P (1998a) Virtual bronchoscopy for directing transbronchial needle aspiration of hilar and mediastinal lymph nodes: a pilot study. AJR 170:1361–1364

McAdams HP, Palmer SM, Erasmus JJ (1998b) Bronchial anastomotic complications in lung transplant recipients: virtual bronchoscopy for noninvasive assessment. Radiology 209:689–695

Mehnert F, Pereira PL, Dammann F (2000) High resolution multislice CT of the lung: comparison with sequential HRCT slices. Rofo Fortschr Geb Rontgenstr Nuklearmed 172:972–977

Naidich DP (1996) Invited commentary (editorial comment). Ann Thorac Surg 62:817

Naidich DP, Harkin TJ (1995) Airways and lung: correlation of CT with fiberoptic bronchoscopy. Radiology 197:1–12

Naidich DP, Gruden JF, McGuinness G (1997) Volumetric (helical/spiral) CT (VCT) of the airways. J Thorac Imaging 12:11–28

Neumann K, Winterer J, Kimmig M (1999) Real-time interactive virtual endoscopy of the tracheo-bronchial system: influence of CT imaging protocols and observer ability. Eur J Radiol 33:50–54

Padhani AR (1998) Spiral CT: thoracic applications. Eur J Radiol 28:2–17

Padhani AR, Fishman EK, Heitmiller RF (1995) Multiplanar display of spiral CT data of the pulmonary hila in patients with lung cancer: preliminary observations. Clin Imaging 19:252–257

Perhomaa M, Lahde S, Rossi O (1997) Helical CT in evaluation of the bronchial tree. Acta Radiol 38:83–91

Prokop M (2001) Dose optimization in thoracic computer tomography. Radiologe 3:269–278

Quint LE, Whyte RI, Kazerooni EA (1995) Stenosis of the central airways: evaluation by using helical CT with multiplanar reconstructions. Radiology 194:871–877

Rapp-Bernhardt U, Welte T, Doehring W (2000) Diagnostic potential of virtual bronchoscopy: advantages in comparison with axial CT slices, MPR and MIP? Eur Radiol 10:981–988

Ravin CE (1998) Future directions in pulmonary imaging. Radiology 206:9–10

Remy J, Remy-Jardin M, Artaud D (1997) Multiplanar and three-dimensional reconstruction techniques in CT: impact on chest diseases. Eur Radiol 8:335–351

Remy J, Remy-Jardin M, Bonnel F (2000) Spiral (helical) CT of tracheobronchial diseases. J Radiol 81:201–216

Remy-Jardin M, Remy J, Artaud D (1996a) Diffuse infiltrative lung disease: clinical value of sliding-thin-slab maximum intensity projection CT scans in the detection of mild micronodular patterns. Radiology 200:333–339

Remy-Jardin M, Remy J, Deschildre F (1996b) Obstructive lesions of the central airways: evaluation by using spiral CT with multiplanar and three-dimensional reformations. Eur Radiol 6:807–816

Remy-Jardin M, Remy J, Artaud D (1998a) Tracheobronchial tree: assessment with volume rendering – technical aspects. Radiology 208:393–398

Remy-Jardin M, Remy J, Artaud D (1998b) Volume rendering of the tracheobronchial tree: clinical evaluation of bronchographic images. Radiology 208:761–770

Rogalla P (2001) Virtual Endoscopy of the trachea and bronchi. In: Rogalla P, van Scheltinga J, Hamm B (eds) Virtual endoscopy and related 3D techniques. Springer, Berlin Heidelberg New York, pp 45–75

Rubin GD (2000) Data explosion: the challenge of multidetector-row CT. Eur J Radiol 36:74–80

Rubin GD, Beaulieu CF, Argiro VA (1996a) Perspective volume rendering of CT and MR images: applications for endoscopic imaging. Radiology 199:321–330

Rubin GD, Napel S, Leung AN (1996b) Volumetric analysis of volumetric data: achieving a paradigm shift. Radiology 200:312–317

Rydberg J, Buckwalter KA, Caldemeyer KS (2000) Multisection CT: scanning techniques and clinical applications. Radiographics 20:1787–1806

Salvolini L, Gasparini S, Baldelli S (1997) Virtual bronchoscopy: endoscopic reconstructions versus actual findings. Radiol Med 94:454–462

Salvolini L, Bichi Secchi E, Costarelli L (2000) Clinical applications of 2D and 3D CT imaging of the airways – a review. Eur J Radiol 34:9–25

Sartoni Galloni S, Miceli M, Lipparini M (1999) Comparison of various parameters (pitch 1 and 2) in the study of the lung with spiral computerized tomography. Radiol Med 97:121–125

Schaefer-Prokop C, Prokop M (1996) Spiral CT of the trachea and main bronchi. In: Remy-Jardin M, Remy J (eds) Spiral CT of the chest. Springer, Berlin Heidelberg New York, pp 161–184

Schoepf UJ, Seemann M, Schuhmann D (1998) Virtual and three-dimensional bronchoscopy with spiral and electron beam computed tomography. Radiologe 38:816–823

Storto ML, Migliorato L, Guidotti A (1995) Spiral computed

tomography of the trachea. Technique and clinical applications. Radiol Med 89:233–236

Tanaka M, Takizawa H, Satoh M (1994) Assessment of an ultra-thin bronchoscope that allows cytodiagnosis of small airways. Chest 106:1443–1447

Touliopoulos P, Costello HP (1995) Helical (spiral) CT of the thorax. Radiol Clin North Am 33:843–861

Uffmann M, Prokop M (2001) Multislice CT of the lungs: technique and clinical applications. Radiologe 41:240–247

Vannier MW, Haller JW (1999) Navigation in diagnosis and therapy. Eur J Radiol 31:132–140

Vining DJ (1996) Virtual endoscopy: is it reality? Radiology 200:30–31

Vining DJ, Liu K, Choplin RH (1996) Virtual bronchoscopy: relationships of virtual reality endobronchial simulations to actual bronchoscopic findings. Chest 109:549–553

Vining DJ, Ferretti G, Stelts DR (1997) Mediastinal lymph node mapping using spiral CT and three-dimensional reconstructions in patients with lung cancer: preliminary observations. J Bronchol 4:18–25

Wai-man Lam W, Tam PKH, Chan FL (2000) Esophageal atresia and tracheal stenosis: use of three-dimensional CT and virtual bronchoscopy in neonates, infants, and children. AJR 174:1009–1012

Wang KP (1998) Continued efforts to improve the sensitivity of transbronchial needle aspiration. Chest 114:4–5

14 Aorta

Carlo Bartolozzi, Emanuele Neri, Irene Bargellini, Claudia Gianni

CONTENTS

14.1
Introduction

Traditionally, the study of the aorta has been performed with conventional angiography through intravenous injection of iodinated contrast medium. This method has gained wide acceptance in clinical practice and is still considered the most reliable in terms of spatial resolution. However, as is well known, angiography is invasive for the patient, requires a high dose of contrast and is based on two-dimensional acquisitions. Such reasons have led to the role of angiography in the diagnostic approach to aortic pathology being reconsidered, and to a search for alternative imaging methods that can offer both a minimally invasive approach and a cross-sectional or even volumetric study of the vessel.

Ultrasound, born as a noninvasive cross-sectional technique, is currently the primary approach to the study of aorta. It provides much important information such as lumen caliber, presence of parietal calcification and thrombosis, or even dissection. More recently, the integration of conventional US with color Doppler has allowed the hemodynamic study

of the aorta, combining information on aortic caliber with blood velocity. US has also been upgraded by the introduction of methods for direct volumetric acquisition that exploit both the features of conventional gray-level imaging and color coding of blood movement.

Computed tomography provides a more advanced study of the aorta. Since its introduction into the clinical practice, CT has progressively modified the concept of image acquisition. Initially CT was a purely axial imaging method that required long acquisition times, but in 1989 a revolution occurred with the introduction of spiral or helical technology (Kalender 1990). This new approach provides volumetric acquisition of patient data in a significantly shorter time frame; spiral CT study of aorta and other vessels has been called CT angiography (CTA). More recently spiral CT has been upgraded with faster scanners based on multi-row detectors or multislice technology.

Even MR imaging has undergone a great technological improvement. Traditionally considered a slow imaging method, it has been upgraded in the last 10 years by the increased power of magnets and gradients, and by the elaboration of fast imaging sequences (time-of-flight, phase contrast and spoiled gradient echo recalled) that variously exploit the effects of blood flow and contrast administration; accordingly the selective study of vessels with MR is called MR angiography (MRA).

In parallel to the development of imaging techniques, the generation of new algorithms for three-dimensional (3D) image processing has occurred. Methods for the 3D study of the aorta from any 3D data set include multiplanar reconstruction (MPR), multiplanar volume reconstruction (MPVR), curved planar reconstruction (CPR), maximum intensity projection (MIP), surface rendering and volume rendering. A specific application of 3D study to aortic imaging is represented by virtual endoscopy or virtual angioscopy.

The principles of 3D acquisition with US, CTA and MRA have been discussed in the section of the

C. Bartolozzi, MD, E. Neri, MD, I. Bargellini, MD,
C. Gianni MD
Diagnostic and Interventional Radiology, Department of Oncology, Transplants, and Advanced Technologies in Medicine, University of Pisa, Via Roma 67, 56100, Pisa, Italy

book on technique. The next paragraphs will review the specific acquisition technique for the 3D study of aorta, and the application of 3D image processing.

14.2
3D Image Processing and Imaging Techniques

14.2.1
3D Ultrasound

3D US acquisition is based on two methods: direct 3D acquisition with two-dimensional (2D) US arrays, or 3D reconstruction from a series of 2D images produced with one-dimensional US arrays (von Ramm and Smith 1991; Stetten 1998). One specific acquisition method is from endoluminal US, where circular arrays provide sequential images along the vessel path that can be reconstructed to generate a volumetric model.

During US acquisition, the implementation of the color and power Doppler modules allows the vessels to be highlighted with color coding (Picot 1993; Rickey 1995). This enhances the vessel boundaries and permits discrimination of the lumen from the external space, especially in US images where the noise is a critical factor influencing the image contrast.

Regardless of the method used to obtain 3D data sets, the 3D image processing methods are essentially the same as used in other modalities: MPR, surface rendering and volume rendering.

The application of 3D US to the study of aorta and its branches is still under evaluation to determine its clinical usefulness (Guo and Fenster 1996; Nelson and Pretorius 1998). Although US is limited by a low spatial resolution, 3D US of the aorta will compete with more established applications of 3D imaging in CTA or MRA. The study of aneurysms seems one important area of interest. A patient undergoing treatment for an aneurysm requires a multiplanar evaluation of the aorta to determine the length of the aneurysm neck, the condition of aortic wall, the distance between renal arteries and aortic bifurcation, and the aneurysm's dimensions. These measurements are not easy to perform in a standard examination and US has a low diagnostic accuracy in characterizing aneurysms. In this setting 3D US could be more efficient and promising.

14.2.2
3D CT Angiography

CTA is one of the most advanced and noninvasive techniques available for the study of the aorta and its branches. Imaging protocols for study of the aorta aim to provide a volumetric acquisition in a short time frame to image the aorta during maximum contrast enhancement. To obtain angiographic-like perspectives, contrast administration is optimized with a bolus timing test at specific flow rates; the scan delay is calculated with automatic bolus-triggering software. To achieve the highest quality 3D reconstructions a deliberate attempt is made to combine thinner collimation, maximum scan velocity and reconstruction spacing (see Chap.2).

In our experience the best scanning protocol with single-slice CT for the study of the abdominal aorta consists of collimation 3 mm, pitch 2 and reconstruction spacing 1 mm; 5 mm collimation is used for the study of thoracic aorta (Bartolozzi 1998). Rubin (2000) suggested the following protocol for multislice CT: 2.5 mm nominal section thickness, pitch 6.0, and a table speed of 15 mm per rotation (18.75 mm/s). The same author compared this acquisition protocol with spiral CT and reported that multislice CT is significantly faster (scanning speed is more than double), has a higher spatial resolution (on the longitudinal axis) and requires half the dose of contrast medium needed in single-slice acquisition.

The improvement in spiral CT with the introduction of multislice scanners is having a significant impact in vascular applications, with increased accuracy of CTA in the study of aorta, where maximum contrast enhancement is a prerequisite for imaging. Multislice CT permits the scanning of large volumes in a short time frame; for example, the simultaneous study of the thoracic and abdominal aorta, up to the iliac vessels, can be performed in 30 s, obtaining a CT aortographic acquisition, as in conventional angiography.

The application of 3D image processing to CTA data sets of the aorta has modified the conventional approach to many diseases. MPR has been proposed as a first step in postprocessing; the free-hand orientation of reconstructed planes along the aorta allows the precise analysis of the vessel's path. However, oblique planes are not easy to orient along a curved path, requiring multiple reconstructions at different steps of the aortic lumen. To overcome this limitation, a curvilinear reconstruction method has been introduced. The advantage of MPR and CPR is to display in the same plane the aortic lumen, the wall and the extraparietal compartment with standard gray-level image coding.

MPRs are bi-dimensional planes and therefore do not allow volumetric analysis. To obviate this problem, the use of MPVR (or thick slabs) has been proposed in combination with a maximum intensity projection algorithm. This combined approach allows the acquisition of angiographic-like projections of the aorta where the structures with maximum density are brightest (iodinated contrast within the lumen, calcified plaques, metallic structures).

Moving from reformatted planes to full 3D views of the aorta, shaded surface display (SSD) has been proposed as a surface rendering method. The aorta and its main branches can be displayed after the setting of a segmentation threshold to exclude the surrounding anatomical structures, exploiting the high density of contrast within the aortic lumen. SSD provides an entire view of the aorta but is affected by some intrinsic limitations of surface rendering: the threshold segmentation may cause a significant lack of data, with incomplete representation of the vessel anatomy, and consequent influence on the assessment of pathology; the segmentation is not always sufficiently accurate to separate the aorta from surrounding structures (spine, sternum, ribs, vena cava, left renal vein, etc.); and the segmentation has a significant operator variability.

To overcome these limitations volume rendering has been preferred for the study of the aorta and its branches. This method provides an interactive display of the vessel based on the modulation of voxel visibility on the basis of CT density. The aorta can easily be displayed without data loss, even its small branches (such as the renal arteries) being clearly represented.

Among the latest development in 3D imaging, virtual endoscopy or angioscopy has been reported to have a role in CTA. This provides an endoluminal view of the aorta with details of the inner wall, demonstrating parietal alterations such as thrombosis, calcifications, aneurysms and stenosis. In cases of metallic prosthetic material, this can be visualized from the inside of the aorta as well.

14.2.3
3D MR Angiography

The study of the aorta and its branches with MRA started with the introduction of fast imaging techniques, such as time-of-flight (TOF) or phase contrast sequences (SINGER 1959). TOF takes advantage of the

contrast between inflowing fully magnetized blood and the saturated surrounding tissue, showing the flowing blood as the brightest voxels. On the other hand phase contrast techniques detect the shift in phase that occurs when spins move in the presence of an imaging gradient, and allow measurement of the flow velocity; even in phase contrast techniques the flow is represented by bright voxels (HUSTON and HERMAN 1993). The term MRA was given to these technique because with the integration of the MIP algorithm into the acquired data sets the final 3D reconstruction showed angiographic-like images. To obtain a 3D view of a MIP angiogram multiple perspectives can be created within a 360° rotation and finally a cine-view of the angiogram sequence can be created to simulate the image rotation. Main limitations of non-enhanced MRA are the long acquisition time (5–8 min), the short field of view with lack of kidney visualization and major artefacts.

These technique are still used but mainly proposed as a complement to the most recent methods that use contrast enhancement magnetic resonance angiography (CE-MRA). These techniques, using ultrafast gradient echo sequences, allow (in the same fashion as CTA) the acquisition of volumetric data sets during a single breath-hold (18–25 s) and bolus injection of a gadolinium chelate.

As well as MIP the other image processing techniques described in the CTA section can be applied to CE-MRA data sets.

14.3
3D Imaging of Pathology

14.3.1
Aortic Dissections

An aortic dissection is a tear in the inner layer of the aortic wall. An aortic dissection that does not stop tearing will ultimately become a fatal rupture; this makes it essential to evaluate symptoms that could be related to a dissection and perform the adequate imaging approach. When left untreated, about 33% of patients die within the first 24 h, and 50% die within 48 h. The 2 week mortality rate approaches 75% in patients with undiagnosed ascending aortic dissection (CHEN 1997).

Among the imaging methods available, the role of transesophageal US, CTA and MRA is still under debate, especially in the diagnostic investigation of the acute dissection. Initial application of 3D imaging of thoracic aorta was carried out with MR imaging. The first study was by VALK et al. (1985), who developed an algorithm capable of reconstructing in three dimensions the outline of the aorta (identified as a flow channel); in aortic dissection, the MR images showed the two lumens more completely than did angiography. This work was followed by other reports on the application of MRA to the study of dissections by applying MPR and MIP techniques (LIM et al. 1989). PRINCE (1996) studied eight patients in whom gadolinium-enhanced MRA correctly identified the intimal flap (sensitivity 100%). KRINSKY (1997) reported that gadolinium-enhanced MRA was sensitive (92–96%) and specific (100%) for acute and chronic aortic dissection (n=26), but did not reveal two intramural hematomas.

In the most recent reports on the study of aortic dissection with MRA, the use of gadolinium is considered essential (ALLEY 1998; HO and PRINCE 1998); recently echo planar imaging without contrast enhancement and MIP has also been proposed as a screening method for dissections (NITATORI 1999). Three-dimensional reconstructions such as MIP and MPR can easily be produced during image analysis and are considered part of the MR examination since they allow better display of the complexity of the dissection (WATANABE 2000). Among these techniques, MPR should be preferred since it allows direct visualization of the intimal flap; the intrinsic nature of

MIP causes an average sum of voxels pertaining to the aortic lumen and in the final projection the intimal flap is not displayed (Fig. 14.1).

However, 3D imaging of dissections has found specific applications in CTA, emphasized by the need to properly evaluate patients undergoing surgery. Surgery is indicated in the presence of a proximal dissection (Stanford type A) and in cases where the following conditions occur: evidence of fluid in the pericardial sac, marked enlargement of the dissected aorta (aneurysm formation), blood leakage in the mediastinum, ischemia of vital organs, intramural hematoma. Prospective studies with CTA have shown a sensitivity of 83–94% with a specificity of 87–100% in detecting aortic dissection. The role of CTA in the presence of an aortic dissection is to detect the origin of the intimal flap and define the true and false lumen, and exclude complications such as extension in aortic branches with organ-specific damage (renal or mesenteric ischemia) or rupture with hemopericardium and pleural effusion (CHUNG 1996). In such evaluations 3D imaging can integrate CTA with MPR, MIP, virtual endoscopy and volume rendering techniques.

The contribution of 3D imaging to the diagnosis of aortic dissection was first emphasized by RUBIN (1993), who applied MPR, MIP and SSD to spiral CT data sets. Later studies confirmed this trend. ZEMAN (1995) evaluated the role of MPR, MIP and SSD in

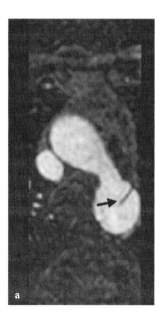 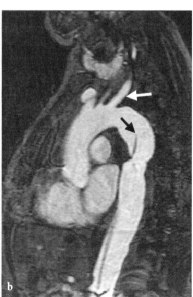 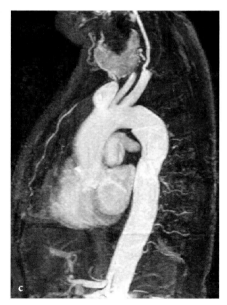

Fig. 14.1a–c. Contrast-enhanced MRA of the thoracic aorta in type B aortic dissection. **a** MPR generated in the axial plane shows the intimal flap (*arrow*). **b** MPR generated along the sagittal-oblique plane (along the main axis of the aortic arc) demonstrates that the flap (*black arrow*) arises in the descending aorta, after the origin of the left subclavian artery (*white arrow*). **c** Thick slab MPR with integration of MIP does not display the intimal flap because of the superimposition of bright voxels

13 patients, and a comparison was made with axial images in seven patients who proved to have documented dissection. In three of seven patients with dissection, axial images did not allow the extent of the intimal flap to be determined; in contrast MPR or the other 3D views clarified the relevant anatomy in all three cases. BRADSHAW (1998) reports the use of oblique or other MPR images and SSD in the study of 21 aortic dissections, the relationship of dissections to major vessels being better shown with 3D reconstruction or oblique reformats. The author reported that there was little additional information from 3D reconstruction or reformats in assessment of type A dissection and an improved spatial orientation was helpful for surgical planning in certain cases of type B dissection.

LU (2000) used SSD, MPR and MIP methods with electron beam computed tomography data sets, and diagnosed 97 cases of aortic dissection (diagnostic accuracy 100%). A similar experience is reported by NAKANISHI (1997) who studied 15 aortic dissections and found MPR useful to demonstrate the intimal flap and entry sites.

Using CT virtual endoscopy, called the "cruising eye view method", HAYASHI (1999) studied 10 patients with aortic dissection. All parietal lesions were identified in this study, and the use of the endoluminal perspective yielded precise information about the relationship between the intimal flap and the epiaortic branches. However, in a study specifically on the performance of virtual endoscopy in detecting aortic dissection by KIMURA (1996), which included 10 patients with aortic dissection evaluated by CTA, the comparison between axial images and virtual endoscopy showed that no additional information on the features of dissection, with respect to native images, was obtained by the use of endoluminal views. SMITH (1998) evaluated various pathologies of the thoracic aorta with "virtual angioscopy" based on volume rendering technique and suggested that it could be a potentially useful technique for the noninvasive evaluation of vascular pathology.

We believe that virtual endoscopy is a useful tool, since it can clearly depict the intimal flap, distinguish between the false and true lumen, and assess the relationships with aortic branches (BARTOLOZZI 1998) (Fig. 14.2).

In summary, CTA of aortic dissection is more valuable and effective if 3D imaging is used.

14.3.2
Aneurysms of the Abdominal Aorta

Aortic aneurysms can develop anywhere along the length of the aorta but the majority are located along the abdominal aorta; 90% of abdominal aneurysms are located below the level of the renal arteries and about two-thirds are not limited to the aorta but extend into one or both of the iliac arteries. The natural history of abdominal aortic aneurysms depends on their size; rupture is uncommon if the maximum diameter is less than 5 cm, but more common if it is over 6 cm. Surgical repair is therefore indicated for all aneurysms over 6 cm wide, and elective repair for those between 4 and 6 cm.

US usually gives a clear picture of the extent and size of an aneurysm and has about 98% accuracy in measuring the size of the aneurysm. However, US cannot clearly demonstrate the aneurysm neck and its relationships with the renal arteries. Moreover in planning surgery concomitant diseases, such as stenosis of the celiac and mesenteric arteries, as well as renal arteries, are not depictable (unless a color Doppler imaging study is also performed).

Since its introduction into clinical routine, CT has gained an important role in the management of patients with abdominal aortic aneurysms, a role that has been strengthened by the advent of singleslice and then multislice spiral CT. CTA has the great advantage of providing in a single session all the information needed to grade the severity of an aneurysm, and even more importantly to analyze all its features, such as dimensions, extension and parietal alterations. Furthermore, the new endovascular treatment options that are alternatives to open surgical repair have a greater requirement for accurate characterization of the aneurysm. The positioning of endoprostheses within the aortic lumen requires the precise knowledge of some important parameters that determine the type of prostheses to be used and allow their successful insertion (Fig. 14.3). Moreover after treatment information about the outcome and presence of complications is essential in the follow-up of the patient. All these evaluations can only be done if CTA is integrated with 3D image processing techniques; therefore 3D imaging has found here an elective application.

A dedicated approach to preoperative imaging for endovascular treatment was made by BROEDERS (1997a, b). Curved linear or planar reconstructions were used for accurate measurement of the diameters and length of the potential attachment zones in the aorta and iliac arteries. The approach proposed in

Fig. 14.2a–d. CTA in a patient with a Stanford type A dissection. **a** Axial CTA crossing through the descending aorta shows the true (*T*) and false (*F*) lumen. **b, c** The shapes of both the true (**b**) and false (**c**) lumen can be recognized in virtual endoscopic views created from the same level. **d** The navigation in the abdominal aorta demonstrates the extension of the flap to the bifurcation and the origin of the celiac artery (*CA*), left renal artery (*LRA*) and left iliac artery (*LIA*) from the false lumen; the "run-off" site of the false lumen is demonstrated as well (*arrows*)

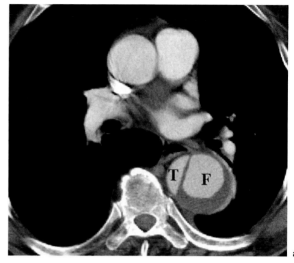

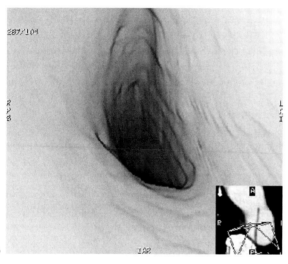

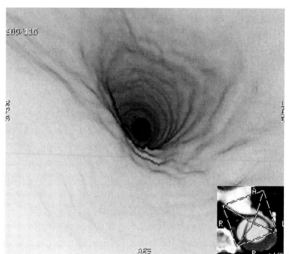

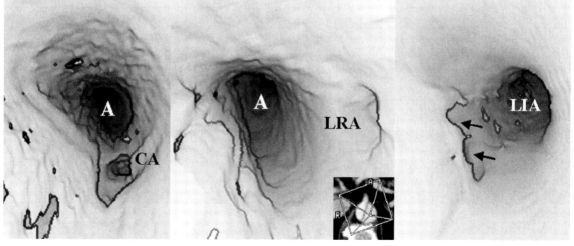

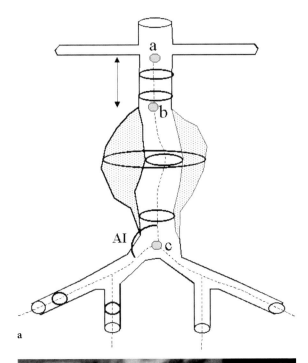

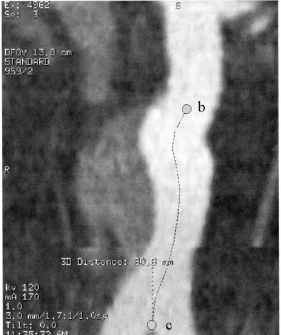

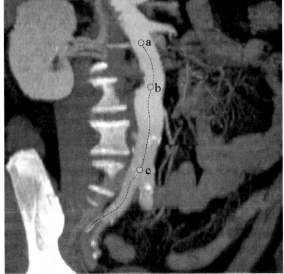

Fig. 14.3a–c. CTA study of an infrarenal aortic aneurysm. a The planning of endoprosthetic treatment requires multiple measurements: length of the neck (from *a* to *b* along the centerline), the distance from neck to bifurcation (from *b* to *c*), the aorto-iliac (*AI*) angle, the circumference of neck, aneurysm and iliac arteries, etc. CTA allows these measurements to be performed. b The use of curved planar reconstructions permits the generation of a centerline and measurements of distance can be taken. c Multiplanar reconstructions are also useful in some instances to measure angles and distances in the study of iliac arteries

this work is quite reasonable since the length measurement of the aorta was performed with curved reconstructions (obtained with markers in the center of the lumen) that allowed the tortuosity of the vessel to be taken into account, and the diameter is measured using many steps of the curved plane; in each step the diameter was measured in a plane perpendicular to the curve, corresponding to a true axial section. The creation of a centerline in the aortic lumen is the most reliable method to measure the true length of the vessel. RUBIN (1998) developed a method to automatically calculate the centerline of

the aorta and multiple diameters. The method also allowed the identification of curvatures and local variations in diameter represented by the origin of the aortic branches.

For a similar purpose we have used virtual reality modeling language (VRML) in 25 patients undergoing endovascular treatment of abdominal aortic aneurysms. Academic software (CRS4 Center for Research, Cagliari, Italy) was used to perform vessel segmentation (by using snakes, elastic contours and region growing methods), extract the centerline (arterial skeleton) and measure the true axial sections

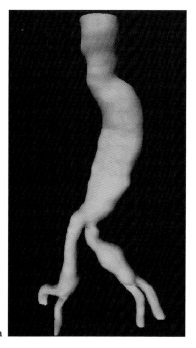

a

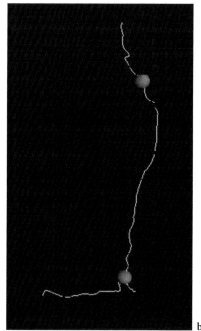

b

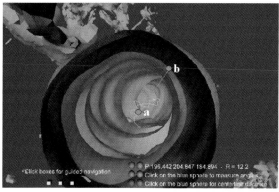

c

Fig. 14.4. a VRML model of the abdominal aorta and iliac arteries in a patient with an infrarenal aneurysm. b Using the centerline of the aortic lumen the distance between the renal artery level and the aortic bifurcation can be calculated. c The aortic lumen can also be displayed from the inside and multiple measurements are obtained along the centerline, such as diameters, area and angles

(Fig. 14.4). Another example of software to facilitate the radiologist in making measurements was proposed by Subasic (2000), who developed a system capable of performing 3D segmentation of CT images and extracting a 3D model of the aortic wall. Once the 3D model of aortic wall is available it is easy to perform all the required measurements for appropriate stent-graft selection.

Not only measurements but also an accurate assessment of parietal alterations and concomitant disease of the renal arteries should be done in these patients. These evaluations are better performed by CTA with 3D imaging. The condition of the aneurysm neck is the main parameter in deciding whether suprarenal clamping should be performed during open surgical repair or whether the proximal portion of an endoprosthesis can be reliably attached. A retrospective analysis of CTA data sets (Neri

1999), obtained in 39 patients who underwent suprarenal cross-clamping for surgical repair of abdominal aortic aneurysms, revealed that preoperative CTA reports following evaluation of axial images correctly predicted juxtarenal aneurysms in 79% of cases; the retrospective consideration of thrombosis, calcifications and vessel tortuosity using MPR and virtual endoscopy further increased the accuracy in predicting suprarenal clamping (100%).

The use of 3D reconstructions and CTA in preoperative evaluation of abdominal aortic aneurysms is advocated by many authors (Gomes 1994; Balm 1994; Chuter 1994; Aarts 1999; Rubin 2000), but CTA with 3D reconstructions is essential also in the follow-up of these patients. Especially in the control of endoprostheses CTA is required to exclude complications (endoleak, migration, tortuosity, increased volume of endograft).

KRAMER (2001) used 3D reconstructions to assess geometric changes in endografts in a 2 year follow-up. The author took angle measurements in the proximal aneurysm neck, the mid-portion of the endograft, and the graft limbs at the origin of the iliac arteries, and observed that lateral changes predominated, i.e., the proximal neck changed by a mean −0.71° in the anteroposterior view and by 4.0° in the lateral projection, while the left limb angles changed by 1.38° in the anteroposterior view and 11.71° in the lateral plane.

The possibility there being either volumetric stability or an increase in volume of an endograft can be seen by measuring the diameter of the prosthesis; it attributed to a phenomenon called "endotension" (WHITE 1999). POLLOCK (2000) calculated the volume of the endograft by summing the 2D areas of the individual slices, including the preoperative thrombosis. He identified five patterns of behavior: shrinkage, no change, initial shrinkage but a later increase, and a progressive increase in volume. Although this approach is precise and reliable, it is time-consuming because of the need to trace graft contours in each slice. Volumetric changes can also be evaluated by segmentation of CTA data sets to obtain direct estimation of the segmented volume; with this approach we followed up 25 patients who underwent treatment of abdominal aortic aneurysm, observing that in those with endoleaks no volumetric reduction occurred.

In the follow-up of these patients virtual endoscopy may have a role. The endoluminal views of the aorta looking caudally from the celiac level allow assessment of the positioning of the proximal portion of the endoprosthesis and its relationship with the origin of the renal arteries. In some difficult cases, this evaluation is quite difficult to do with axial slices, and virtual endoscopy can play the role of a problem-solving tool (Fig. 14.5). Concerning endoleaks, it seems difficult for virtual endoscopy to assess all types of endoleaks, especially those arising from patent inferior mesenteric or lumbar arteries. For type 1 endoleaks, arising from the attachment site, virtual endoscopy can demonstrate the separation between prosthetic web and aortic wall (Fig. 14.6).

To demonstrate the morphology of the endoprosthesis, CTA data sets can be processed with MIP and volume rendering. These methods allow the metallic component of the prosthesis to be distinguished from the contrast-enhanced lumen, and therefore to assess the tortuosity and even the relationship with the aortic branches. This latter element is particularly important in studying the nature of type 2 endoleaks, aris-

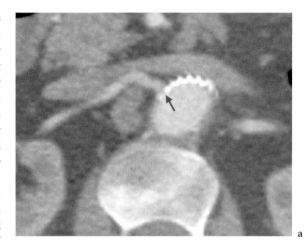

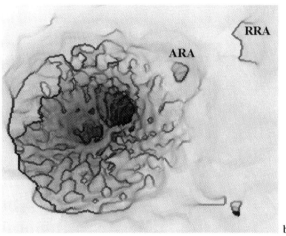

Fig. 14.5a, b. CTA follow-up of an Aneurix endoprosthesis positioned just below the renal arteries. **a** Axial image crossing through the right renal artery (*arrow*) does not clearly exclude the involvement of the ostium. **b** Endoluminal view demonstrates the presence of an accessory renal artery (*ARA*) just below the right renal artery (*RRA*), not involved by the proximal portion of the endoprosthesis

ing from patent branches. Thick slab MIPs (also called MPVRs) allow the orientation of the thick plane along the vessel path and therefore are useful for recognizing the course of thin vessels (such as the lumbar arteries) that arise from the aortic wall. The same principle can be applied to volume rendering, which seems to provide better performance than MIP.

14.3.3
Aortic Branch Diseases: Renal Arteries

Stenosis of the renal artery accounts for less than 1% of all hypertension in people who have moderately increased blood pressure, the main cause being the

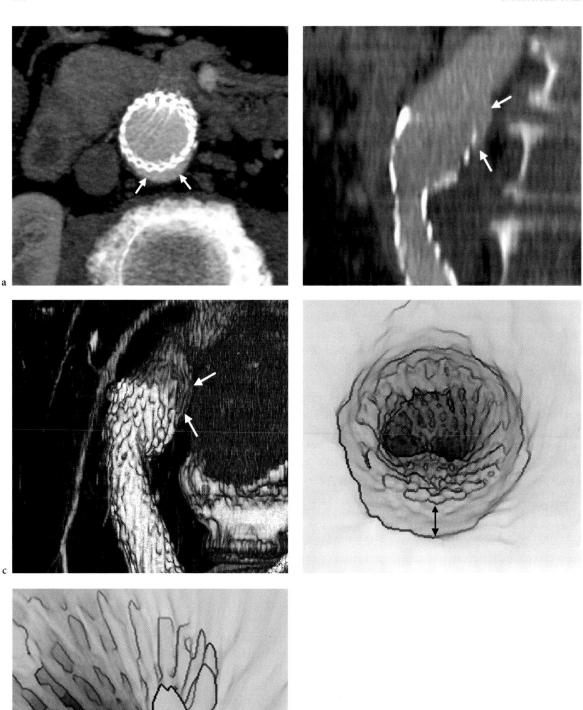

Fig. 14.6. a This proximal type 1 endoleak (*arrows*) occurred 1 month after endoprosthetic treatment of abdominal aortic aneurysm. MPVR with MIP (**b**) obtained along the sagittal plane, and volume rendering (**c**) demonstrate the posterior location of the endoleak (*arrows*). **d, e** Virtual endoscopy generated from the renal arteries level and looking downward shows the detachment of the proximal portion of the endoprosthesis (*arrows*)

presence of atherosclerotic plaques; another cause of stenosis is fibromuscular dysplasia, which occurs almost exclusively in women aged 30–40 years. Renovascular hypertension occurs when stenosis of the renal artery produces a critical narrowing of the lumen. Critical stenosis is defined as at least 70% narrowing of the renal artery (at angiography, CTA or MRA) accompanied by an increase in flow velocity detected at Doppler US; Doppler criteria for a significant stenosis include a peak systolic velocity >180 cm/s with a renal/aortic ratio >3.5.

Three-dimensional image processing has found elective application in postprocessing CTA or MRA data sets.

The imaging strategies in CTA have been discussed by many authors in the last 10 years and in summary the basic principle of all investigators was to use thin collimation (2–3 mm) with an adequate contrast injection, optimizing scan delay (20–30 s for the renal arteries) and flow rate (3–5 ml/s). In MRA the strategy moved from unenhanced to contrast-enhanced acquisition with gadolinium, the latter providing images that are almost comparable to angiography. Most authors agree that in both CTA and MRA native images are sufficient to detect the presence of renal artery stenosis but not to estimate the degree of narrowing. For this purpose an angiographic-like perspective is advocated, and 3D postprocessing is required.

The possibilities for image processing of CTA and MRA have been discussed in Sect. 14.2, and certainly in renal artery stenosis the role of MPR (with thin and thick slabs) and MIP is well accepted. MPR allow multiple oblique planes to be created along the renal artery path with selective study of the arterial segments. In general there are no standardized reconstruction planes or a specific reconstruction protocol, but in our experience the use of MPR starts with a coronal view of the renal arteries to identify the ostium. From the same level the plane can be rotated and moved along the artery path to study the proximal, middle and distal portion of the vessel. In this framework MPR thickening can be increased to generate a subvolume of the data sets and visualize the data with MIP or volume rendering (Fig. 14.7).

The initial interpretation of CTA or MRA examinations is done by an interactive viewing of native images (Berg et al. 1998), but the accurate assessment of the degree and length of stenosis can be done by taking advantage of postprocessing methods. MIP has been widely used in this framework, with either MRA or CTA (Napel et al. 1992; Rubin et al. 1994). More recently Johnson et al. (1999) compared volume rendering of CTA with MIP in assessing renal artery stenosis, and reported that although there was no significant difference in sensitivity, volume rendering led to a significantly higher specificity than MIP (99% vs 87%). The author found the characterization of stenosis to be more reliable in volume rendering than in MIP. This is partly because the former allows the calculation of a weighted sum of voxel values crossing through the ray cast, with inclusion in the final image of even volume-averaged voxels, which are not displayed by MIP. As consequence MIP tends to overestimate stenoses. Another inherent limitation of MIP is the superimposition of structures in the final projection. This specifically affects the evaluation of stenoses caused by calcified plaque; with MIP the hyperdense voxels representing the calcification are difficult to separate from those pertaining to the endoluminal contrast medium, even using multiple projections viewed in a cine mode (Rubin et al. 1994).

Display of calcified plaques and thrombosis (useful in planning angioplasty or renal stenting), and reduced costs for the examination, are the main advantages of CTA over MRA. However, for many reasons the competition between these technique is still open, especially with the recent introduction of CE-MRA. After data acquisition, image processing can be performed with MIP and MPVR images of each renal artery. Normal findings, pitfalls and anatomical variants can be evaluated in detail. It is important to be aware of the existence of accessory or aberrant renal arteries, which are detected by CE-MRA with 3D reconstructions in 75–100% of the cases. Three-dimensional enhanced MRA has good sensitivity and specificity in the detection of proximal renal artery stenosis (88–100% and 71–100%, respectively). No data exist on the use of volume rendering for evaluating renal artery stenosis from CE-MRA data sets, but presumably the contribution of this method is consistent and should be equivalent to that in the case of CTA. In this framework even virtual endoscopy can contribute to defining the severity of a stenosis, although the cause can not be demonstrated as in the case of CTA (Fig. 14.8).

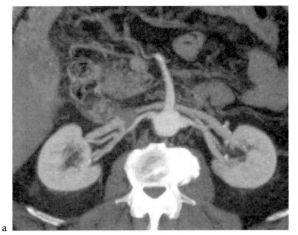

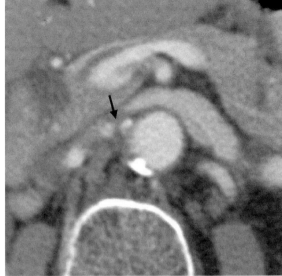

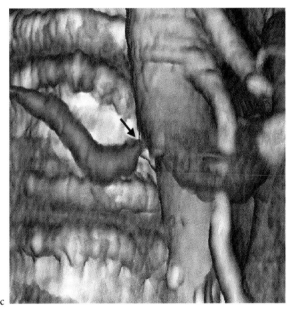

Fig. 14.7a–c. CTA study of the renal arteries. **a** MPVR with MIP generated along the axial plane allows the display of both renal arteries from the origin to the renal hilum, and the exclusion of a stenosis. **b** The use of axial slices alone is enough to detect a stenosis (*arrow*), but the assessment of degree can only be performed by 3D tools. **c** Volume rendering, here represented with color coding, is effective in demonstrating the stenosis (*arrow*) and allows the estimation of its severity

References

Aarts NJ (1999) Abdominal aortic aneurysm measurements for endovascular repair: intra- and interobserver variability of CT measurements. Eur J Vasc Endovasc Surg 18:475–480

Alley MT (1998) Ultrafast contrast-enhanced three-dimensional MR angiography: state of the art. Radiographics 18:273–285

Balm R (1994) Spiral CT-angiography of the aorta. Eur J Vasc Surg 8:544–551

Bartolozzi C (1998) CT in vascular pathologies. Eur Radiol 8:679–684

Berg MH, Manninen HI, Vanninen RL (1998) Assessment of renal artery stenosis with CT angiography: usefulness of multiplanar reformation, quantitative stenosis measurements, and densitometric analysis of renal parenchymal enhancement as adjuncts to MIP film reading. J Comput Assist Tomogr 22:533–540

Bradshaw KA (1998) Multiplanar reformatting and three-dimensional reconstruction: for pre-operative assessment of the thoracic aorta by computed tomography. Clin Radiol 53:198–202

Broeders IA (1997a) Preoperative sizing of grafts for transfemoral endovascular aneurysm management: a prospective comparison study of spiral CT angiography, arterial angiography and conventional CT imaging. J Endovasc Surg 4:252–261

Broeders IA (1997b) Multiplanar reconstructions of spiral CT data: a valuable tool in preoperative sizing of grafts for transfemoral endovascular aneurysm management (TEAM). In: Lemke HU (ed) Computer assisted radiology and surgery. Elsevier Science, Amsterdam. pp 812–817

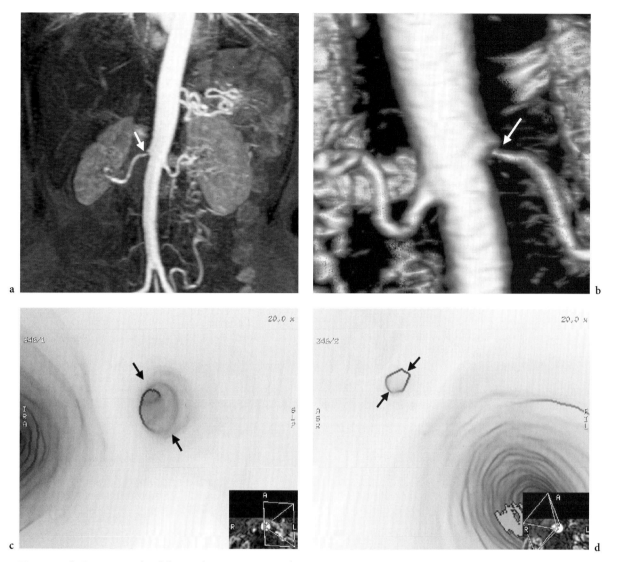

Fig. 14.8a–d. CE-MRA study of the renal arteries. **a** MIP shows a severe stenosis of the right renal artery (arrow). **b** This is confirmed in the posterior view (arrow) by volume rendering and is further demonstrated by virtual endoscopy, comparing left (**c**) and right (**d**) ostia of the renal arteries (arrows), where the right appears significantly smaller

Chen K (1997) Acute thoracic aortic dissection: the basics. J Emerg Med 15:859–867

Chuter TA (1994) Infrarenal aortic aneurysm structure: implications for transfemoral repair. J Vasc Surg 20:44–49

Chung JW (1996) Spiral CT angiography of the thoracic aorta. Radiographics 16:811–824

Gomes MN (1994) Preoperative assessment of abdominal aortic aneurysm: the value of helical and three-dimensional computed tomography. J Vasc Surg 20:367–375

Guo Z, Fenster A (1996) Three-dimensional power doppler imaging: a phantom study to quantify vessel stenosis. Ultrasound Med Biol 22:1059–1069

Hayashi H (1999) Three-dimensional CT angiographic assessment of vascular diseases using various postprocessing techniques: the voxel transmission and cruising eye view methods and their respective merits. Int Angiol 18:113–121

Ho VB, Prince MR (1998) Thoracic MR aortography: imaging techniques and strategies. Radiographics 18:287–309

Huston J III, Heman RL (1993) Comparison of time of flight and phase contrast MR neuroangiographic techniques. Radiographics 13:5–19

Johnson PT, Halpern EJ, Kuszyk BS, Heath DG, Wechsler RJ, Nazarian LN, Gardiner GA, Levin DC, Fishman EK (1999) Renal artery stenosis: CT angiography – comparison of real-time volume-rendering and maximum intensity projection algorithms. Radiology 211:337–343

Kalender WA (1990) Spiral volumetric CT with single-breath-hold technique, continuous transport, and continuous scanner rotation. Radiology 176:181–183

Kimura F (1996) Thoracic aortic aneurysm and aortic dissection: new endoscopic mode for three-dimensional CT display of aorta. Radiology 198:573–538

Kramer SC (2001) Geometric changes in aortic endografts over a 2-year observation period. J Endovasc Ther 8:34–38

Krinsky GA (1997) Thoracic aorta: comparison of gadolinium-enhanced three-dimensional MR angiography with conventional MR imaging. Radiology 202:183–193

Lim TH, Saloner D, Anderson CM (1989) Current applications of magnetic resonance vascular imaging. Cardiol Clin 7:661-683

Lu B (2000) Electron beam tomography with three-dimensional reconstruction in the diagnosis of aortic diseases. J Cardiovasc Surg 41:659–668

Nakanishi T (1997) Electron-beam CT angiography for thoracic aortic aneurysm and dissection: application of continuous volume scan and electrocardiographically triggered scan. Radiat Med 15:155–161

Napel S, Marks MP, Rubin GD (1992) CT angiography with spiral CT and maximum intensity projection. Radiology 185:607–610

Nelson TR, Pretorius DH (1998) Three-dimensional ultrasound imaging. Ultrasound Med Biol 24:1243–1270

Neri E (1999) CT 3D angiography of abdominal aortic aneurysms for predicting intraoperative suprarenal aortic cross-clamping. Radiology 213:S438

Nitatori T (1999) Clinical application of single shot GRE-EPI as non-enhanced MRA (EPI-MRA) for aortic aneurysm and dissection. Radiat Med 17:393–397

Picot P (1993) Three-dimensional colour Doppler imaging. Ultrasound Med Biol 19:95–104

Pollock JG (2000) Volumetric analysis of abdominal aortic aneurysms following endovascular repair. Cardiovasc Intervent Radiol 23 (Suppl 1):120

Prince MR (1996) Three-dimensional gadolinium-enhanced MR angiography of the thoracic aorta. AJR 166:1387–1397

von Ramm OT, Smith SW (1990) Real time volumetric ultrasound imaging system. J Digit Imaging 3:261–266

Rickey D (1995) A wall-less vessel phantom for Doppler ultrasound studies. J Ultrasound Med Biol 21: 1163–1176

Rubin GD (1993) Three-dimensional spiral CT angiography of the abdomen: initial clinical experience. Radiology 186:147–152

Rubin GD (1998) Measurement of the aorta and its branches with helical CT. Radiology 206:823–829

Rubin GD (2000) Aorta and iliac arteries: single versus multiple detector-row helical CT angiography. Radiology 215:670–676

Rubin GD, Dake MD, Napel S (1994) Spiral CT of renal artery stenosis: comparison of three-dimensional rendering techniques. Radiology 190:181–189

Singer JR (1959) Blood flow rates by nuclear magnetic resonance measurements. Science 130:1652–1653

Smith PA (1998) Virtual angioscopy using spiral CT and real-time interactive volume-rendering techniques. J Comput Assist Tomogr 22:212–214

Stetten GD (1998) Real-time 3D ultrasound: a new look at the heart. J Cardiovasc Diagn Proc 15:73–84

Subasic M (2000) 3-D image analysis of abdominal aortic aneurysm. Stud Health Technol Inform 77:1195–2000

Valk PE, Hale JD, Kaufman L (1985) MR imaging of the aorta with three-dimensional vessel reconstruction: validation by angiography. Radiology 157:721–725

Watanabe Y (2000) Dynamic subtraction contrast-enhanced MR angiography: technique, clinical applications, and pitfalls. Radiographics 20:135–152

White GH (1999) Endotension: an explanation for continued AAA growth after successful endoluminal repair. J Endovasc Surg 6:308–315

Zeman RK (1995) Diagnosis of aortic dissection: value of helical CT with multiplanar reformation and three-dimensional rendering. AJR 164:1375–1380

15 Peripheral Vessels

Carlo Catalano, Francesco Fraioli, Alessandro Napoli, Federica Pediconi,
Massimiliano Danti, Andrea Laghi, Roberto Passariello

CONTENTS

15.1
Introduction

Obstructive arterial disease of the lower extremities is an extremely common disease in Western countries (Dormandy et al. 1999a; Tierney et al. 2000) that requires an accurate diagnosis for correct treatment planning (Dormandy et al. 1999b; Semba et al. 2000). The examination of choice for the assessment of patients with obstructive arterial disease is X-ray angiography, which correctly demonstrates the arterial anatomy; nevertheless, its invasiveness has led to the development of noninvasive examinations. In many arterial districts X-ray angiography has been progressively substituted by noninvasive examinations, among which are magnetic resonance angiography (MRA) and computed tomography angiography (CTA) (Dillon et al. 1993; Schmiedl et al. 1996).

Contrast-enhanced MRA provides excellent results in the assessment of the runoff vessels; continuous developments have significantly improved the technique, which requires a short acquisition time and has become extremely reliable in the evaluation not only of large vessels but also of distal trifurcation vessels. The typical features of the MRA acquisition do not require a sophisticated three-dimensional rendering algorithm and therefore make this technique

straightforward. As a result, contrast-enhanced MRA has increasingly substituted in several centers for X-ray angiography.

In the assessment of the peripheral arterial district, due to the length of the volume to be examined, CTA could not previously be used because of technical limitations. However, the recent development of multi-row detector computed tomography (MRDCT) has completely revolutionized and improved the technique of CTA (Hu 1999), and the possibility of scanning large volumes allows the routine examination of arterial districts which could not previously be examined with single-slice spiral CTA (Rubin et al. 1999). Furthermore in multi-row detector CTA some of the disadvantages of single-slice spiral CTA, such as the use of large doses of iodinated contrast agent and the high X-ray dose to the patient, are being reduced due to the speed of acquisition (smaller amount of contrast agent) and technical improvements (reduction of the X-ray dose to the patient).

The rapid development of scanners and software has resulted in exciting new applications in medical practice. Different reconstruction algorithms for three-dimensional (3D) acquisitions of CTA and MRA is now a major area of clinical and academic interest. Three-dimensional reconstructions generate clinically accurate and immediately available images from the full computer tomography (Rubin et al. 1993) and magnetic resonance data set without extensive editing. In contrast to the growing problem of information overload presented by the large acquisition rates of modern scanners, rendering techniques have the potential to simplify the standard radiological study.

The advent of MRDCT, MRA and 3D rendering has allowed the noninvasive, detailed investigation of the entire vasculature, running down to more distal vessels (Fig. 15.1). The combination of powerful gradients, non-nephrotoxic contrast agents and moving tables has made contrast-enhanced MRA part of the investigation of patients with peripheral vascular disease. The combination of intravenously administered nonionic contrast material, multidetector array CT assemblies, X-ray tubes with higher heat capacity,

C. Catalano, MD, M. Danti, MD, F. Fraioli, MD, A. Laghi, MD, A. Napoli, MD, R. Passariello, MD, F. Pediconi, MD
Department of Radiology, University of Rome "La Sapienza", Policlinico Umberto I, Viale Regina Elena 324, 00161 Rome, Italy

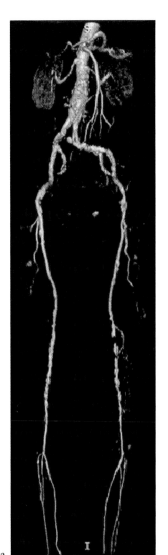

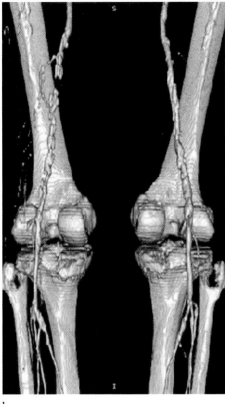

b

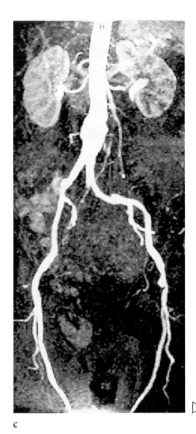

c

Fig. 15.1. a The large volume of multi-row detector CT allows the coverage of arterial segments from the celiac trunk down to the ankles. b A back view 3D volume rendered image, without bone editing, correctly shows the distal vessels. c, d In the same patient MRA provides the same information but needs two different acquisitions

a

faster helical rotation times (McCollough and Zink 1999), more powerful computers and advanced reformation algorithms has led to the acceptance of CTA as an alternative to conventional angiography.

15.2
Magnetic Resonance Angiography

A fast 3D spoiled gradient echo MR imaging sequence with minimum repetition time and echo time is needed to achieve a contrast-enhanced MRA study of the runoff vessels (Klingenbeck-Regn et al. 1999). By using this type of sequence, intrinsic tissue contrast is low and vascular contrast is achieved with high intravascular concentrations of paramagnetic contrast agent, which is injected intravenously as a bolus with an automatic injector. The first pass of the contrast material bolus provides a brief temporal window of high intravascular concentration, which in turn generates high signal intensity by means of T1 shortening of the blood. As venous filling reduces image quality, timing is very important; the best images are obtained when acquisition of the central portion of k space corresponds with the maximum concentration of contrast material in the vessels of interest.

The method of choice is the timing bolus (Maki et al. 1998), in which a small amount of contrast agent is injected along with saline solution for flushing and the vessel of interest is scanned approximately once per second. The circulation time can be directly observed and then used to calculate the correct scan delay. This method almost always yields MR angio-

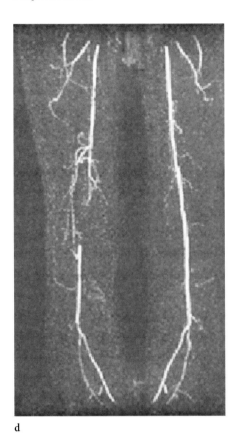

d

grams with excellent contrast. Disadvantages of this technique include residual contrast material in the renal collecting systems from the test bolus, which can obscure visualization of branch vessels of the renal arteries during MRA, as well as the additional time required for the test bolus sequence.

Contrast-enhanced peripheral MRA can be performed with good results with almost any medium to high field strength equipment; powerful gradients are required to reduce the scan time and improve the signal-to-noise ratio. The examination can be performed by means of three separate acquisitions at the level of the aorta and ilio-femoral vessels, the thigh vessels, and the popliteal and calf vessels. By using this method of acquisition three different boluses of contrast agent must be injected, after calculation of a delay time for the first volume; an empirically determined further 10 s delay, based on the delay time of the first acquisition, provides excellent results in most cases. If three separate acquisitions and contrast agent injections are utilized, a precontrast sequence should be acquired in the second and third stations in order to perform a subtraction and eliminate venous signal and background noise arising from prior contrast administration. By doing so, excellent arterial enhancement is achieved also in the thigh and calf vessels (Fig. 15.2). An entire runoff study requires nevertheless a relatively long acquisition time. More recently the development of moving tables (LEINER et al. 2000) has allowed acquisition of an entire peripheral MRA study after injection of a single bolus of contrast agent. In addition to moving tables a significant improvement in signal-to-noise ratio and image quality is provided by dedicated extremity coils which are adapted to the size of the volume to be examined.

A further improvement in signal enhancement and signal-to-noise ratio can be achieved by means of high-relaxivity paramagnetic contrast agents, which appear particularly useful in the assessment of small peripheral arterial branches.

15.2.1
Data Processing

Data processing is an important aspect of 3D contrast-enhanced MRA. A variety of reconstruction techniques are now available to the radiologist, and it is important to be well versed in as many of these as possible. Each technique has its own strengths and weaknesses, which can lead to pitfalls and artefacts in inexperienced hands.

Maximum intensity projection (MIP) imaging is the most common means of displaying data. With this technique, a ray is projected along the data set in the desired direction, and the highest voxel value along the ray becomes the pixel value of the two-dimensional MIP image. This method is well suited to contrast-enhanced MRA, particularly arterial-phase imaging, in which background signal is low and arterial contrast is high. Nevertheless, MIP images obtained from the entire data set are almost always contaminated somewhat by wraparound or edge artefacts, which can limit the visibility of vessels. Image quality can almost always be improved by obtaining subvolume MIP images or by manually editing the entire data set. Standard coronal and oblique views are often sufficient for diagnosis; if not, additional projections can easily be obtained.

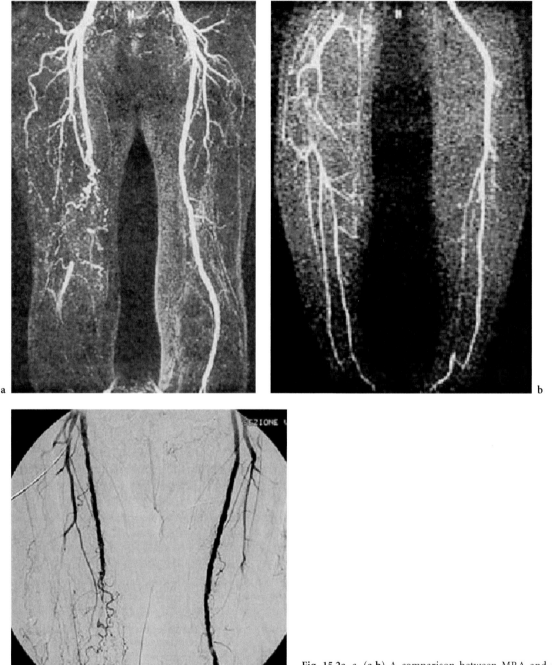

Fig. 15.2a–c. (a,b) A comparison between MRA and digital subtraction angiography (c) allows a good depiction of obstruction of the vessels of the thigh and popliteal vessels

MIP images are useful and are generally preferred by clinicians. However, source images or thin-section reconstructed images should be examined routinely because severe stenosis and non-occlusive thrombus can easily be missed on MIP images, which may be a cause of error due to overestimation.

Subtraction of a precontrast data set from the arterial-phase data is widely used in 3D contrast-enhanced MRA of the lower extremities (RUEHM et al. 2001), as previously mentioned, to eliminate background noise and provide better visualization of smaller vessels.

An important tool in contrast-enhanced MRA is vessel tracking, which allows vessels to be followed along their course and therefore facilitates the reconstruction process and eliminates superimposition of other structures such as the veins (LEINER et al. 2000). Vessel tracking appears particularly useful if intravascular contrast agents are used. In fact these types of contrast agents produce opacification of all vascular structures and difficulties in their differentiation. In this respect, volume rendering might be useful, allowing separation of arterial and venous structures by perspective view. Volume rendering, surface rendering and virtual endoscopy are alternative techniques that may be useful in certain applications. Volume rendering in particular is now widely available on most new MR workstations, although it currently has limited applications, mainly as the consequence of the excellent results with MIP and selective MIP reconstructions. Although all reconstruction techniques provide excellent results in contrast-enhanced MRA, raw data must still be analyzed, especially when information on peripheral distal branches, which may be obscured in the reconstruction process, is needed.

Three-dimensional contrast-enhanced MRA is not without its limitations. Many patients are not candidates for MRA because of pacemakers, aneurysm clips or claustrophobia. Others may not be capable of performing breath-holds sufficient to obtain a diagnostic angiogram. Metallic clips, stents and embolization coils can cause considerable artefact and obscure important structures. Even when the study is optimal, the resolution of contrast-enhanced MRA is relatively low compared with that of conventional angiography (Fig. 15.3), and visualization of small peripheral arteries is very limited. Contrast-enhanced MRA, although less expensive than conventional angiography, is still an expensive examination.

15.3 CT Angiography

Vascular arterial assessment by means of spiral CTA is made possible by very thin collimation and increased speed of acquisition (HU et al. 2000), which allow scanning of relatively large volumes during the arterial pass of iodinated contrast agents. Although spiral CT is ubiquitous in clinical practice and there is always a larger demand for 3D rendering, single-slice spiral CT data sets are characterized by differences between axial and longitudinal resolution (POLACIN et al. 1992; RUBIN et al. 1996); as a consequence isotropic voxels cannot be obtained (RUBIN et al. 1999).

Spiral CT has been completely revolutionized by the recent introduction of multidetector technology,

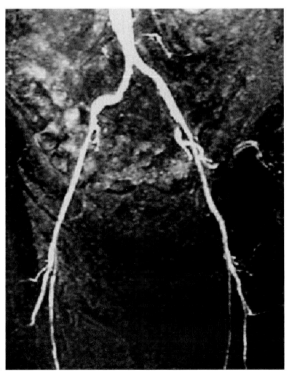

a

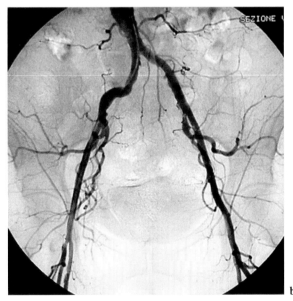

b

Fig. 15.3a,b. The low resolution of MIP MRA examination (**a**) in comparison with digital subtraction angiography (**b**), especially in the peripheral arteries

which allows the acquisition, per single rotation of the gantry, of four slices (and very soon a larger number of slices); furthermore the gantry rotation time has been reduced to 0.5 s compared with 0.75–1 s for single-slice spiral CT. The combination of the acquisition of four slices per gantry rotation and increased speed of rotation has led to a significant reduction in the acquisition time per volume – up to 8 times compared with single-slice spiral CT scanners. Improvements in the capacity of the generator and X-ray tube allow the acquisition to be prolonged and therefore large volumes to be studied (KLINGEN-BECK-REGN et al. 1999). MRDCT scanners therefore allow the examination of large volumes, something not achievable with single-slice CT scanners; high resolution volumes (thin collimation) with improvement of longitudinal resolution (FISHMAN 1997); and near-isotropic voxels. This last feature permits high-quality data sets for excellent diagnosis and 3D rendering (Fig. 15.4).

Single-slice scanners do not allow runoff studies to be performed and therefore this application of CTA represent a real innovation with multislice technology (RUBIN et al. 2000).

Patient Positioning. Patients can be positioned either feet-first or head-first; however, a wider volume can be examined by positioning the patient supine with the feet first. Furthermore when the patient is positioned head-first the table movement does not allow examination of the distal tract of the thigh vessels and the ankles, even if the patient is not particularly tall. On the contrary if the patient is positioned with the feet first it is possible to widen the examination volume down to the ankles, and if necessary down to the pedal circulation. It is furthermore important, exactly as it is advisable in conventional arteriography, to fix the patient's feet in introversion in order to separate the tibia from the fibula and as a consequence the trifurcation vessels, which have a course parallel to the bony structures. The separation of vessels from bony structures is essential to simplify the 3D reconstructions following the acquisition. In order to avoid even minimal motion artefacts during the acquisition it is advisable to fix the patient's feet.

Scanning Protocol. After a 1024 mm initial topogram, the acquisition volume is positioned in such a way as to comprise all arterial structures from the suprarenal abdominal aorta down to the ankles, reaching, if possible, the feet also. The largest volume achievable is currently 120 cm, which is sufficient in most cases. The limitation, in terms of examination volume, is

related to the motion of the table, which can be exploited to the maximum, as mentioned previously, if the patient is positioned feet-first. The protocol we use consists of a 4×2.5 mm collimation with a slice thickness of reconstructed images of 3 mm. The reconstruction interval is 3 mm. This enables 120 cm to be covered in a scanning time of 40 s, during which approximately 400 images are produced. If necessary the acquired volume can then be reconstructed at different slice thicknesses and/or different reconstruction intervals. In particular, in order to obtain greater detail, especially at the level of the origin of the renal arteries and of the distal trifurcation vessels, images are reconstructed with a slice interval of 1 mm, which means an overlap of 2 mm.

Intravenous Administration of the Contrast Agent. In order to obtain a good CTA examination of the peripheral arteries, correct intravenous administration of iodinated contrast agent is crucial (FLEISCHMANN et al. 2000). A 17–18 gauge intravenous cannula must be inserted in an antecubital vein; its patency is verified by flushing with saline solution. Different types of iodinated contrast agents can be utilized in CTA. In our experience the best results are obtained using an agent with a high iodine concentration (400 mg I/ml). In fact the comparison with contrast agents with a lower concentration of iodine (300 and 350 mg I/ml) has shown an increase in arterial enhancement directly proportional to the concentration of iodine in the contrast agent, while maintaining the same overall amount of iodine injected (40 g I/examination).

Regarding the flow velocity, the best results are obtained with a flow rate of 4 ml/s, with a uniphasic injection. In our early experience with MRDCT no technique for calculation of the patient delay time (test bolus or bolus chasing) was available, and therefore it was decided empirically, based on previous experiences with single-slice-spiral CT and MRA, to utilize a fixed delay time in all patients of 25–28 s. Of more than 120 patients examined to date with this method, in less than 5% was the arterial opacification inadequate. In young patients the delay time can be reduced to a few seconds; in general in patients with obstructive arterial disease and claudication, a fixed delay time can be satisfactorily utilized. Nevertheless if the clinical suspicion is aneurysmal disease (i.e. popliteal artery aneurysm) (Fig. 15.5), the delay time may be prolonged at the level of the dilatation and it can be considered to use a longer delay time or to calculate the delay time by means of a test bolus if available.

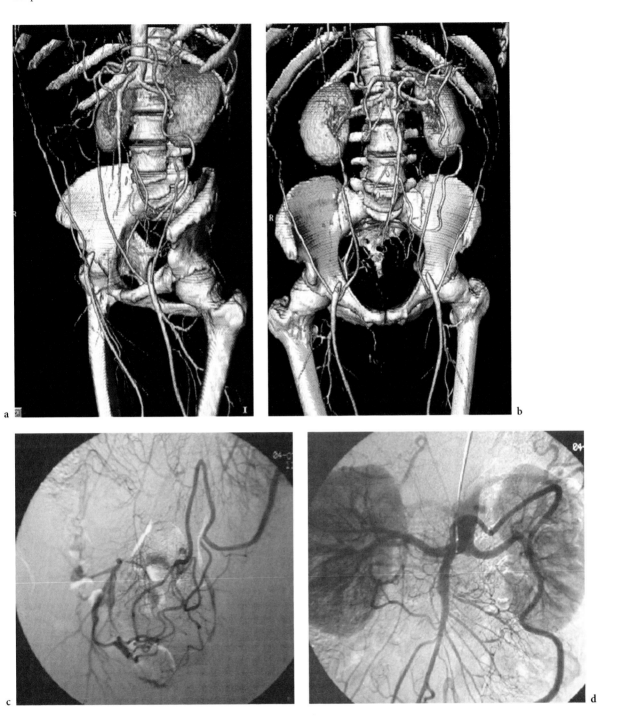

Fig. 15.4a–d. Three-dimensional volume rendered CTA (**a,b**) shows the obstruction of the aorta and iliac arteries in a patient with Leriche's syndrome, with excellent delineation of the collateral vessels, superior to digital subtraction angiography (**c,d**)

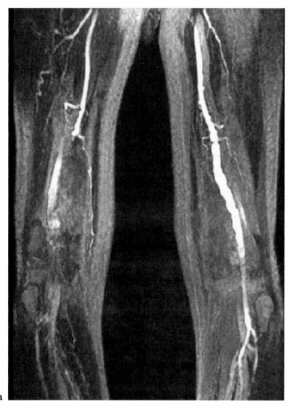

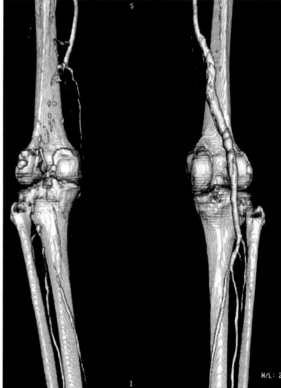

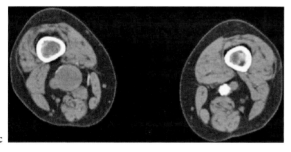

Fig. 15.5a–c. The thrombus responsible for this obstruction of the popliteal artery is well seen in the axial plane (c), while is not visualized either on coronal MIP MRA (a) or on volume rendered CTA techniques (b)

In no case have we found venous enhancement overlying arterial segments that impaired the image quality.

15.3.1
Data Processing

In contrast to contrast-enhanced MRA, which is based on 3D acquisition along the longitudinal axis of the vessel (i.e. the coronal plane in runoff studies), in multi-row detector CTA the volume is acquired in the transverse axis, which means dealing with a large quantity of images and a data set much greater than that obtained with MRA.

Again in contrast to MRA, in which most of the reconstructions are performed simply using the MIP algorithm, with CTA several different algorithms are used (Hayashi et al. 1999) and useful, each of them providing important information (Fig. 15.6).

The development of MRDCT provides, for the first time, true volume data sets; it means that scrolling all data sets is unsatisfactory, as the volume data set grows from 50 to 100 to 200 to 500 to 1000 images per patient study. The information seen on axial CT alone is very limited for some applications and totally unsatisfactory for many others; while axial images are fine for detecting an aortic aneurysm, they might not be ideal for defining its relationship with, for instance, the renal arteries, or whether the aneurysm

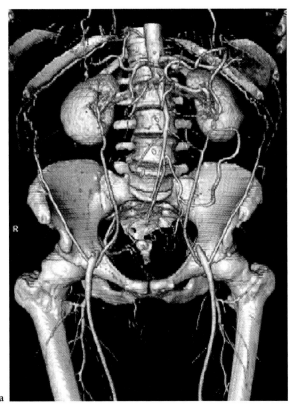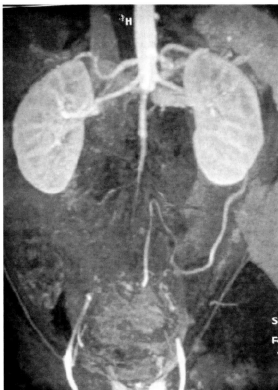

a   b

Fig. 15.6a,b. Three-dimensional volume rendered CTA (a) compares well with MIP MRA (b)

needs surgery or can be treated with an endovascular approach. Axial images are limited for the radiologist, but even more for the vascular surgeon. The limitation of axial display only is obvious from the magnetic resonance paradigm, one of its key values being its multiplanarity. While CT was able to present axial images reformatted into coronal, sagittal or oblique planes, the reconstructions were limited in quality, especially due to anisotropy. The introduction of MRDCT now allows excellent 3D reconstructions in any plane, with image quality similar, and in many cases clearly superior, to the direct multiplanar acquisitions of MR imaging (HONG and FREENY 1999). It must be clear, therefore, that the display can no longer be based on axial images but must be a true volume display.

We must therefore move towards a concept of real-time 3D interaction, taking advantage of all available reconstruction algorithms; it becomes possible to display and select any portion of the scan volume interactively, and what is even more important, instantaneously (KIM et al. 2000).

Multiplanar reconstruction (MPR) is very useful for rapidly obtaining all the information needed and for rapidly scrolling the 3D data set in either coronal, sagittal or oblique views (Fig. 15.7). MPR provides the best results if contemporaneous information on vascular structures and parenchymal organs is needed (COLL et al. 2000).

MIP is the most common means of displaying vascular data. With this technique, the highest voxel value along a ray projected in the data set becomes the pixel value of the two-dimensional MIP image. This method provides excellent results in MRDCT angiography (Fig. 15.8), particularly if thin MIPs are utilized and modulated in order to avoid bony structures.

Volume rendering is the representation, visualization and manipulation of objects represented as sampled data in three or more dimensions. Volume rendering, unlike standard reconstruction algorithms, does not distort objects (MASUTANI et al. 2001); the perspective information is the main feature of volume rendering.

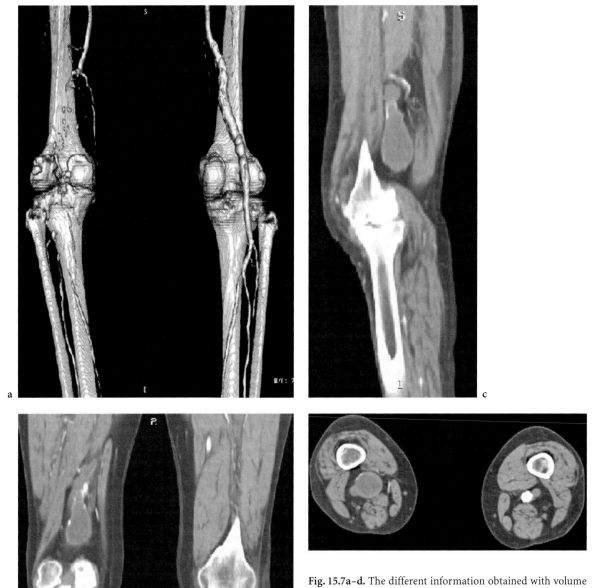

Fig. 15.7a–d. The different information obtained with volume rendering, MPR and axial plane imaging. **a** Volume rendering allows good delineation of the extent of the obstruction and vessel calcification. **b, c** MPR in different planes provides perfect visualization of the morphology and length of the popliteal thrombus. **d** Axial plane imaging confirms the findings

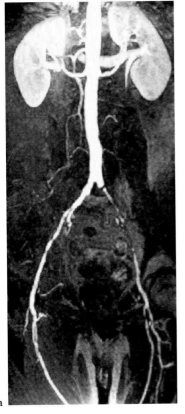

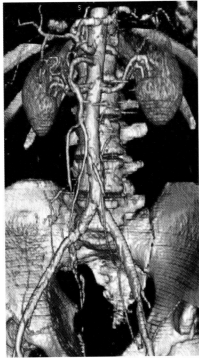

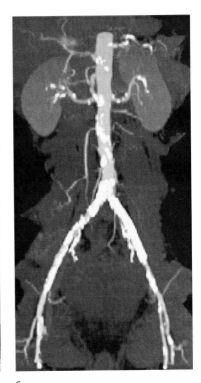

b

c

Fig. 15.8a–c. The left iliac stent responsible for the signal void in MRA (**a**) is well visualized with both volume rendering (**b**) and MIP (**c**) techniques

a

References

Coll DM, Herts BR, Davros WJ (2000) Preoperative use of 3D volume rendering to demonstrate renal tumors and renal anatomy. Radiographics 20:431–438

Dillon EH, van Leeuwen MS, Fernandez MA (1993) Spiral CT angiography. AJR 160:1273–1278

Dormandy J, Heeck L, Vig S (1999a) Predictors of early disease in the lower limbs. Semin Vasc Surg 12:109–117

Dormandy J, Heeck L, Vig S (1999b) Peripheral arterial occlusive disease: clinical data for decision making. Introduction. Semin Vasc Surg 12:95

Fishman EK (1997) High-resolution three-dimensional imaging from subsecond helical CT data sets: applications in vascular imaging. AJR 169:441–443

Fleischmann D, Rubin GD, Alexander A (2000) Improved uniformity of aortic enhancement with customized contrast medium injection protocols at CT angiography. Radiology 214: 363–371

Hayashi H, Kobayashi H, Takagi R (1999) Three-dimensional CT angiographic assessment of vascular diseases using various postprocessing techniques: the voxel transmission and cruising eye view methods and their respective merits. Int Angiol 18:113–121

Hong KC, Freeny PC (1999) Pancreaticoduodenal arcades and dorsal pancreatic artery: comparison of CT angiography with three-dimensional volume rendering, maximum intensity projection, and shaded surface display. AJR 172:925–931

Hu H (1999) Multi-slice helical CT: scan and reconstruction. Med Phys 26:5–18

Hu H, He D, Dennis W, Foley WD (2000) Four multidetector-row helical CT: image quality and volume coverage speed. Radiology 215: 55–62

Kim TH, Kim YM, Suh CH (2000) Helical CT angiography and three-dimensional reconstruction of total anomalous pulmonary venous connections in neonates and infants. AJR 175:1381–1386

Klingenbeck-Regn K, Schaller S, Flohr T (1999) Subsecond multi-slice computed tomography: basics and applications. Eur J Radiol 31:110–124

Leiner T, Ho KY, Nelemans PJ (2000) Three-dimensional contrast-enhanced moving-bed infusion-tracking (MoBI-track) peripheral MR angiography with flexible choice of imaging parameters for each field of view. J Magn Reson Imaging 11:368–377

Maki JH, Chenevert TL, Prince MR (1998) Contrast-enhanced MR angiography. Abdom Imaging 23:469–484

Masutani Y, MacMahon H, Doi K (2001) Automated segmentation and visualization of the pulmonary vascular tree in spiral CT angiography: an anatomy-oriented approach based on three-dimensional image analysis. J Comput Assist Tomogr 25:587–597

McCollough CH, Zink FE (1999) Performance evaluation of a multi-slice CT system. Med Phys 26:2223–2230

Polacin A, Kalender WA, Marchal G (1992) Evaluation of section sensitivity profiles and image noise in spiral CT. Radiology 185:29–35

Rubin GD, Walker PJ, Dake MD (1993) 3D spiral CT angiography: an alternative imaging modality for the abdominal aorta and its branches. J Vasc Surg 18:656–666

Rubin GD, Napel SA, Ringl H (1996) Assessment of section profile and clinical images in helical CT with pitch values of 0.5–3.0 by using 180° linear extrapolation and segmented reconstruction. Radiology 201(P):246

Rubin GD, Shiau MC, Schmidt AJ (1999) Computed tomographic angiography: historical perspective and new state-of-the-art using multi detector-row helical computed tomography. J Comput Assist Tomogr 23(Suppl 1):83–90

Rubin GD, Shiau MC, Leung AN (2000) Aorta and iliac arteries: single versus multiple detector-row helical CT angiography. Radiology 215:670–676

Ruehm SG, Nanz D, Baumann A (2001) 3D contrast-enhanced MR angiography of the run-off vessels: value of image subtraction. J Magn Reson Imaging 13:402–411

Schmiedl UP, Yuan C, Nghiem HV (1996) MR angiography of the peripheral vasculature. Semin Ultrasound CT MR 17:404–411

Semba CP, Murphy TP, Bakal CW (2000) Thrombolytic therapy with use of Alteplase (rt-PA) in peripheral arterial occlusive disease: review of the clinical literature. The Advisory Panel. J Vasc Interv Radiol 11(P1):149–161

Tierney S, Fennessy F, Hayes DB (2000) ABC of arterial and vascular disease. Secondary prevention of peripheral vascular disease. BMJ 320:1262–1265

16 Esophagus and Stomach

Andrea Laghi, Valeria Panebianco, Isabella Baeli, Riccardo Iannaccone,
Franco Iafrate, Roberto Passariello

CONTENTS

16.1
Introduction

Although the introduction of double-contrast radiographic techniques has reduced the comparative advantage of endoscopy over barium studies (LEVINE et al. 1987), most papers suggest that upper gastrointestinal endoscopy is more accurate (KETO et al. 1979), particularly regarding the evaluation of inflammatory mucosal abnormalities, bleeding lesions (THOENI and CELLO 1980) and the postoperative stomach (OMINSKY and MOSS 1979).

Upper gastrointestinal endoscopy is a safe and effective technique, which not only has diagnostic advantages but also provides the opportunity to perform interventional procedures (biopsy, sclerotherapy, etc.). A very important limitation is that upper gastrointestinal endoscopy displays only the inner surface of hollow organs, thus preventing evaluation of the transmural extent of tumors (LEVINE et al. 1987). Fur-

I. BAELI, MD, F. IAFRATE, MD, R. IANNACCONE, MD, A. LAGHI, MD, V. PANEBIANCO, MD, R. PASSARIELLO, MD
Department of Radiology, University of Rome "La Sapienza", Policlinico Umberto I, Viale Regina Elena 324, 00161 Rome, Italy

thermore, disease extension to surrounding anatomical structures cannot be detected. These limitations are the major impetus in the search for an inexpensive technique that would provide both endoscopic and exoscopic information simultaneously (GONVERS and BURNAND 1996; SCHMID et al. 1999).

Both CT and MR imaging have proven to be valuable adjuncts to barium studies and endoscopy in the evaluation of gastric and esophageal diseases because of their ability to delineate the primary pathological condition and demonstrate how far the disease has extended to adjacent or distant organs. The continuing development of helical CT equipment, with the ultimate progress represented by multislice technology, has improved the quality of volumetric data sets by diminishing respiratory misregistration artefacts and allowing data collection of larger volumes with a narrower collimation, thus ensuring higher-resolution images (JOHNSON and HEATH 1996). In the case of MR imaging, the availability of high-performance gradient systems, together with fast scanning techniques, has allowed acquisition of complex three-dimensional (3D) data sets within the confines of a comfortable breath-hold (LEUNG and MCKINNON 1996). The further advantage of MR imaging is its ability to perform multiplanar acquisition, which is particularly useful when evaluating the esophagus and the stomach to detect the longitudinal extension of a lesion.

Thus, currently, both spiral CT and MR imaging are able to provide volumetric data sets suitable for 3D reconstructions using dedicated software. The utility of 3D images provides improved evaluation of the anatomical relationships between different organs, especially when extramural invasion is suspected. Moreover, conventional slice-to-slice presentation of data sets precludes contiguous viewing of the inner wall, forcing radiologists to create a mental picture of anatomical continuity, which can be faulty. The most recent development in volumetric analysis is virtual reality imaging, a form of interactive 3D imaging that provides computer-rendered intraluminal views of any hollow viscera, comparable to fiberoptic viewing. Virtual endoscopy enables the operator to virtually navigate inside the organs using data sets extracted from CT scans or MR images (JOLESZ and LORENSEN 1997).

In this chapter, we will review the specific technical requirements necessary to obtain adequate studies of the esophagus and stomach and the clinical applications of 3D imaging techniques.

16.2
Study Techniques

Specific techniques are necessary to acquire data sets suitable for 3D reconstructions. Together with the optimization of acquisition parameters, luminal distension of hollow viscera is also mandatory if evaluation of the parietal wall and virtual endoscopy images are required. Different techniques for optimizing both CT and MR studies have been proposed, all of which aim to minimize patient discomfort and increase the quality of image data sets. Following the acquisition of the data set, images must be reconstructed using dedicated software, which uses different algorithms to generate 3D reconstructions.

16.2.1
Computed Tomography

Optimal 3D image rendering requires high-resolution data acquisition, both in-plane (X- and Y-axis) and through-plane (Z-axis). For this reason, voxels should be isotropic, i.e., have the same dimensions along the three axes, and be as small as possible, in order to increase spatial resolution. With single-slice spiral CT, however, the effective slice thickness is greater than the collimation width, and this is directly proportional to pitch value, thereby reducing the longitudinal spatial resolution along the Z-axis. On the other hand, a high pitch value is also necessary to increase the volume coverage. Thus, a compromise between volume to be acquired and longitudinal spatial resolution is necessary, the primary goal being the acquisition of the entire volumetric data set within a single breath-hold to avoid respiratory misregistration artefacts. The longitudinal resolution is considered adequate when the effective slice thickness is less than or equal to the lesion diameter.

Longitudinal resolution can be maximized, however, when images are overlapped. For imaging applications that require maximal longitudinal resolution,

single-slice spiral CT images should be reconstructed with at least 60% overlap relative to the effective slice thickness. The use of highly overlapping source images (87–90%) is not necessary to generate 3D images and it increases the time of image reconstruction and the size of the volumetric data set, thus mandating the need for more powerful workstations.

Scan protocols should be optimized in conjunction with the specific technical features of different spiral CT scanners, especially in terms of gantry rotation time and volume coverage with a single spiral scan. However, a routine scan protocol, achievable on several types of equipment, should be based on 3 mm collimation thickness, 2 mm image reconstruction and a pitch less than 2, with the value depending strictly on gantry rotation time. Such a protocol should allow coverage of the entire anatomical region under evaluation, either the esophagus or the stomach, with a longitudinal resolution compatible with good-quality 3D reconstructions.

An optimal study technique for multi-row detector spiral CT equipment remains to be established. With multi-row detector spiral CT, however, either the scan time can be reduced dramatically compared with conventional spiral CT, with a consequent reduction in radiation dose, or the volume to be investigated can be extended. The volume coverage speed of a four-slice multidetector spiral CT can be at least twice as fast with fully comparable image quality or, in many cases, three times as fast with diagnostically comparable image quality. Thus, a high-resolution study of the upper abdomen can be performed using 1 mm slice collimation and image reconstruction, which provides near-isotropic resolution along the longitudinal axis. On the other hand, if the speed of the acquisition must be maximized, but still preserving a data set compatible with image manipulation and 3D reconstructions, 3 mm slice collimation with subsequent 2 mm image reconstruction could be an appropriate choice.

16.2.1.1
Esophagus

The esophagus is a hollow organ and may appear collapsed on routine CT. Its nondistended wall, even if normal, may appear thickened, nodular and irregular, thus simulating a tumor. Furthermore, it is difficult to judge the superior and inferior extent of esophageal tumors on standard CT examinations (LYANG and CHAN 1996). When the esophagus is adequately distended prior to examination, 3D image reconstruction of the esophageal lumen is possible.

In the evaluation of esophageal diseases, the use of an antiperistaltic drug suppresses normal peristalsis, which may simulate tumor thickening of the esophageal wall. Realistic 3D reconstruction of esophageal tumors is dependent on good gaseous distension of the esophagus above and below the tumor, which can be obtained by oral administration of effervescent granules prior to examination.

Griffith and Kew (1999) evaluated 70 patients with known esophageal cancer. The study technique included the oral administration of a capsule of effervescent granules mixed with water immediately prior to scanning, together with an intravenous injection of an antispasmodic drug; intravenous injection of iodinated contrast medium was also performed to evaluate the liver parenchyma. The imaging protocol included a scan of the thorax and upper abdomen with the patient in the prone position during a single breath-hold, with beam collimation of 10 mm and a pitch of 1.5. However, the scan time of 20–25 s was sometimes too long for frail esophageal tumor patients and insertion of a breath interval was necessary; the location of this breath interval was chosen away from the esophageal tumor. Alternatively, the pitch was increased to 2, thus reducing the scan time by one-quarter.

In our experience with multi-row detector spiral CT, we perform a single scan acquisition with the patient in the supine position beginning 20–25 s after intravenous administration of iodinated contrast medium; to maximize mucosal detail and to proceed with a realistic detailed view of lesions, we acquire images with a collimation thickness of 3 mm, a pitch of 1.0 and image reconstruction of 1 mm. Prior to examination, esophageal luminal distension is obtained with the oral administration of effervescent granules.

16.2.1.2
Stomach

For the stomach as well as the esophagus, luminal distension and reduction of peristaltic motion are mandatory in order to obtain high-quality 3D data sets (Lee and Ko 1996, 1999a). The required contrast difference between the gastric wall and its lumen can be enhanced by ingestion of positive or negative contrast materials. Positive oral contrast materials are diluted water-soluble contrast materials or barium sulfate, and they are not suitable for performing virtual navigation. Negative contrast media include either tap water or air. Compared with air, on two-dimensional (2D) axial images, water has the advantage of generating no beam-hardening effects, but with virtual CT gastroscopy, water may show artefacts that can mimic polyps, erosions or flat ulcers.

The best results are obtained with the oral administration of effervescent powders. In any case, attention must be given to the fact that extensive gastric fluid may produce an air-fluid level that prevents the reconstruction of the underlying mucosa. Consequently, the patient should be properly prepared with a 12 h fast and ingestion of a very small amount of water with the effervescent powder, and two spiral acquisitions, with the patient in both the supine and prone position, should be acquired (Bielen et al. 2001). To maximize mucosal detail and to proceed with a realistic detailed intraluminal view of lesions, a narrow beam collimation is the most crucial factor. Typical parameters are reported in Tables 16.1 and 16.2. Depending on the parameters, artefacts such as smoothing, stair-step, longitudinal blurring and distortion may be minimized.

During the second spiral acquisition, to assess the stage of gastric carcinoma, if present, intravenous administration of iodinated contrast medium is required with acquisition of images during the portovenous phase.

16.2.2
Magnetic Resonance Imaging

The availability of high-performance gradient systems has allowed the acquisition of 3D MR data sets in a single breath-hold. On the basis of these MR data, virtual angioscopy has been performed in the aorta as well as the pulmonary artery. This technique has also been applied to the endoluminal

Table 16.1. CT parameters suggested to maximize mucosal detail

Author	Oral contrast medium	kV	mAs	Collimation	Pitch	Recon.
Springer	Effervescent granules	120	220	5 mm	1	1 mm
Lee	Effervescent granules	120	233	3 mm	1.3–2	1 mm
Ogata	Effervescent granules	120	180–220	3 mm	1.2	1 mm

Table 16.2. Parameters evaluated by virtual gastroscopy

Location
Dimensions and size
Morphology (according to Bormann classification)
Extraparietal involvement
Lymphadenopathy
Metastasis

evaluation of colonic disorders, and was recently adapted to obtain endoscopic and exoscopic views of the stomach. MR evaluation of esophageal lesions is relatively limited, and currently no experience exists concerning the acquisition of 3D MR data sets.

For the evaluation of the stomach prior to examination, an antiperistaltic drug is injected to reduce motion artefacts. Adequate gastric distension can be obtained by oral administration of water. Recently, a new oral contrast medium has proven to be useful for gastric distension, namely blueberry juice, which is characterized by T1 and T2 relaxation times of 32 ms and 8 ms, respectively, and which provides a bright signal on T1-weighted images and a dark signal on T2-weighted images (SCHMID et al. 1999).

A 3D study is based on the acquisition of a T1-weighted 3D gradient echo sequence with short TR (repetition time) and short TE (echo time), which provides a near-isotropic voxel. Three-dimensional Fourier transform gradient recalled echo (GRE) imaging has potential advantages over 2D imaging. Compared with traditional 2D GRE sequences, properly structured 3D GRE sequences have the capacity to provide thinner sections, no gaps, fat saturation, higher signal-to-noise ratio and comparable image contrast in the same breath-hold time frame. Furthermore, with appropriately thin sections and accurate timing, the same data set could be used to generate high-quality MR angiograms and thus provide added value. Therefore, 3D GRE imaging has the potential to yield a comprehensive evaluation of the upper abdomen (ROFSKY et al. 1999).

16.2.3
Data Processing and Viewing

After data acquisition, images are transferred to a dedicated workstation over an Ethernet or an Intranet network to be postprocessed.

Three-dimensional data sets can be examined using different 2D and 3D reconstruction techniques, starting with multiplanar reconstructions along three orthogonal axes and on oblique planes. Three-dimensional reconstructions can be obtained by using both surface rendering and volume rendering algorithms.

Using an adequate threshold value, all the pixels other than this value are automatically removed. Contiguous pixels at the boundary of a predefined threshold value are modeled as surfaces. In shaded surface display (SSD), only the first voxel encountered along the projection ray that is above a user-defined threshold is selected as an inner surface of the gastric lumen. Computer-produced imaginary sources of illumination depict surface reflections that are encoded in the image gray scale.

With volume rendering, more flexible management of the 3D data set is possible, with generation of surface views (similar to surface rendering), 3D models, and tissue transition projection images, which resemble a "double-contrast" barium study (Fig. 16.1). The major advantage of volume rendering is that the entire data set is preserved, with either no or very limited data segmentation, and tissue reconstruction using different opacity levels.

Using both surface and volume rendering algorithms, virtual endoscopic images resembling conventional endoscopic views are rendered. Color can be assigned to simulate expected normal tissue color in vivo. In addition, "fly-through" sequences within the lumen can be produced by creating a "flight path." The camera position along the endoscopic path must be defined by an interactive display of correlated 2D and 3D data sets in a multiwindow format, thus assisting the virtual endoscopist in establishing the relation of anatomical structures located outside the surfaces.

16.3
Clinical Applications

16.3.1
Esophagus

Most esophageal tumors are diagnosed by endoscopy, with thoraco-abdominal axial CT used to stage tumor spread; acquisition of 3D data sets permits acquisition of 3D modeling, virtual endoscopic images and conventional axial CT information within a single examination.

Realistic 3D reconstructions of the esophageal lumen are dependent on good gaseous distension of the esophagus above and below the tumor. Three-

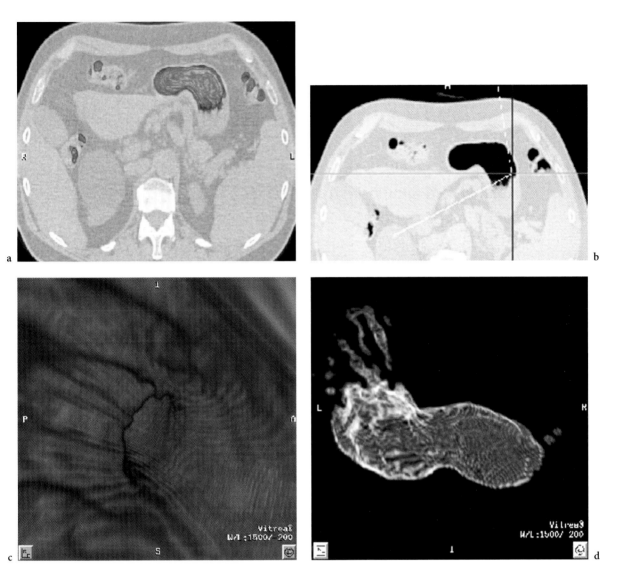

Fig. 16.1a–d. Volume-rendered images of the stomach. **a** Three-dimensional axial reformatted image showing the distended gastric lumen. **b** Two-dimensional axial image with reference lines showing the position of the virtual camera. **c** Endoscopic view of the internal surface of the stomach with evidence of longitudinal plicae. **d** Tissue transition projection image ("virtual double-contrast" evaluation of the stomach) showing a well-distended gastric lumen with clear evidence of the mucosal surface of the gastric antrum

dimensional display of the esophagus provides a readily recognizable image depicting tumor length and location with respect to other mediastinal structures and the gastroesophageal junction, and provides an estimation of longitudinal tumor extension (Fig. 16.2); this is useful additional information, particularly for stenosing tumors that do not allow passage of an endoscope.

The analysis of multiplanar images permits definition of the degree of perivisceral extension and metastatic involvement.

The disadvantages of 3D CT of esophageal tumors are related to suboptimal distension of the lumen, which leads to unsatisfactory reconstructions and an inability to differentiate between a nondistended normal lumen and a malignant stricture.

Although not the examination of choice, volumetric CT might show esophageal diverticula, with images comparable to conventional barium studies.

As already mentioned, no experience exists about the use of volumetric acquisition of the esophagus using an MR scanner.

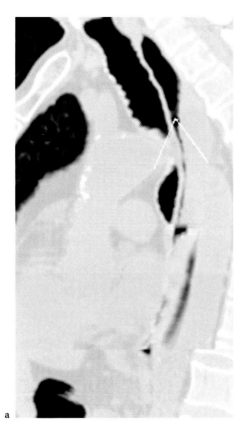

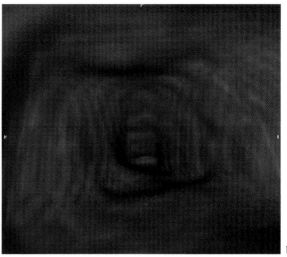

Fig. 16.2. a Sagittal multiplanar reformation of the esophagus showing a neoplastic stricture with poor distention of the esophageal lumen. **b** Virtual endoscopy view showing progressive narrowing of the esophageal lumen

16.3.2
Stomach

Virtual endoscopy is a valuable technique for detecting gastric lesions and, when malignancy is suspected, for establishing locoregional and distant involvement within a single examination. Compared with axial 2D CT, virtual endoscopy has the advantage of displaying gastric lesions as they are seen with conventional gastroscopy, thus allowing an accurate categorization according to the Bormann classifications (Tables 16.3, 16.4). Moreover, with the ability to display virtual endoscopic images, there is an increased rate in the detection of early gastric cancer, as reported by LEE and KO (1998). Compared with conventional endoscopy, virtual gastroscopy presents several advantages. Because of its larger field of view, virtual endoscopy enables a more accurate evaluation of lesion size; simultaneous availability of endoscopic, multiplanar, and axial 2D images permits, at the same time, local staging of gastric lesions, including the depth of parietal and perivisceral extension and the detection of lymph node and distant metastasis.

It should also be noted that 3D CT is a noninvasive technique, with minimum patient discomfort related to gastric distension; consequently, it is associated with higher patient compliance. However, compared with colonoscopy, fiberoptic gastroscopy is easier to perform and this is one of the reasons MR or CT imaging of the stomach are not considered ideal methods for detecting primary tumors. In addition, when a neoplastic lesion is detected during fiberoptic

Table 16.3. Bormann classification of early gastric cancer

I	Polypoid
II	Superficial
	IIa Elevated
	IIb Flat
	IIc Depressed
III	Excavated

Table 16.4. Bormann classification of advanced gastric cancer

I	Intraluminal protruding mass
II	Central ulcer within the tumor mass
III	Infiltrative tumor surrounding the ulcer
IV	Luminal narrowing

endoscopy, the lesion is biopsied and the patient can be scheduled for surgical treatment without the need for other diagnostic examinations.

Virtual endoscopy has several limitations, primarily concerning its inability to detect flat or small lesions or to obtain histological results. An additional limitation is related to ionizing radiation if CT is used, but because acquisition time is short and so much extra useful information is obtained, this disadvantage is negligible.

In any case, virtual gastroscopy should be considered a natural complement to a CT or MR study of the upper abdomen when a gastric disease is suspected or when a known neoplastic lesion must be staged. There is currently no indication to use this imaging technique as a primary method for evaluation of the gastric lumen.

In the next sections, different clinical results for gastric pathologies will be reviewed.

16.3.2.1
Gastric Carcinoma

The role of CT in advanced gastric cancer is to detect the primary lesion and to stage the tumor accurately. However, assessment of endoluminal morphology is limited when using axial images alone.

Three-dimensional images depict gastric wall surfaces in continuity and allow interactive, operator-initiated exploration, navigation, and maneuvering within the inner space of the organ, thus demonstrating the tumor mass as seen with gastroscopy. At the same time, the relation to anatomical structures located outside the surfaces is continuously maintained and displayed with reference to the position of the segment being viewed. The use of 3D or 2D pointers assists the operator to locate the lesion precisely, which could be also useful for mapping the tumor before a surgical resection.

In addition, this technique makes it possible to record accurately the maximum volume of the mass without magnification and the resulting image distortion; as a consequence, virtual endoscopy may be more accurate for measuring gastric lesions than conventional endoscopy because of its wider field of view (LEE and Ko 1998).

When virtual endoscopy reconstructions are performed, it is also possible to define tumor morphology according to the Bormann classification (Table 16.4).

Displaying multiplanar and 3D reconstructions allows an accurate evaluation of perigastric tumor involvement; likewise, the simultaneous availability of axial 2D images is mandatory for detecting lymphatic involvement as well as distant metastasis.

The detection of early gastric cancer (EGC) on axial CT is generally low (LEE and Ko 1998). With the use of 3D CT, not only is the detection rate of EGC over 90%, but it is also possible to obtain accurate categorization according to the Bormann classification (Table 16.3; Figs. 16.3–16.5). In general, 3D CT images of EGC I and IIa are excellent but those of EGC IIb and IIc are poor (LEE and Ko 1999b).

16.3.2.2
Other Gastric Lesions

Spiral CT of gastric leiomyoma discloses a well-demarcated, smooth, round, uniformly attenuated endogastric mass. The characteristic indication of submucosal tumor on an upper gastrointestinal series or gastroscopy is the presence of bridging folds over the tumor mass. This sign is not detected on the tumor surface with axial CT scanning. On virtual endoscopy, bridging folds may be detected around the protruding mass. Three-dimensional CT produces excellent images of gastric leiomyoma (LEE and Ko 1996; LEE 1998) (Fig. 16.6).

Spiral CT of gastric lymphoma discloses a less enhanced and a markedly thickened wall or discrete masses. Three-dimensional reconstructions also provide an accurate depiction of these features.

Finally, a controversial application for virtual endoscopy is the benign gastric ulcer, as reported by LEE (1998). In this case, spiral CT is not used to detect merely the ulcer crater but also may be performed in cases of suspected perforation or in cases of difficult differentiation from malignant ulcer by gastroscopy or barium study. Indeed, 3D imaging of the benign ulcer provides good-quality images and, often, ulcer craters are well visualized.

16.4
Conclusions

In conclusion, 3D imaging of the esophagus and stomach represents a valuable adjunct to conventional cross-sectional imaging, which can be easily obtained from both CT and MR data sets using dedicated workstations and commercially available software. Virtual endoscopy images offer a more comprehensive evaluation of the disease process from an inner perspective, representing a potentially interesting complement to conventional endoscopy.

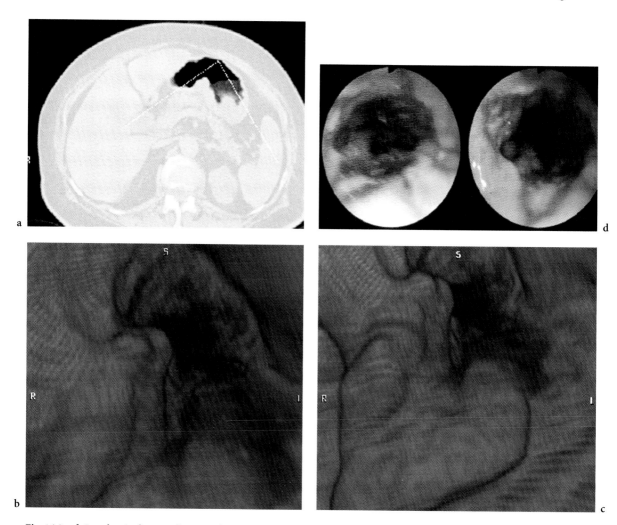

Fig. 16.3a–d. Intraluminal protruding gastric carcinoma (Bormann type I). **a** The vegetating lesion is observed on the axial CT image. **b, c** Two different endoluminal views of the same lesion; 3D image shows the morphological features of the lesion with a bulky appearance. Virtual gastroscopy findings are confirmed at conventional gastroscopy (**d**)

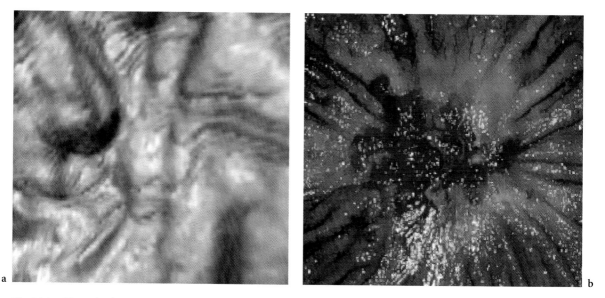

Fig. 16.4. a Ulcerative lesion (Bormann type II) demonstrated on a virtual endoscopy image; radiated folds are clearly evident. **b** Pathological specimen shows similar findings for the gastric ulcer

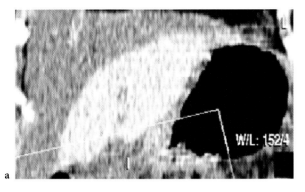

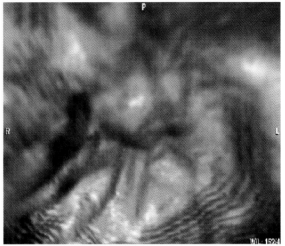

Fig. 16.5a, b. Bormann type III lesion. **a** The infiltrative tumor surrounding the ulcer is evident on the sagittal multiplanar reformatted image. **b** Virtual endoscopy view shows the lesion with elevated margins

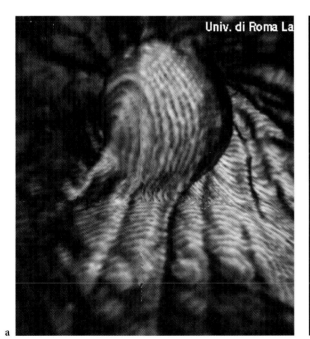

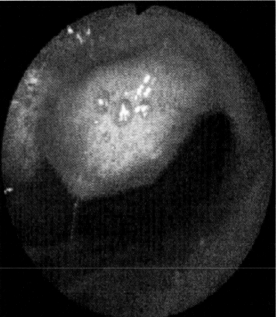

Fig. 16.6. a Virtual endoscopy view of a pedunculated gastric leiomyoma; the rounded lesion, with smooth margins and a long pedicle, is clearly demonstrated. **b** The same lesion as observed on conventional gastroscopy

References

Bielen D, Vanbeckevoort D, Thomeer M (2001) Virtual endoscopy, in multislice CT: a practical guide. Proceedings of the 5th international SOMATOM CT scientific user conference, Zurich, June 2000, pp 204–215

Gonvers J, Burnand B (1996) Appropriateness and diagnostic yield of upper gastrointestinal endoscopy in an open-access endoscopy unit. Endoscopy 28:661–666

Griffith JF, Kew J (1999) 3D CT imaging of oesophageal carcinoma. Eur J Radiol 32:216–220

Johnson P, Heath D (1996) Three dimensional CT: real-time interactive volume. AJR 167:761–766

Jolesz F, Lorensen W (1997) Interactive virtual endoscopy. AJR 169:1229–1235

Keto P, Suoranta H, Ihamaki T (1979) Double contrast examination of the stomach compared with endoscopy. Acta Radiol Diagn 20:762–768

Lee DH (1998) Three dimensional imaging of the stomach by spiral CT. J Comput Assist Tomogr 22:52–58

Lee DH, Ko YT (1996) The findings and the role of axial CT imaging and 3D imaging of gastric lesion by spiral CT. J Korean Radiol Soc 35:731–738

Lee DH, Ko YT (1998) The role of 3D spiral CT in early gastric carcinoma. J Comput Assist Tomogr 22:709–713

Lee DH, Ko YT (1999a) The role of three-dimensional and axial imaging in advanced gastric carcinoma by spiral CT. Abdom Imaging 24:111–116

Lee DH, Ko YT (1999b) Advanced gastric carcinoma: the role of three-dimensional and axial imaging by spiral CT. Abdom Imaging 24:111–116

Leung DA, McKinnon GC (1996) Breath hold, contrast-enhanced, three dimensional MR angiography. Radiology 201:569–571

Levine MS, Creteur V, Kressel HY (1987) Benign gastric ulcers: diagnosis and follow-up with double contrast radiography. Radiology 164:9–13

Lyang EY, Chan A (1996) Short communication. Oesophageal tumour volume measurement using spiral CT. Br J Radiol 69:344–347

Ominsky SH, Moss AA (1979) The postoperative stomach: a comparative study of double-contrast barium examinations and endoscopy. Gastrointest Radiol 4:17–21

Rofsky NM, Lee VS, Laub G (1999) Abdominal MR imaging with a volumetric interpolated breath-hold examination. Radiology 212:876–884

Schmid MR, Hany TF, Debatin JF (1999) 3D MR gastrography: exoscopic and endoscopic analysis of the stomach. Eur Radiol 9:73–77

Thoeni RF, Cello JP (1980) A critical look at the accuracy of endoscopy and double-contrast radiography of the upper gastrointestinal (UGI) tract in patients with substantial UGI hemorrhage. Radiology 135:305–308

17 CT Colonography

Darren Brennan, John Bruzzi, Helen M. Fenlon

17.1
Introduction

Colorectal cancer (CRC) is the second most common cancer in Western countries and the third most frequent cancer worldwide (SILVERBERG et al. 1990). It is estimated that 140,000 adults in the United States will be diagnosed with CRC each year, representing a total of 11–14% of all cancer cases (LANDIS et al. 1999). Many lifestyle risk factors are associated with CRC including a sedentary lifestyle, obesity and an increased waist-to-hip ratio (GIOVANNUCCI et al. 1995). Conversely, a diet high in fibre is thought to be protective (BURKITT 1971), although this belief has recently been questioned (BONITHON-KOPP et al. 2000). The incidence of CRC increases with age and there is an almost equal incidence in males and females. The role of chemoprevention in CRC has recently been extensively investigated and it would

appear that aspirin and other agents that act as cyclo-oxygenase inhibitors confer a reduced risk of up to 40% (SJODAHL 2001).

17.2
The Adenoma-Carcinoma Sequence

The adenoma-carcinoma sequence was first described in 1951 by JACKMAN and MAYO. Since then, a large volume of evidence has accrued indicating that CRC is almost inevitably preceded by an adenomatous polyp, although a very small proportion of CRCs arise from normal mucosa, so-called flat carcinomas. Evidence that supports the adenoma-carcinoma theory includes the facts that it is unusual to discover CRC in the absence of other associated adenomas (TURRELL and BROADMAN 1959; MORSON 1966), that malignant foci occur with increasing frequency in larger adenomatous polyps (GRINNELL and LANE 1958) and that the distribution of cancers and polyps is similar (JACKMAN and MAYO 1951). Further support for the adenoma-carcinoma sequence is found in the molecular genetic literature, where stepwise sequential mutations prescribe a molecular progression from adenoma through to carcinoma that mirrors the histological changes seen at pathology (FEARSON and VOGELSTAIN 1990). The inherited cancer syndrome of familial adenomatous polyposis in which innumerable polyps invariably lead to frank CRC also provides evidence of the premalignant potential of neoplastic polyps (DEBINSKI et al. 1996).

Because the premalignant potential of adenomatous polyps has long been recognized and the accepted policy is to remove these precursor polyps, few longitudinal studies describing their natural history have been reported. STRYKER et al. (1987) reported a series of 226 patients with polyps larger than 10 mm found at single-contrast barium enema that were followed for a mean of 68 months. They found that 37% of polyps enlarged and that 21 invasive CRCs developed at the site of the index polyp

D. BRENNAN, MB, BCh, MRCPI, J. BRUZZI, MB, BCh, MRCPI, H.M. FENLON, MB, BCh, MRCPI, FFRRCSI
Department of Radiology, Mater Misericordiae Hospital, Eccles Street, Dublin 7, Ireland

during the follow-up period. They calculated the cumulative risk of CRC at the polyp site at 5, 10 and 20 years as 2.5%, 8% and 24%, respectively. It is of note that CRC at a site remote from the index polyp was discovered in 11 patients during the follow-up period.

While these studies strongly support the widely held belief that CRC arises from polyps, it is also clear that only a proportion of polyps will actually develop into cancers. Polyps are common (35% of patients >50 years) whereas the lifetime risk of developing CRC in patients with no specific risk factor is approximately 6%. Small hyperplastic polyps are common, particularly in the distal colon, and are not associated with an increased risk of CRC. Adenomatous polyps are subdivided histologically into tubular, villous and tubulovillous types. The likelihood of a polyp becoming malignant depends primarily on its size (MUTO et al. 1975) and also on the amount of villous tissue it contains. Studies have shown that a polyp less than 1 cm in size has a less than 1% chance of being malignant whereas the risk rises to 10% for larger polyps (WINAWER et al. 1987; WAYE et al. 1988). It is also clear that progression from polyp into frank carcinoma proceeds at a leisurely rate, with most authors suggesting a time period of 10 years as an average, based on the observed protective effect of polypectomy. Polypectomy has been shown to reduce mortality from CRC, and is the basis of CRC screening programmes (SELBY et al. 1992; WINAWER et al. 1993). Although universal polypectomy would appear logical, in practice it is not feasible and may not be necessary due to the slow progression of the adenoma-carcinoma sequence. Selective removal of medium and large polyps would produce a similar reduction in CRC mortality to universal polypectomy, but with less risk (WAYE et al. 1998; GLICK et al. 1998). The importance of detecting and removing small polyps therefore remains doubtful.

17.3
Colorectal Cancer Screening

Because CRC is associated with precursor polyps and has a long subclinical phase that renders it suitable for screening, the American Cancer Society has recently produced guidelines for screening of average-risk individuals (BYERS et al. 1997). Furthermore, approved screening guidelines are now reimbursable by Medicare, and many European countries follow similar guidelines. Current US guidelines for the average-risk patient (described as any individual >50 years of age without other specific risk factors) include annual faecal occult blood testing (FOBT), with colonoscopic follow-up of positive cases. The sensitivity of this technique has been reported as 92% by the Minnesota Group (MANDEL et al. 1989), which translated into a 40% reduction in mortality at 14 years for the screened group when compared with a control group. However, this was at the expense of a false-positive rate of 38%, corresponding to many unnecessary colonoscopies. Furthermore, this was not a true screening population and the investigators used rehydrated stool specimens, which are not commonly used in clinical practice. Other large trials of FOBT have shown more modest reductions in mortality (HARDCASTLE et al. 1996). However, the single greatest limitation of FOBT as a screening test is that it detects only 10% of polyps, thus missing a unique opportunity to identify these potentially premalignant lesions at a stage where polypectomy would offer a cure.

17.3.1
Flexible Sigmoidoscopy

Flexible sigmoidoscopy has also been recommended on a 5-yearly basis as a potential screening technique. Case-control studies suggest that sigmoidoscopic screening can reduce the mortality from CRC by 30%, and also provide a benefit extending up to 10 years (SELBY et al. 1992). However, because it is not a total colon examination, sigmoidoscopy is inherently flawed, particularly in the African-American population where there is a higher percentage of proximal cancers (DAMERS et al. 1997; NELSON et al. 1997). Furthermore, it has been shown that sigmoidoscopy also misses up to 10% of neoplasms located in the distal colon within reach of the sigmoidoscope.

17.3.2
Colonoscopy

Colonoscopy, although providing a total colon examination, has never been evaluated in randomized controlled trials or case-control studies in a screening population. However, colonoscopy was used as the method of follow-up in the three largest FOBT trials and in the National Polyp Study (WINAWER et al. 1993), where a reduction of CRC incidence of 76–90% compared with historical controls was achieved. These studies suggest that colonoscopy can result in a marked reduction in CRC mortality as a consequence of prophylactic polypectomy, and it is currently recommended on a 10-yearly basis as a screening technique. Despite its appeal as both a diagnostic and a therapeutic tool, colonoscopy is invasive, requires sedation, is expensive and is associated with a perforation rate of approximately 1 in 1500. Furthermore, colonoscopy is not an irrefutable gold standard, with significant discrepancies in polyp detection rates reported. In one study (REX et al. 1997), 27% of adenomas <5 mm, 13% of adenomas 6–9 mm and 6% of adenomas >1 cm were missed, with an overall miss rate of 24%. Colonoscopy also fails to examine the proximal colon in up to 10% of patients (OBRECHT et al. 1984). Further studies have demonstrated that where a discrepancy exists between colonoscopy and double-contrast barium enema studies, approximately half the lesions that were overlooked on colonoscopy were ultimately verified as neoplastic (WEYMAN et al. 1981).

17.3.3
Double-Contrast Barium Enema

Double-contrast barium enema (DCBE) is safer, easier, cheaper and more acceptable to patients than colonoscopy and also offers the potential of a total colon examination. It is also more accurate for localizing lesions in the colon. Over 25 studies regarding the efficacy of DCBE in symptomatic patients show a sensitivity rate of approximately 85% for CRC. The published sensitivity of DCBE for large adenomas (>1 cm) is approximately 70%, although rates as low as 44% were reported in the National Polyp Study (WINAWER et al. 2000). A more recent study showed that DCBE was the most effective method, in monetary terms, for screening for CRC (McMAHON et al. 2001).

Because the various methods available for screening and diagnosis of CRC have individual drawbacks, there is considerable interest in developing a technique that can deliver a safe, reliable total colon examination that identifies both carcinomas and premalignant polyps. Recognizing that size is the greatest predictor of malignancy in polyps, it seems reasonable that a technique that will detect these large polyps (>1 cm) with a high sensitivity, even at the expense of missing smaller polyps, will be effective in screening for CRC. A new technique, CT colonography, first described in 1994, fulfils many of

these requirements and promises to challenge existing techniques as both a diagnostic and screening tool for CRC in the near future.

17.4
CT Colonography

First described in 1994 (VINING et al. 1994), CT colonography has quickly captured the imagination of both the imaging and gastrointestinal communities. Diverse terms such as "virtual colonoscopy", "3D colonoscopy", "CT pneumocolon", "CT colonoscopy" and "CT colography" were initially proposed, but "CT colonography" has been general accepted as the most suitable term (JOHNSON et al. 1998). Notwithstanding the different nomenclature, all techniques describe a similar method of volumetric CT image acquisition of a prepared colon with variable rendering of images for review by the radiologist.

17.4.1
Patient Preparation

17.4.1.1
Bowel Preparation

Most authors currently advocate a clean colon for CT colonography. Standard preparations include polyethylene glycol electrolyte solutions such as Klean-Prep (Helsinki Birex Pharmaceuticals, Dublin), which induce osmotic diarrhoea and are commonly favoured by colonoscopists, and phospho-soda preparations such as Picolax (Ferring Pharmaceuticals, Berkshire, UK) and Fleet Prep, which are favoured for barium enema examinations. These latter preparations result in a drier colonic mucosa than polyethylene glycol electrolyte solutions but are contraindicated in those with renal or cardiac failure because of their high sodium content. Experience suggests that a drier colonic mucosa is more beneficial for CT colonography, as residual fluid (which can be aspirated at colonoscopy) can obscure polyps. In a recent study (MACARI et al. 2001), semi-quantitative analysis of residual colonic fluid revealed that phospho-soda preparations produce a statistically significantly drier colonic mucosa compared with polyethylene glycol preparations. In addition, no difference in the amount of faecal residue was noted between the two preparations.

Other authors have concentrated on "faecal tagging" methods as an alternative to bowel purgation, which is perceived by many patients to be the worst part of a colon examination. In one study where patients were randomized to undergo either conventional bowel catharsis with polyethylene glycol or reduced cleansing with or without use of a faecal tagging agent (a specially designed barium suspension), GRYSPEERDT et al. (2000) found that despite the fact there was increased faecal residue in the unprepared group, there was less residual fluid and greater confidence in differentiating polyps from residual stool. Another study also demonstrated the feasibility of faecal tagging, although the regimen used was somewhat onerous: seven separate doses of oral faecal tagging preparation over 48 hours (CALLSTROM et al. 2000). Some researchers have examined postprocessing algorithms for the digital removal of tagged faecal residue and fluid (ZALIS and HAHN 2001). The authors describe two methods for removal of material of high attenuation that involve either calculation of mathematical gradients (matrix method) or interrogation of neighbouring pixels (raster method). Both methods take volume averaging of pixels into account. The authors noted that a simple threshold technique, based on attenuation alone, would be susceptible to partial volume artefact. Other researchers have used "segmentation rays" to travel through the data set in search of residual faecal material and partially volumed voxels are then removed (WAX 2000). Both methods appear to be feasible and have shown promising early results but require further evaluation. Use of faecal tagging with or without electronic bowel cleansing would have a major impact on screening uptake and also in the evaluation of elderly and infirm patients. The technique might also obviate the need to perform both prone and supine scans as is currently standard practice.

17.4.1.2
Spasmolytics

Initial studies of CT colonography involved routine use of a spasmolytic, either glucagon or N-butylbromide, the former been favoured in the United States and the latter in Europe. Glucagon is expensive, up to $130-$170 per dose (PRESTON 2001) and N-butylbromide has many contraindications because of its anticholinergic effects. Furthermore, two separate studies have demonstrated that glucagon does not improve colonic distension for CT colonography (YEE et al. 1999; MORRIN et al. 1999a). Because of its hypotonic action on the ileocaecal valve, glucagon may facilitate reflux of air through the valve, thus lessening colonic distension and

increasing the likelihood of shine-through artefact and artefacts from external compression by the distended small bowel. We have abandoned the use of spasmolytics in our practice.

17.4.1.3
Colon Insufflation

Adequate colon distension is the cornerstone on which successful CT colonography is built. The patient is placed in a decubitus position and a soft-tipped enema tube is inserted into the rectum. Because the rectum is a relative blind spot for CT colonography, digital rectal examination is advocated prior to tube insertion. The bowel is then insufflated with either room air or CO_2. Monitored CO_2 delivery allows a controlled amount of gas to be delivered. Furthermore, CO_2 is absorbed more rapidly across the lipid layer of the intestinal mucosa than room air, thus potentially lessening patient discomfort. Some authors have suggested that CO_2 is superior to room air (ROGALLA et al. 1999), but their results did not reach statistical significance. Other authors have not found a difference in image quality between the two methods (HARA et al. 1997). CO_2 adds to cost and inconvenience, and in our practice we use room air, insufflated gently to patient tolerance.

17.4.1.4
Intravenous Contrast

Most initial studies of CT colonography did not involve the use of intravenous contrast, as it was felt that the air–soft tissue interface offered sufficient contrast to permit detection of pathology. However, several recent reports have advocated its use (MORRIN et al. 2000a; NERI et al. 2000; LUZ et al. 2000; FLETCHER et al. 2000; ROGALLA et al. 2000a; AMIN et al. 2000). The rational is that because polyps and carcinomas enhance with contrast and faecal material will not, intravenous contrast administration will improve the performance characteristics of CT colonography.

MORRIN et al. (1999b), in a series of 200 patients, reported an improved sensitivity for medium-sized (6–9 mm) polyps following intravenous contrast, with a sensitivity of 75% compared with 58% for non-contrast studies. However, the authors conceded that improved user expertise might have accounted for some of this improved sensitivity. Contrast studies produce a significant increase in the attenuation of polyps when compared with the adjacent colonic wall, with a mean polyp to wall contrast of 82% (LUZ et al. 2000). Other authors have reported that intravenous contrast administration allows detection of local disease spread and evaluation for distant metastases (AMIN et al. 2000; ROGALLA et al. 2000b; NERI et al. 2000), thus allowing for accurate preoperative staging and optimization of treatment when a CRC is present. Two authors have also used contrast-enhanced CT in an effort to correlate the degree of enhancement with histological grade, with widely divergent results: MORRIN et al. (2000a) described a highly significant correlation between enhancement values in lesions >1 cm while TAYLOR et al. (1999) calculated a perfusion index for colorectal neoplasms and failed to show any significant correlation with Duke's staging. The use of intravenous contrast in the setting of CT colonography and as an adjunct to predicting histological grade requires further evaluation.

Despite the appeal of contrast enhancement, disadvantages such as increased cost, patient discomfort and the potential risk of adverse reactions need to be considered. The current trend would appear to reserve contrast enhancement for people strongly suspected of having CRC and who inevitably will require a staging contrast-enhanced CT examination.

17.4.2
Image Acquisition

The basic principle of CT colonography is rapid acquisition of a thin-section volumetric data set using helical (spiral) CT. This information is then reformatted with slice overlap providing gapless image information. Initial work was performed using single-slice helical CT systems, but with the ever-increasing availability of multirow detector computed tomography (MRDCT) it is likely that this will become the dominant method for data acquisition. Most authors perform CT scanning in a cranio-caudal direction (HARA et al. 1997; JOHNSON et al. 1997; ROYSTER et al. 1997; FENLON et al. 1998), to minimize artefact from breathing. Motion is less of a problem with MRDCT, where the whole abdomen and pelvis can be examined in a single 15 s breath-hold, well tolerated by most patients. With single-slice CT a typical protocol would be as follows: image slice thickness 5 mm, overlap 3 mm, pitch 1–2, kV 120. These figures are not arrived at arbitrarily but rather reflect both in vivo and laboratory work by a number of authors (SPRINGER et al. 2000; WHITING et al. 2000; POWER et al. 2000). As with most imaging techniques, these parameters represent a compromise between image noise, acquisition time, sensitivity and radiation burden. The radiation dose (calculated to be approximately the same as for a standard barium enema examination: approximately 6–8 mSv), can be reduced by using a low mAs, as the high contrast at the air–soft tissue interface precludes the need for higher tube outputs (VAN GELDER et al. 2000).

Many authors have described imaging parameters for CT colonography using MRDCT (GILLAMS et al. 2000; ROGALLA et al. 2000b; LAGHI et al. 2000). MRDCT has the benefit of high Z-axis resolution making isotropic voxel acquisition possible, thus improving image quality. Acquisition time is vastly reduced with subsecond gantry rotation times. All authors have concluded that MRDCT has excellent potential for CT colonography. Although a slice thickness of 1 mm is possible, most agree that the added radiation dose makes such thin slices unsuitable. ROGALLA et al. (2000b) described a sensitivity and specificity of 100–89% for large polyps and 96–87% for small (3–5 mm) polyps using images reconstructed in 1 mm slices with 50% overlap. Although this is impressive, the authors question the relevance of finding such small polyps and whether the increased radiation and computing burden warrant such thin-section imaging. They advocate an image reconstruction interval of 2 mm as a compromise. We currently use the following parameters: 4×2.5 cm collimation, pitch 1.25, 100 mAs, kVp 120.

Most authors concur that imaging in prone and supine positions improves the accuracy of CT colonography (FENLON et al. 1998; CHEN et al. 1999; FLETCHER et al. 2000; MORRIN et al. 2000a, b). FLETCHER et al. (2000) showed that prone positioning resulted in increased sensitivity for identification of large and medium-sized polyps with no decrease in specificity. Repositioning facilitates examination of segments of colon that were previously collapsed and also allows differentiation of mobile faecal residue from immobile polyps. Whether the use of faecal tagging agents will make this practice redundant in the future is the subject of investigation.

17.4.3
Image Rendering

After data acquisition images may be viewed in either two-dimensional (2D) axial or multiplanar reconstructed images or as three-dimensional (3D) endoluminal images (Fig. 17.1). For endoluminal images both volume and surface rendering may be used, with a general preference for perspective volume rendered images. Volume rendered images offer the advantage of using the whole data set and thus more accurately represent the acquired information than surface rendered images, which use only about 10% of the available information.

17.4.3.1
Image Segmentation and Navigation

Image segmentation (sculpturing) is a useful post-processing technique for isolating voxels from a particular area of interest. This reduces the time required for 3D rendering and navigation of endoluminal images, and troublesome artefacts such as shine-through are removed. Most image segmentation is currently done via a mouse-driven function, but automated methods have been developed. Most rely on the high contrast between the air-filled lumen and soft tissue interface to segment data of interest. However, as small bowel, lung and stomach also meet this criterion, seed points have to be placed in discrete locations along the colonic lumen to spatially isolate the colon. Areas of incompletely distended bowel (whether due to spasm or tumour) also cause difficulties with segmentation. Nonetheless, these semi-automated methods of bowel segmentation promise to improve the speed of 3D reconstruction (BITTER et al. 2000). More recently, fully automated methods of bowel segmentation have been developed (WYATT et al. 2000). Automated navigation relies on an ability to calculate a midline flight-path through the colonic lumen. Some software also includes collision avoidance functions.

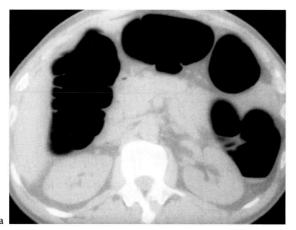

a

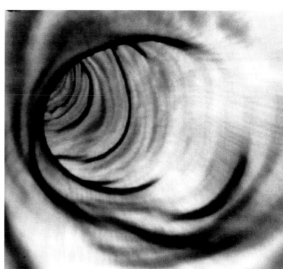

b

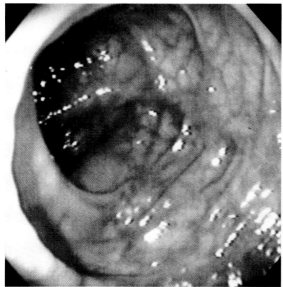

c

Fig. 17.1a–c. Normal colon on CT colonography and conventional colonoscopy. Axial CT image (**a**) demonstrates a normal clean and well-distended colon. The normal splenic flexure is seen on CT colonography (**b**) and conventional colonoscopy (**c**)

17.4.3.2
Automated Polyp Detection

Computer-aided diagnosis is not a new concept and much research in CT colonography has focused on automated polyp detection. To date, these techniques have largely been based on shape analysis. Studies in computer-generated and human polyp models have shown promising results (Paik et al. 2000a; Summers et al. 2001; Yoshida et al. 2000), but at the moment high sensitivity is at the expense of many false positives as the software programs cannot differentiate between polyps, residual faecal material, mucosal folds and artefacts such as the stair-step artefact.

17.4.3.3
3D Projection Techniques

Numerous techniques have been developed to review perspective rendered endoluminal images. Most authors currently use cine mode review at a variable frame rate of 5–30/s to virtually navigate the colon. The images can be reviewed separately in both antegrade and retrograde directions (Macari et al. 2000a), in both directions simultaneously with the use of a rear-view mirror facility, or with other more complicated image manipulations. Rogalla et al. (2000c) used a hybrid fusion of both 2D and 3D images, while others have demonstrated the feasibility of synchronized combinations of an endoluminal image with a multiplanar reformatted image vertical to the viewing vector (Minami et al. 2000). Other authors have attempted to produce panoramic endoscopic views, which they argue allow for more complete visualization of the colon. Using stereographic techniques or Mercator map projections, a perspective rendered image of a laid-out flat colon is generated, similar to a cut lumen at pathology. They report greater sensitivity for polyp detection with these techniques than with conventional endoluminal views (Paik et al. 2000b). For instance, using the Mercator map projection (named after the Dutch Renaissance cartographer), they reported significantly improved sensitivity for polyp detection compared with conventional endoluminal 3D CT colonography (87.5% versus 67.5%).

17.4.4
Image Interpretation and Pitfalls

Whatever the chosen method for image rendering and review, in practice, most authors base their interpretation on a review of the supine and prone 2D axial images with 3D reconstructions reserved for problem-solving. Axial 2D images are readily interpreted by most radiologists and allow accurate localization of pathology by reference to adjacent landmarks. Using a method termed "colon-tracking" by Fenlon, images are viewed at an interactive workstation in a retrograde fashion from rectum to caecum. The images are reviewed at "lung windows" (window level –750, width 1500). It is imperative that any areas of underdistended bowel are also reviewed at "soft tissue" windows (level 40, width 400), as areas of collapsed bowel can be due to stenosing carcinomas, a fact that may be overlooked at lung window settings. It is widely accepted that 2D and 3D images are complementary (Hara et al. 1996; Royster et al. 1997; Dachman et al. 1998; Macari et al. 2000b). Many authors have commented on the usefulness of 3D images for problem-solving. Dachman et al. (1998) found that endoluminal images, used to supplement primary review of axial 2D images, increased reader confidence, with a minimal impact on interpretation time, while Macari et al. (2000b) concluded that axial 2D colonography was comparable, in performance terms, with complete 2D and 3D CT colonography. When a potential abnormality is seen on 2D images, 3D rendered images may be used to determine if its morphology is linear or polypoid. The differentiation of polyps from folds is often easier on 3D images as a more global view of the fold and adjacent mucosa is achieved with endoluminal techniques (Fenlon and Ferrucci 1997). Flat sessile polyps and carcinomas are easier seen on axial 2D images as they may obscured by smoothing algorithms on endoluminal images.

17.4.5
The Normal Colon

On 2D and 3D images the rectum has the three mucosal folds: the valves of Houston. The rectum is usually well distended and easy to navigate. The more tortuous sigmoid colon is more difficult to evaluate and due to its high tone is often partially collapsed. Diverticular disease is frequently present here also, making evaluation more difficult. The sigmoid colon is usually better distended on prone images. The descending colon is relatively featureless and easy to evaluate. The splenic flexure can vary from a gradual 90° turn to a complex series of loops and bends (Fig. 17.1). The transverse colon can be recognized by its triangular shape, with three prominent taeniae coli identified as longitudinal bands orientated along the long axis of the bowel. The hepatic flexure is usually easier to traverse than the splenic, and it leads to the ascending colon, which can be recognized by its triangular shape (similar to the transverse colon). Recognition of the caecum, by the confluence of three taeniae coli at its base and the presence of appendiceal and ileal orifices, is the key to a complete evaluation on 3D images. The ileocaecal valve can vary in appearance from a labial-type structure with a patulous orifice to a prominent polyp type, and it should not be mistaken for a neoplastic lesion.

17.4.6
Pathology

Polyps are seen as well-defined round or oval smooth intraluminal projections. They are best appreciated in profile (Figs. 17.2, 17.3). CRCs are recognized as larger intraluminal masses (Figs. 17.4, 17.5). Their appearance at 2D and 3D endoluminal CT colonography varies from a polypoid mass to a fungating annular or ulcerated mass, reflecting the morphology observed at colonoscopy and surgery. Finer mucosal detail, such as ulceration, is often obscured due to partial volume

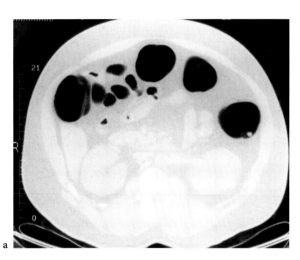
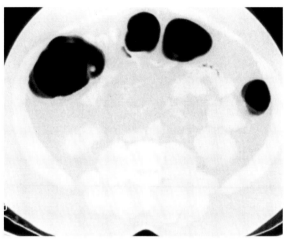

Fig. 17.2a,b. Axial CT images from a CT colonography study demonstrate a 6 mm polyp in the descending colon (**a**) and a 6 mm polyp in the ascending colon (**b**)

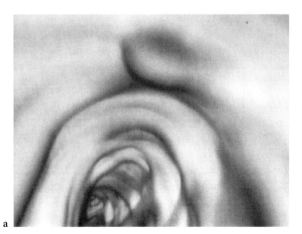
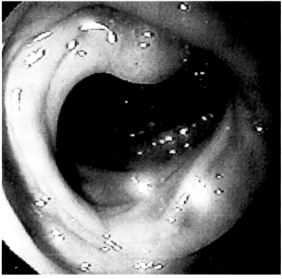

Fig. 17.3a,b. A 10 mm polyp is demonstrated on CT colonography (**a**) and conventional colonoscopy (**b**)

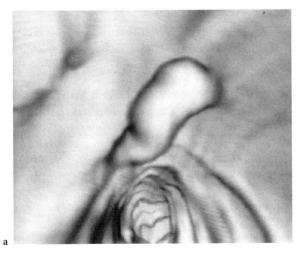

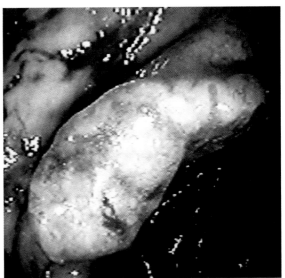

Fig. 17.4a,b. A 20 mm caecal carcinoma is demonstrated on
CT colonography (a) and conventional colonoscopy (b)

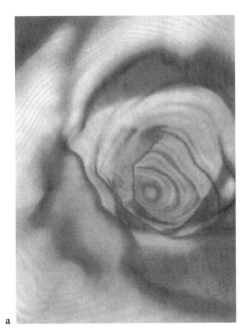

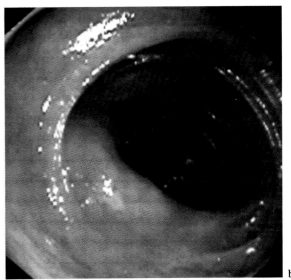

Fig. 17.5a,b. A 30 mm sessile carcinoma is demonstrated on
CT colonography (a) and conventional colonoscopy (b)

averaging and smoothing effects. Flat sessile lesions are difficult to detect but careful scrutiny of the axial 2D images increases their pick-up rate. In the future, programs that calculate bowel wall thickness may improve detection of these difficult carcinomas.

Diverticula are readily identified on axial images and on 3D images are characteristically seen as sharply defined circumferential dark rings (similar to the appendiceal orifice). A polyp does not have a complete circumferential ring as it is a raised structure. An impacted or inverted diverticulum can cause diagnostic difficulty, but referral to the axial 2D image

will reveal the lesion to have portions that extend outside the colonic wall.

Normal haustral folds are identified as variably thin translucent structures, the degree of translucency being a function of the opacity settings (Fig. 17.6). Complex folds may simulate polyps but again combined use of 2D and 3D images is useful in this setting. Retrograde tracking or use of "rear-view mirror" techniques allows visualization of polyps on the blind side of a fold.

Residual stool may simulate polyps, but they can often be differentiated by reviewing both prone and

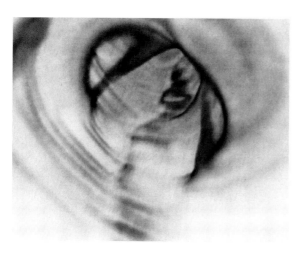

Fig. 17.6. An endoluminal image of the descending colon demonstrates normal semi-translucent colonic folds and a small volume of retained intraluminal fluid

17.4.7
CT Colonography Performance

17.4.7.1
Polyp Detection

CT colonography has been evaluated for polyp detection by many authors, with conventional colonoscopy as the gold standard. The sensitivity of the technique is dependent on lesion size and many authors have emphasized the steep learning curve involved in interpretation of images. The first reported study on CT colonography for polyp detection was by HARA et al. (1996).They reported sensitivities of 100% for polyps >1 cm, 71% for polyps of 5–9 mm and 26% for polyps smaller than 5 mm. Numerous other authors have also reported their results and Table 17.1 summarizes the findings of the largest series reported to date. As user expertise grows the performance characteristics of CT colonography are likely to improve. Retrospective review of examinations has shown that many polyps are missed due to correctable human and technical factors (CHEN et al. 1999; FLETCHER et al. 2000).

With the more widespread availability of MRDCT, it is also anticipated that the performance of CT colonography will approximate that of conventional colonoscopy in the detection of smaller polyps. HARA et al. (2001) recently reported the first large series of 160 patients examined with MRDCT, and although they did not report a statistical improvement in polyp detection, they did report that MRDCT resulted in reduced artefact and improved bowel distension. Other authors (ROGALLA et al. 2000a) have reported higher sensitivity and specificity for the detection of smaller polyps using MRDCT, but the clinical relevance of these small lesions remains questionable.

supine images. Polyps are immobile whereas faecal residue will assume a dependent position. Faecal material often contains air, thus further aiding its differentiation from polyps. Fluid can obscure polyps and its presence makes the acquisition of both prone and supine images important.

Extrinsic compression may appear as an endoluminal projection that can be misinterpreted as a polyp or mass on 3D images. The extrinsic compression may arise from adjacent viscus (liver, spleen, kidney), vessels (aorta) or bowel loops. Reference to the axial 2D images is a simple solution to this problem.

Stair-step artefact appears as concentric mucosal rings, and can be kept to a minimum by using a slice overlap of at least 50% with pitch of less than 2 (SPRINGER et al. 2000). Use of a smoothing algorithm reduces stair-step artefact but at the expense of mucosal detail.

Table 17.1. Published results of CT colonography

Authors	No. patients	Use of intravenous contrast	Sensitivity for polyps >1 cm	Sensitivity for polyps 6–9 mm	Sensitivity for polyps <6 mm
HARA et al.(1997)	70	No	75%	66%	45%
DACHMAN et al. (1998)	44	No	83% for polyps>8 mm	NA	NA
FENLON et al. (1999)	100	No	91%	82%	55%
MORRIN et al. (2000b)	200	Yes	100%	65%	33%
FLETCHER et al. (2000)	180	No	75%	47%	NA
YEE et al. (1999)	155	No	93.9%	82%	59%
MIAO et al. (2000)	201	No	73%	NA	NA
MENDELSON et al. (2000)	100	No	73%	19% for polyps <1 cm	NA

17.4.7.2
Carcinoma Detection

The ability of CT colonography to demonstrate CRC has been evaluated in many similar studies. CRCs tend to be larger than polyps and high detection rates are reported. FENLON et al. (1999) reported a 100% detection rate for CRC, whilst similar success has been reported by other authors (HARA et al. 1997). As in conventional colonoscopy, flat sessile polyps and carcinomas appear to cause diagnostic difficulty. The Mayo Clinic group reported a disappointing sensitivity for these lesions on careful review of 617 CT colonography examinations, but more encouragingly showed that review by two radiologists raised the sensitivity to 68%. These large flat lesions also cause considerable difficulty in conventional colonoscopy (JARAMILLO et al. 1995; MITOOKA 2000).

17.4.7.3
Incomplete Colonoscopy

CT colonography has been shown to be a very useful method of imaging the colon following failed or incomplete colonoscopy. It is preferable to barium enema in patients immediately following colonoscopy as the proximal colon will be distended with air. It has also been shown to be a useful test for evaluating the proximal colon in patients with distal occlusive cancers that cannot be passed endoscopically. Between 1.5% and 9% of patients with CRC have a second synchronous cancer (DASAMAHAPATRA and LOPYAN 1989). Preoperative endoscopic or barium evaluation of synchronous tumours is often restricted due to the occlusive nature of the index tumour.

FENLON et al. (1998) performed CT colonography on 29 patients with occlusive CRC. Conventional colonoscopy and barium examination of the proximal bowel failed in all cases. CT colonography demonstrated the proximal colon in 26 of 29 patients (90%). All 29 occlusive CRCs, two synchronous carcinomas and 24 polyps were identified in this study. Other authors have similarly used CT colonography for evaluation of the proximal bowel in similar cases (MORRIN et al. 1999b; NERI et al. 2000; MACARI et al. 2000a) and have uniformly reported similar technical and overall success. Furthermore, these authors conclude that CT colonography is better tolerated than conventional colonoscopy or barium enema and is highly accurate for tumour staging when intravenous contrast is given. Because these patients have a very high clinical suspicion or proven diagnosis of CRC,

the administration of intravenous contrast, use of a higher mAs values and review at soft tissue window settings is particularly appropriate. AMIN et al. (2000) reported their experience with 201 patients who underwent CT colonography followed by conventional endoscopy and found CT colonography to have a sensitivity of 100% and specificity of 99% for the diagnosis of invasive carcinoma. They also detected three colorectal carcinomas not identified at conventional colonoscopy because of incomplete examination, metastases in six patients and extracolonic malignancies in a further seven patients.

17.4.7.4
Incidental Findings

Besides the ability to offer a "total colon" examination, CT colonography also has the capability to evaluate the extracolonic abdomen and pelvis. Because these examinations are often carried out in the elderly, "incidental" findings are frequent. ROSEN et al. (2000) reported extracolonic findings in 24% of 224 patients. While many of these were of limited clinical significance (e.g. gall stones), diseases classified by the authors as "major findings" were discovered in 36%. These included non-cystic liver lesions, pancreatic masses, solid renal masses, lytic bone lesions and abscesses. HARA et al. (2000) reported that 11% of 264 patients had "significant" extracolonic findings including aortic aneurysms. In their series, 18 patients underwent further abdominal imaging and six underwent surgery based on extracolonic findings. It would appear, therefore, that in a significant minority of patients CT colonography offers potential health benefits beyond its primary brief of colorectal polyp and carcinoma detection.

17.4.8
Screening

Since its inception, CT colonography has been touted as a potential screening tool for CRC. Although polyp screening reduces mortality from CRC and is cost-efficient, debate about the best method of screening still persists. The relative merits of the available techniques have already been discussed. Like all screening tests, if CT colonography is to be considered, it must be proved accurate, safe, reliable, readily available and acceptable to patients. Uptake in colorectal carcinoma screening programmes to date has been uniformly poor, as healthy people are generally hesitant to undergo invasive colon examinations. CT colonography is perceived by many patients to be preferential to conventional colonoscopy, and it is likely that this acceptance will become more established if faecal tagging agents can eliminate the need for bowel purgation.

Nearly all studies done to date with CT colonography have been in high-risk patient groups, and as such it is difficult to extrapolate the published results directly to an asymptomatic, average-risk population. In one study of 46 asymptomatic patients, CT colonography resulted in findings that would have led to conventional colonoscopy in 75% of patients with an adenoma >2 cm, in 83% of patients with an adenoma of 1–2 cm and in 43% of patients with an adenoma of 6–9 mm (REX et al. 1999). If one selected a polyp size threshold of 1 cm, these findings are extremely promising, but this study also had a biased population, and again extrapolation to a general population is difficult. Large-scale studies on asymptomatic populations are necessary to assess the use of CT colonography in a screening population. Multicentre trials are currently under way in the United States and are planned for Europe. Their results are eagerly awaited.

17.5
Conclusion

CT colonography is a nascent technology, barely 7 years old. In this short time, however, CT colonography has rapidly evolved as a powerful diagnostic tool. With improvements in scanner and computer technology, image quality will improve. Much research is under way to improve and facilitate image reconstruction and interpretation. Optimal parameters for scanning are not yet fully defined nor are they standardized. With increasing experience with this technique, the future looks bright for CT colonography in colorectal polyp and cancer detection.

References

Amin Z, Miao YM, Healy JC (2000) A prospective single centre study comparing CT pneumocolon against colonoscopy in detection of colorectal neoplasms. Eleventh annual conference of the European Society of Gastrointestinal and Abdominal Radiology (ESGAR) 2000. Eur Radiol 10:D2

Bitter I, Sato M, Bender MA (2000) Automatic, accurate and robust colon centreline algorithm. Eighty-sixth annual meeting and scientific assembly of the Radiological Society of North America (RSNA). Radiology 217:370

Bonithon-Kopp C, Kronborg O, Giacosa A (2000) Calcium and fibre supplementation in prevention of colorectal adenoma recurrence. A randomised intervention trial. European cancer prevention organization group. Lancet 356 :1300–1306

Burkitt DP (1971) Epidemiology of cancer of the colon and rectum. Cancer 28:3–13

Byers T, Levin B, Rothenberger D (1997) American Cancer Society guidelines for screening and surveillance for early detection of colorectal polyps and cancer: update 1997. CA Cancer J Clin 47:154–160

Callstrom MR, Johnson CD, Fletcher JG (2000) A feasibility study of CT colonography of the unprepped colon. Eighty-sixth annual meeting and scientific assembly of the Radiological Society of North America (RSNA). Radiology 217:371

Chen SC, Lu DSK, Hecht JR (1999) CT colonography; value of scanning in both the supine and prone positions. AJR 172:595–599

Dachman AH, Kuniyoshi JK, Boyle CM (1998) CT colonography with 3-D problem solving for detection of colonic polyps. AJR 171:989–995

Damers RY, Severson RK, Schottenfeld D (1997) Incidence of colorectal adenocarcinoma by anatomic subsite: an epidemiologic study of time trends and racial differences in the Detroit, Michigan area. Cancer 79:441–447

Dasamahapatra CS, Lopyan K (1989) Rationale for aggressive colonoscopy in patients with colorectal neoplasia. Arch Surg 124:63–66

Debinski HS, Love S, Sipigelman AD (1996) Colorectal polyp counts and cancer risk in familial adenomatous polyposis. Gastroenterology 110:1028–1030

Fearson ER, Vogelstein BA (1990) Genetic model for colorectal tumorigenesis. Cell 61:759–767

Fenlon HM, Ferrucci JT (1997) Virtual colonoscopy: what will the issues be? AJR 169:453–457

Fenlon HM, Clarke PD, Ferrucci JT (1998) Virtual colonoscopy: imaging features with colonoscopic correlation. AJR 170:1303–1309

Fenlon HM, McAneny DB, Nunes DP (1999) Occlusive colon carcinoma: virtual colonoscopy in the preoperative evaluation of the proximal colon. Radiology 210:423–428

Fletcher JG, Johnson CD, Krueger WR (2000) Contrast-enhanced CT colonography: simultaneous evaluation for metastatic disease, local recurrence and metachronous neoplasia in recurrent colorectal carcinoma. Eighty-sixth annual meeting and scientific assembly of the Radiological Society of North America (RSNA). Radiology 217:230

Gillams AR, Lees WR, Bhardwaj R (2000) Protocol optimization for multislice CT colography. Eighty-sixth annual meeting and scientific assembly of the Radiological Society of North America (RSNA). Radiology 217:370

Giovannuci E, Ascherio A, Rimm EB (1995) Physical activity, obesity and risk for colon cancer and adenoma in men. Ann Intern Med 1222:327–334

Glick S, Wagner JL, Johnson CD (1998) Cost-effectiveness of double-contrast barium enema in screening for colorectal cancer. AJR 170:629–636

Grinnell RS, Lane N (1958) Benign and malignant adenomatous polyps and papillary adenomas of the colon and rectum. An analysis of 1,856 tumors in 1,335 patients. Int Abstr Surg 106:519–538

Gryspeerdt SS, Lefere PP, Van Holsbeech BG (2000) Dietary faecal tagging enables reduced colon cleansing and improves diagnosis in virtual CT Colonoscopy. Eighty-sixth annual meeting and scientific assembly of the Radiological Society of North America (RSNA). Radiology 217:170

Hara AK, Johnson CD, Reed JE (1996) Detection of colorectal polyps by computed tomographic colography: feasibility of a novel technique. Gastroenterology 110:284–290

Hara AK, Johnson CD, Reed JE (1997) Colorectal polyp detection using computed tomographic colography: initial assessment of sensitivity and specificity. Radiology 205:59–65

Hara AK, Johnson CD, MacCarty RL (2000) Incidental extracolonic findings at CT colonography. Radiology 215:353–357

Hara AK, Johnson CD, MacCarty RL (2001) CT colonography: single versus multi-detector row imaging. Radiology 219:461–465

Hardcastle JD, Roginson MHE, Moss SM (1996) Randomized Controlled trial of faecal occult screening for colorectal cancer. Lancet 348:1472–1477

Jackman RJ, Mayo CW (1951) The adenoma-carcinoma sequence in cancer of the colon. Surg Gynecol Obstet 93:327–330

Jaramillo E, Watanabe M, Slezak P (1995) Flat neoplastic lesions of the colon and rectum detected by high-resolution video colonoscopy and chromoscopy. Gastrointest Endosc 42:114–122

Johnson CD, Hara AK, Reed JE (1997) Computed tomographic colonography (virtual colonoscopy): a new method for detecting colorectal neoplasms. Endoscopy 29:454–461

Johnson CD, Hara AK, Reed JE (1998) Virtual endoscopy: what's in a name? AJR 171:1201–1202

Laghi A, Panebianco V, Baeli I (2000) Multislice spiral CT colography technique optimization. Eleventh annual scientific assembly and meeting of the European Society of Gastrointestinal and Abdominal Radiology (ESGAR) 2000. Eur Radiol 10:D2

Landis SH, Murray T, Bolder S (1999) Cancer statistics, 1999. CA Cancer J Clin 49:18–31

Luz O, Luboldt WW, Heuschmid M (2000) Enhancement of colonic polyps in high resolution CT colonography following bolus injection of intravenous contrast. Eighty-sixth annual meeting and scientific assembly of the Radiological Society of North America (RSNA). Radiology 217:583

Macari M, Milano A, Lavelle M (2000a) Comparison of time-efficient CT colonography with two- and three-dimensional colonic evaluation for detecting colorectal polyps. AJR 174:1543–1549

Macari MJ, Milano A, Berman P (2000b) Prospective comparison of CT colonography and barium enema in patients with incomplete colonoscopy. Eighty-sixth annual meeting and scientific assembly of the Radiological Society of North America (RSNA). Radiology 217:341

Macari M, Lavelle M, Pedrosa I (2001) Effect of different bowel preparations on residual fluid at CT colonography. Radiology 218:244–247

Mandel JS, Bond JH, Bradley M (1989) Sensitivity, specificity and positive predictivity of the Haemoccult test in screening for colorectal cancers: the University of Minnesota's colon cancer control study. Gastroenterology 97:597–600

McMahon PM, Bosch JL, Gleason S (2001) Cost-effectiveness of colorectal cancer screening. Radiology 219:44–50

Mendelson RM, Foster NM, Edwards JT (2000) Virtual colonoscopy compared with conventional colonoscopy: a developing technology. Med J Aust 173:472–475

Miao YM, Amin Z, Healy J (2000). A prospective single centre study comparing computed tomography pneumo-colon against colonoscopy in the detection of colorectal neoplasm. Gut 47:832–837

Minami M, Miyazawa M, Akahane M (2000) Diagnosis of CRC using new virtual CT endoscopy: computed sectional probe method. Eighty-sixth annual meeting and scientific assembly of the Radiological Society of North America (RSNA). Radiology 217:230

Mitooka H (2000) Flat neoplasms in the adenoma-carcinoma sequence in Japan. Semin Gastrointest Dis 11:238–247

Morrin MM, Kruskal JB, Farrell RJ (1999a) Does glucagon improve colonic distension and polyp detection during CT colonography? Eighty-fifth annual meeting and scientific assembly of the Radiological Society of North America (RSNA). Radiology 213:341

Morrin MM, Kruskal JB, Farrell RJ (1999b) Endoluminal CT colonography after an incomplete endoscopic colonoscopy AJR 172:913–918

Morrin MM, Farrell RJ, Kruskal JP (2000a) Utility of intravenously administered contrast medium at CT colonography. Radiology 217:768–771

Morrin M, Kruskal JB, Farrell RJ (2000b) Clinico-pathological correlation of colorectal lesions detected at intravenous enhanced CT colonography. Proceedings from the 2nd international symposium on virtual colonoscopy, 16–17 Oct 2000, Boston

Morson BC (1966) Factors influencing the prognosis of early cancer of the rectum. Proc R Soc Med 59:607–608

Muto T, Bussey HJR, Morson BC (1975) The evolution of cancer of the colon and rectum. Cancer 36:2251–2270

Nelson RL, Doller T, Freels S (1997) The relation of age, race and gender to the subsite location of colorectal carcinoma. Cancer 80:193–197

Neri E, Giusti P, Battolla L (2000) Contrast-enhanced CT colonoscopy after incomplete fibreoptic colonoscopy in the preoperative management of colorectal cancer. Eighty-sixth annual meeting and scientific assembly of the Radiological Society of North America (RSNA). Radiology 217:582

Obrecht WF, Wu WC, Gelfand DW (1984) The extent of successful colonoscopy: a second assessment using modern equipment. Gastrointest Radiol 9:161–162

Paik DS, Beaulieu CF, Jeffrey RB Jr (2000a) Computer aided detection of polyps in CT colonography: method and free-response ROC evaluation of performance. Eighty-sixth annual meeting and scientific assembly of the Radiological Society of North America (RSNA). Radiology 217:370

Paik DS, Beaulieu CF, Jeffrey RB Jr (2000b) Visualization modes for CT colonography using cylindrical and planar map projections. J Comput Assist Tomogr 24:179–188

Power N, Pryor M, Martin A (2000) Optimization of scanning parameters for spiral CT pneumocolon. Eighty-sixth annual meeting and scientific assembly of the Radiological Society of North America (RSNA). Radiology 217:583

Preston BM (2001) Rethinking the use of glucagon: consider the cost (letter). AJR 176:546–547

Rex DK, Cutler CS, Lemmell GT (1997) Colonoscopic miss rates of adenomas determined by back to back colonoscopies. Gastroenterology 112:24–28

Rex DK, Vining D, Kopecky KK (1999) An initial experience with screening for colon polyps using spiral CT with and without CT colography (virtual colonoscopy). Gastrointest Endosc 50:309–313

Rogalla P, Schmidt E, Korves M (1999) Optimal colon distension for virtual colonoscopy: room air versus CO_2 insufflation. Eighty-fifth annual meeting and scientific assembly of the Radiological Society of North America (RSNA). Radiology 213:342

Rogalla P, Hein E, Vogel F (2000a) Impact of multislice CT on polyp detection in virtual colonoscopy. Eighty-sixth annual meeting and scientific assembly of the Radiological Society of North America (RSNA). Radiology 217:369

Rogalla P, Hein E, Vogel F (2000b) Virtual endoscopy of the preoperative colon: diagnostic accuracy for tumour staging. Eleventh annual conference of the European Society of Gastrointestinal and Abdominal Radiology (ESGAR) 2000. Eur Radiol 10:D3

Rogalla P, Hein E, Vogel F (2000c) Hybrid visualization in colon imaging: combining axial slices and virtual endoscopic views. Eighty-sixth annual meeting and scientific assembly of the Radiological Society of North America (RSNA). Radiology 217:371

Rosen MP, Morrin MM, Raptopoulos VD (2000) Prevalence of findings unrelated to the colon detected during CT colonography. Eighty-sixth annual meeting and scientific assembly of the Radiological Society of North America (RSNA). Radiology 217:583

Royster AP, Fenlon HM, Clarke PD (1997) CT colonoscopy of colorectal neoplasms: two-dimensional and three-dimensional virtual reality techniques with colonoscopic correlation. AJR 169:1237–1242

Selby JV, Friedman GD, Quesenberry CP (1992) A case control study of screening sigmoidoscopy and mortality from colorectal cancer. N Engl J Med 326:653–657

Silverberg E, Boring CE, Squires TS (1990) Cancer statistics 1990. CA Cancer J Clin 40:9–26

Sjodahl R (2001) Nonsteroidal anti-inflammatory drugs and the gastrointestinal tract: extent, mode and dose dependence of anticancer effects. Am J Med 110:66S–69S

Springer P, Stohr B, Giacomuzzi SM (2000) Virtual computed tomography colonoscopy: artifacts, image quality and radiation dose load in a cadaver study. Eur Radiol 10:183–187

Stryker SJ, Wolff BG, Culp CE (1987) Natural history of untreated colonic polyps. Gastroenterology 93:1009–1013

Summers RM, Johnson CD, Pusniak LM (2001) Automated polyp detection at CT colonography: feasibility assessment in a human population. Radiology 219:51–59

Taylor SA, Renfrew ID, Gillams AR (1999) Are CT derived perfusion measurements of value in assessing colorectal tumours detected by CT colonography? Eighty-fifth annual

meeting and scientific assembly of the Radiological Society of North America (RSNA). Radiology 213:341

Turrell R, Brodman HR (1959) Adenomas of the colon and rectum. In: Turrell R (ed) Diseases of the colon and anorectum. Saunders, Philadelphia, p 326

Van Gelder RE, Stoker J, Venema HW (2000) Feasibility of radiation dose reduction for virtual colonscopy. Eighty-sixth annual meeting and scientific assembly of the Radiological Society of North America (RSNA). Radiology 217:583

Vining DJ, Shiffrin RY, Grishaw EK (1994) Virtual colonoscopy. Radiology 194:446

Wax MR (2000) Virtual colonoscopy-CT contrast agents. Proceedings from the 2nd international symposium on virtual colonoscopy, 16–17 Oct 2000, Boston

Waye JD, Lewis BS, Frankel A (1988) Small colon polyps. Am J Gastroenterol 83:120–122

Weyman PJ, Koehler RE, Zuckerman GR (1981) Resolution of radiographic-endoscopic discrepancies in colon neoplasms. J Clin Gastroenterol 3:89–93

Whiting BR, McFarland EG, Brink JA (2000) Influence of image acquisition parameters on CT artifacts and polyp depiction in spiral CT colonography: in vitro evaluation. Radiology 217:165–172

Winawer SJ, Zauber A, Diaz B (1987) Temporal sequence of evolving colorectal cancer from the normal colon. Gastrointest Endosc 33:167

Winawer SJ, Zauber AG, Ho MN (1993) Prevention of colorectal cancer by colonoscopic polypectomy. N Engl J Med 329:1981–1997

Winawer SJ, Stewart ET, Zauber AG (2000) A comparison of colonoscopy and double-contrast barium enema for surveillance after polypectomy. National Polyp Study Work Group. N Engl J Med 342:1823–1824

Wyatt CL, Ge Y, Vining DJ (2000) Automatic segmentation of the colon for virtual colonoscopy. Comput Med Imaging Graph 24:1–9

Yee J, Hung RK, Akenker GA (1999) The usefulness of glucagon hydrochloride for colonic distension in CT colonography. AJR 173:169–172

Yoshida H, Masutani Y, MacEneaney PM (2000) Detection of colonic polyps in CT colonography based on geometric features. Eighty-sixth annual meeting and scientific assembly of the Radiological Society of North America (RSNA). Radiology 217:582

Zalis ME, Hahn PF (2001) Digital subtraction bowel cleansing in CT colonography. AJR 176:646–648

18 Virtual Dissection of the Colon

Erich Sorantin, Emese Balogh, Anna Vilanova Bartrolì, Kálmán Palágyi,
Làzlò G. Nyùl, Sven Loncaric, Marco Subasic, Domagoj Kovacevic

CONTENTS

18.1
Introduction and Medical Background

Colorectal cancer represents the third most commonly diagnosed cancer and is the second leading cause of cancer deaths in the United States (Gazelle

E. Sorantin, MD
Department of Radiology, University Hospital Graz, Auenbruggerplatz 34, 8036 Graz, Austria
E. Balogh, MSc
Department of Applied Informatics, University of Szeged, Árpád tér 2, 6720 Szeged, Hungary
A. Vilanova Bartrolì
Institute of Computer Graphics and Algorithms, Vienna University of Technology, Karlsplatz 13/186/2, 1040 Vienna, Austria
K. Palágyi, PhD, L.G. Nyùl, MSc
Department of Applied Informatics, University of Szeged, Árpád tér 2, 6720 Szeged, Hungary
S. Loncaric, PhD, M. Subasic, D. Kovacevic, MD
Department of Electronic Systems and Information Processing, Faculty of Electrical Engineering Computing Zagreb, Unska 3, HR-10000 Zagreb, Croatia

et al. 2000). In addition, colorectal cancer is responsible for about 11% of all new cancer cases per year (Gazelle et al. 2000). Five-year prognosis is about 90% for patients with localised disease compared with 60% if there is a regional spread, and drops to 10% in patients with distant metastasis (Gazelle et al. 2000). There is a widely accepted medical opinion that most colorectal cancers arise from pre-existent adenomatous polyps (Johnson 2000). Therefore, various societies such as the American Cancer Society have proposed screening for colorectal cancer (Byers et al. 1997; Winawer et al. 1997). Different options exist for the detection of colorectal cancer, including digital rectal examination, faecal occult blood testing, flexible and rigid sigmoidoscopy, barium enema and its variants, colonoscopy and, recently, computed tomography or magnetic resonance based virtual colonography (Gazelle et al. 2000). All have their inherent advantages and disadvantages. Colonoscopy is regarded as the gold standard for colonic investigations, but unfortunately it can only be completed in about 85–95% of cases. But at colonoscopy only the retrograde viewing direction is possible, thus making detection of small polyps on the aboral side of colonic folds difficult. In addition, the anatomical distribution of colorectal cancer has changed over the years. In the 1940s cancer of the rectum and sigmoid colon accounted for 65–80% of all colorectal cancers compared with 52–61% in the last 30 years. Over the same period the number of cancers in the proximal colon has increased, which may be related to the increasing number of cholecystectomies (Gazelle et al. 2000).

If screening for colorectal cancer is to be considered, the chosen investigation should allow assessment of the whole colon in all patients, as well as the inspection of the whole colonic surface. Cross-sectional imaging modalities such as helical CT or MR tomography together with appropriate image postprocessing could represent a perfect screening tool, fulfilling all the above-mentioned criteria. As early as 1994 Vining and Gelfand reported their experience of applying methods of virtual reality to helical CT in order to produce endoluminal views similar to colonoscopy (JOHNSON 2000). Today CT colonography refers to a helical CT investigation where the colon is fully prepared and distended by room air or carbon dioxide (JOHNSON 2000). Afterwards offline postprocessing of the axial CT data is done by generating two-dimensional (2D) and three-dimensional (3D) reconstructions including virtual endoluminal views of the colonic surface (JOHNSON 2000). In order to overcome the problem of missed polyps on the oral side of the colonic folds antegrade and retrograde views are generated. Alternative names such as virtual colonoscopy, virtual endoscopy and 3D endoscopy have been abandoned in favour of CT colonography (JOHNSON 1998). Since the generation of all these views is a time-consuming task, new and faster image-processing algorithms as well as alternative display techniques such as virtual pathology, Mercator map projection and panoramic projections have been developed and are under evaluation (JOHNSON 2000).

The technical background and image reconstruction for another display technique called *virtual dissection* will be described in this chapter. Using this technique the colonic surface is automatically extracted from the CT data, stretched and flattened. Example images derived from an artificial and a cadaveric phantom will be shown. All image reconstructions were computed from multi-row detector computed tomography (MRDCT) data. The individual steps are described within the section workflow. Two different image-processing approaches will be presented as well as the preliminary results, conclusions and the direction of further work.

18.2
Methods

18.2.1
Workflow

Different steps have to be undertaken in order to obtain a virtual dissection of the colon. After MRDCT scanning the reconstructed, overlapping slices were transferred to the graphics laboratory computers via the hospital network. At the segmentation step (Sect. 18.2.2.1) the structure of interest within the abdomen, i.e. the colon, was defined. The following skeletonisation (Sect. 18.2.2.2) enabled the extraction of the colonic central path. Using the central path two different approaches were used in order to perform a

virtual dissection: 2D flattening (Sect. 18.2.2.3) and a 3D local flattening approach (Sect. 18.2.2.4). A workflow schema can be seen in Fig. 18.1.

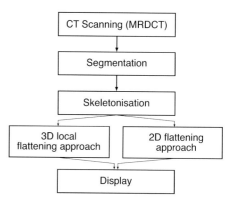

Fig. 18.1. Workflow scheme

18.2.2
Image Processing

18.2.2.1
Segmentation – Fuzzy Connectedness

A vast amount of literature exists on image segmentation techniques. Many different approaches have been investigated for segmenting images of different body regions from different imaging modalities. Their accuracy and reproducibility in some applications is not satisfactory or may not even be known. These are, however, very important factors that need to be taken into account when devising a method for practical use.

After some quick experiments with "simple" techniques (a 3D generalisation of region growing and manual drawing augmented by splines) we found that, although the object of our study (i.e. the colon) is clearly defined in the CT images for the human eye, the results produced by these techniques were not well reproducible and the processes were inefficient (in terms of the amount of human interaction necessary and the way human input is required). Since this is the very first postprocessing step, everything depends on the segmentation results. Therefore, a validated, accurate and highly reproducible method should be used to avoid problems later in the process. This is what made us decide on utilising the segmentation method using fuzzy connectedness (UDUPA et al. 1994; UDUPA and SAMARASEKERA 1996).

Images are inherently fuzzy. Their inhomogeneity is partly due to the graded composition of the material being imaged and to the imaging process (e.g. blurring, partial volume effects). Fuzzy connectedness captures this fuzziness as well as the spatial coherence of the voxels in a well-defined manner. It has a mathematically formulated theory proving its robustness. This framework and the algorithms have now been successfully applied extensively on thousands of 3D volumes in several routine clinical applications (UDUPA et al. 2000).

The fuzzy connectedness method has a proven high reproducibility and is very efficient regarding user intervention as well as its computational requirements. In our case (i.e. segmenting the colon from a 3D CT image volume), air has a well-defined range of Hounsfield units so the parameters for fuzzy affinities required by the method may be set once and used for all studies without in-study training. The user specifies the rectangular volume of interest (VOI) using a graphical user interface (GUI), as well as a "seed point" within the colon for seeding the fuzzy connected objects. The VOI operation is to reduce the data volume to be processed by the fuzzy connectedness method, as well as to exclude unwanted regions from the processing volume that would otherwise make several additional postprocessing steps necessary. The seed points are specified by clicking on voxels "deeply" inside the colon in order to avoid the uncertain regions near the boundary. Generally a single seed point is sufficient; however, several points may be specified if necessary.

Fuzzy connectedness is an extremely robust segmentation technique that very effectively handles inhomogeneity (resulting from both tissue properties and the imaging procedure). It is also robust against the selection of seed points, provided boundaries are avoided. Since the only user input (apart from the VOI selection) is the seed point specification, and all other parameters are fixed, our segmentation inherits the reproducibility and efficiency of the fuzzy connectedness method. Since we use absolute fuzzy connectedness and a single object is segmented, the uncertain boundary regions (due to partial volume effects) are not captured by the fuzzy objects; therefore, the segmentation was initially too tight (uniformly along the entire object) in the physician's opinion. A 3D dilation using a 3×3×3 structuring element is applied to the segmented fuzzy connected object, thus making it better fit the observer's expectations. Finally, the segmented binary 3D volume is transformed into cubic voxels by linear interpolation, because some

of the later steps (e.g. skeletonisation) require isotropic data.

18.2.2.2
Skeletonisation

The notion of the skeleton was introduced by BLUM (1964) as a region-based shape feature descriptor which summarises the general form of objects or shapes. A very illustrative definition of the skeleton is given by the prairie-fire analogy: the object boundary is set on fire and the skeleton is formed by the loci where the fire fronts meet and quench each other. This definition can be naturally extended to any dimension.

During the last two decades skeletonisation (i.e. extracting a skeleton from digital binary images) has become a challenging research field. Three major skeletonisation techniques have been proposed: the distance transform method, the method based on Voronoi diagrams, and the iterative object reduction called thinning.

We prefer thinning, since it is fairly fast and capable of producing a good approximation to the skeleton in a topology-preserving way (KONG and ROSENFELD 1989). It is based on digital simulation of the fire front propagation: border points (i.e. 1s that are "adjacent" to 0s) of a binary object that satisfy certain topological and geometrical constraints are deleted in iteration steps. The entire process is repeated until only the "skeleton" is left.

In 3D imaging there are two major types of thinning: surface thinning produces the medial surface of an object (by preserving surface end-points) while curve thinning can extract the medial lines of an object (by preserving line end-points) (PALÁGYI and KUBA 1999). It is easy to see that the skeleton of a 3D object may contain surface patches; therefore, surface thinning produces a better approximation to the skeleton than curve thinning does. Despite this fact, in the case of "near-tubular" 3D objects (e.g. airway, blood vessel or gastrointestinal tract) medial lines provide more reasonable shape features.

A recently published sequential 3D thinning algorithm (PALÁGYI et al. 2001) is applied to extract the medial lines from the segmented colon.

18.2.2.3
2D Flattening Approach

As a first approach to colonic virtual dissection a transformation of the problem from 3D to 2D was done in the following way. After obtaining the central path by skeletonisation (as described in Sect. 18.2.2.2) the 3D cross-sectional profile orthogonal to the central path is calculated. Care is taken to sample enough cross-sections along the central path; in our experience 1.0 mm is sufficient. Because of the tortuous structure of the colon adjacent cross-sections may intersect and, as a result, polyps may be missed or counted multiple times. WANG et al. (1999) tried to solve this problem using electrical field lines generated by a locally charged path (WANG et al. 1998, 1999). In order to avoid this conflict the angle between two intersecting cross-sections was interpolated and recalculated iteratively until no intersection occurred. Then, the segmented colon is remapped into a new grey-level 3D data volume. Data at every degree of the cross-section were put into a new 3D volume (constant angle sampling).

The result is a virtually stretched and flattened colon. Fig. 18.2 shows an orthogonal cross-section of the colon before flattening, and the same cross-section after flattening. The 3D data volume obtained contains the virtually stretched and flattened colon. For visualisation of the colonic surface after stretching and flattening, both volume and surface rendering techniques were implemented.

18.2.2.4
3D Local Flattening Approach

The method presented in this section (BARTROLÍ et al. 2001) does not generate a flat model of the whole colon, but allows inspection of locally flattened regions in such a way that double counting of polyps does not occur. The method involves moving a camera along the central path of the colon. The central path is calculated using a thinning algorithm. Afterwards, the path is approximated by a B-spline curve.

For each camera position, a small cylinder tangential to the path is defined. The middle point of the cylinder axis corresponds to the camera position. Rays starting at the cylinder axis and orthogonal to the cylinder surface are traced (Fig. 18.3). For each ray, direct volume rendering is used to calculate the colour that corresponds to the cylinder point where the ray was projected. Finally, the coloured cylinder with the sampled rays is mapped onto a 2D image by simply unfolding the cylinder. The cylinder axis must be short enough not to penetrate the surface of the colon. This can be done by taking the distance of the path to the organ surface into account.

Fig. 18.2a,b. An orthogonal cross-section (a) before flattening and (b) after flattening

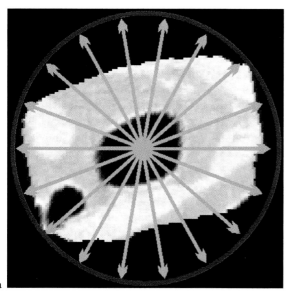

a

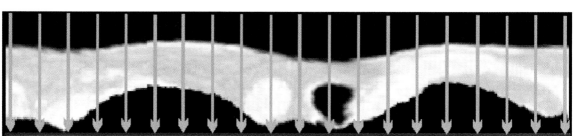

b

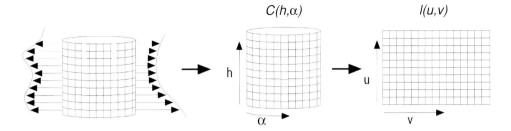

Fig. 18.3. Illustration of the projection procedure. A region of the surface is projected to the cylinder $C(h, \alpha)$. Then the cylinder is mapped to the image

The result is a video where each frame shows the projection of a small part of the inner surface of the organ onto the cylinder. If the camera is moved slowly enough the coherence between frames will be high and the observer will be able to follow the movement of the surface. In this method possible double sampling of polyps emerges only between frames. However, it does not cause a double counting of polyps since the human brain is able to track the polyp movement due to the coherence between frames. Moving along the central path in a high curvature area a polyp might move up and down (due to double sampling) but is clearly identified as a single object.

The proposed projection is illustrated in Fig. 18.3. A cylinder $C(h, \alpha)$ is defined for each camera position. This cylinder is coloured by tracing rays orthogonal to the cylinder surface (i.e. projecting a region of the surface onto the cylinder). Then the cylinder is mapped to the final image $I(u, v)$ by a simple mapping function $f : (h, \alpha)\alpha \rightarrow (u, v)$.

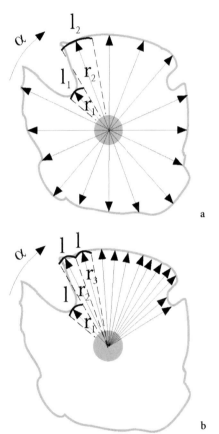

Fig. 18.4. a Constant angle sampling: it is shown that different surface lengths are represented by the same length in the cylinder. **b** Perimeter sampling: same length but different angle

18.2.2.5
Constant Angle Sampling

The sampling distance (i.e. the distance between two consecutive rays) in the h-direction is constant, and it must be at most half the size of a voxel (Fig. 18.4a). In this way the Nyquist frequency in the h-direction is preserved.

For each h-value the rays are traced in radial directions with respect to the cylinder axis. The rays are diverging from each other, so the volume data is not sampled uniformly if the incremental angle is constant. Furthermore, features can be missed.

18.2.2.6
Perimeter Sampling

Perimeter sampling represents another possibility for sampling the surface uniformly (Fig. 18.4b). In this method, a constant sample length l is defined. l must

be at most half the size of a voxel to maintain the Nyquist frequency and therefore not to miss any important feature. l should have the same value as the sampling distance in the h-direction to preserve the ratio, or proportion, in the final mapping.

The algorithm incrementally calculates the ray directions that are in the plane defined by a certain value of h. The angle between the current ray and the next one is computed such that the length of the surface sample that the current ray represents equals l in the α-direction. The first ray is traced along an arbitrary angle α_0, which must be the same for all camera positions. r_i is defined as the distance from the cylinder axis to the surface point hit by the ray. The surface sample length in the α-direction that a ray represents is approximated by the arc with radius r_i. Therefore, the value of the angle increment for the next ray is estimated as l/r_i radians.

In this case, the mapping function f maps the contours and also the surface of the generalised cylinder uniformly. Moving along the central path, contours of varying length are represented by varying numbers of rays. This results in the fact that in the v-direction (horizontal scan lines) typically only part of the pixels are covered by an unfolded contour in the mapping to the image plane. The projected points that correspond to the rays at angle 0 are positioned on a vertical line in the centre of the image. Then, from left to right the ray values are mapped to the image until the perimeter length is reached.

This projection has the property of area preservation, i.e. the relative sizes of surface elements are preserved in the image plane and do not depend on the proximity of the cylinder axis to the surface. On the other hand, a distortion is introduced with respect to the h- and α-direction, so the angles are no longer preserved. There is no distortion at the vertical centre line of the image, but the distortion increases progressively on moving to the left and right.

18.2.2.7
Image Enhancement

Using the distance from a point on the surface to the cylinder axis r_i a depth image can be generated. This depth image together with the shaded image represent a height field, similar to a landscape in topography. A good way to visualise landscapes in topographical maps is to show contour lines, where each line corresponds to a particular depth. The contour lines improve the perception of depth and surface changes of the map. They are also drawn as an enhancement of the shaded flattened image. They are generated based on the technique described by SAITO and TAKAHASHI (1990).

18.2.3
Phantoms

To test the algorithm, an artificial and a cadaveric phantom were created. Both phantoms were scanned using MRDCT (GE Lightspeed QXI, GE Medical Systems). A collimation of 2.5 mm and a high-quality pitch were selected. Scans were reconstructed using the manufacturer's standard reconstruction program with a slice thickness of 1.25 mm, an increment of 0.5 mm and a matrix of 512×512. Thus the resulting in-plane pixel size was 0.585 mm.

18.2.3.1
Artificial Phantom

An artificial phantom was created by putting small Plasticine beads into a plastic tube so as to create six "polyps". Photographs of each end of the tube are shown in Fig. 18.5.

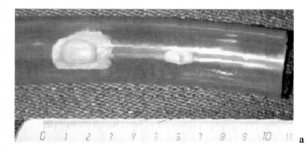

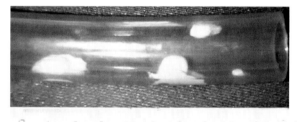

Fig. 18.5a, b. The ends of the tube phantom with embedded Plasticine beads

18.2.3.2
Cadaveric Phantom

The second phantom consisted of a 50 cm long part of a normal, cadaveric colon. The bowel was cleansed and 13 artificial polyps were created using fat tissue. After inflation with room air the specimen was placed in a 5 l water bath containing 5 ml Gastrografin (Schering, Austria) solution. In this way the attenuation of the human abdomen was simulated. A photograph of the phantom can be seen in Fig. 18.6. After CT scanning a real dissection was performed and compared visually with the computed virtual dissection.

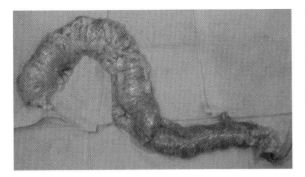

Fig. 18.6. The cadaveric phantom

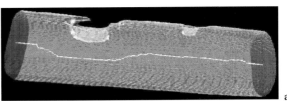

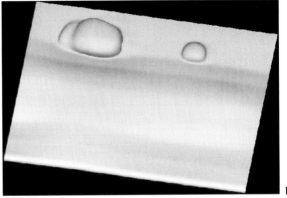

Fig. 18.7a,b. One end of the artificial phantom. a Transparent 3D model with the central path. b The inner surface after virtual dissection using the 2D flattening approach

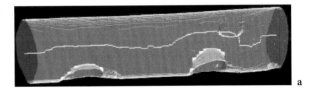

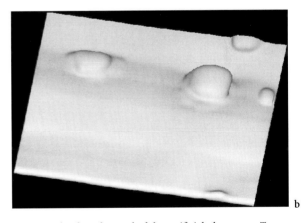

Fig. 18.8a, b. The other end of the artificial phantom. a Transparent 3D model with the central path. b The inner surface after virtual dissection using the 2D flattening approach

18.3
Results

18.3.1
Artificial Phantom

The artificial phantom contains six simulated polyps placed in the ends of the plastic tube. The result after segmentation with its central path and the computed virtual dissection using the 2D flattening approach is shown in Fig. 18.7 for one end of the phantom. The two polyps at this end can be clearly seen. The other end of the phantom, containing four polyps, is presented in a similar way in Fig. 18.8. All the polyps can be clearly detected on the images after virtual dissection (Figs. 18.7, 18.8). The polyps appeared on virtual dissection as bumps.

18.3.2
Cadaveric Phantom

In the case of the cadaveric phantom a total of 13 artificial polyps were created using fat tissue, with a size (in transverse, coronal and sagittal directions) between 4.1×5.2×2.1 mm and 12.9×15×11.4 mm. Fig. 18.9 shows the surface rendered 3D reconstruction of the segmented colon, and the same binary object with its central path as a transparent 3D model. In Fig. 18.10 the appearance of the created polyps on axial (upper row) and virtual endoscopic views (lower row) can be seen.

After scanning, a real dissection of the colon was performed and the polyps were marked (Fig. 18.11). Fig. 18.12 shows the inner surface of the cadaveric colon after virtual dissection had been performed using the 2D flattening approach. Fig. 18.13 shows a frame obtained by the 3D local flattening approach using the two presented sampling techniques. An example of image enhancement achieved by the contour lines method is shown in Fig. 18.14.

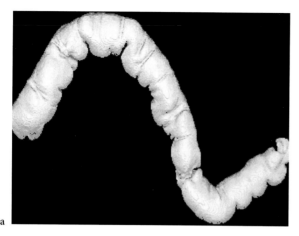

a

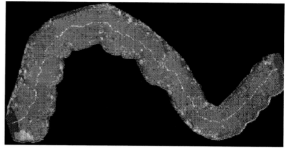

b

Fig. 18.9a, b. The cadaveric phantom. a Surface rendered image of the segmented colon. b Transparent 3D model showing the central path obtained by skeletonisation

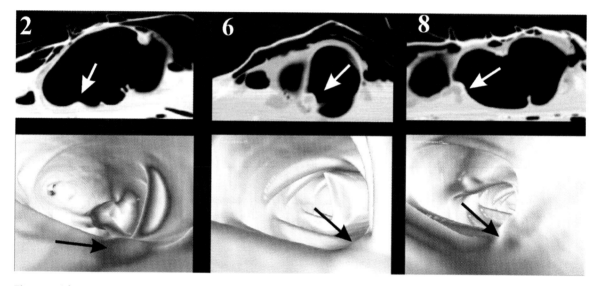

Fig. 18.10. Three representative polyps (*arrows*) shown on axial CT scans (*upper row*) and the same polyps presented on virtual endoscopic views (*lower row*)

With both techniques, the 2D flattening approach and the local 3D flattening approach, all 13 artificially created polyps appeared as a broadening of folds or bumps and could be identified by visual inspection. In our preliminary experience, the polyps could be seen more easily on surface rendered views. The time required for generation of the virtual dissection views was 10 min for the operator and about 2 h of offline computing for the workstation.

In addition an application has been developed for the 3D local flattening approach as presented in Sect. 18.2.2.4. The result of the method is a video where each frame corresponds to a flattened area of the colon. The application allows the physician to easily associate the frames of the video with its correspond-ing region in the original volume data. The application consists of different visualisation techniques shown in separate but related windows.

One window shows the consecutive flattened frames of the video. The current camera position corresponds with the frame shown at the time. An overview image is generated using the horizontal centre lines of each frame. In the overview image, the current camera position is indicated by highlighting its corresponding horizontal centre line. The overview image is incorrect since the cross-sections that correspond to each line intersect each other, but the image gives enough context information to orient the user. Furthermore, there are three windows that show the three orthogonal planes corresponding to the three

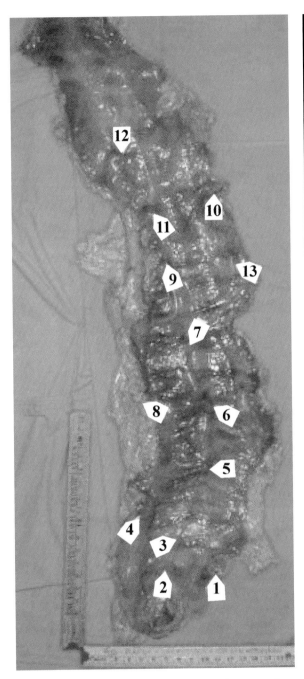

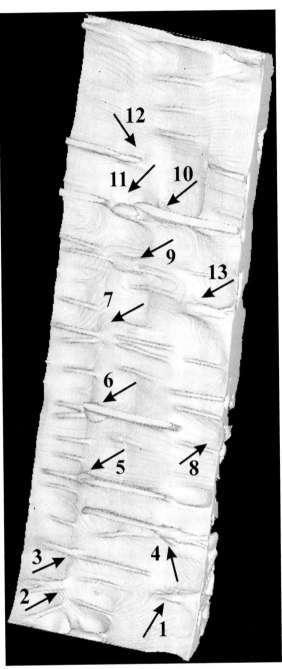

Fig. 18.11. Dissection of the cadaveric colon phantom. Polyps are numbered *1–13*

Fig. 18.12. Virtual dissection of the cadaveric colon phantom using the 2D flattening approach

coordinate planes of the current camera frame. These planes are generated using multiplanar reconstruction.

A window showing a common perspective view of the data set is also present. This window is updated with the current camera frame each time the frame changes. If the user clicks on an area of the flattened frame an update of the perspective view camera is done. The camera of the perspective view points to the same area that has been clicked in the flattened frame. The relationship between windows and different visualisation techniques provides a usable tool for inspection of the data set. An example screenshot can be seen in Fig. 18.15.

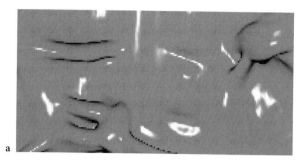

Fig. 18.13a, b. A frame derived from the 3D local flattening approach. **a** Resulting image of the projection technique using constant angle sampling. **b** Same camera position as **a** but with perimeter sampling

a

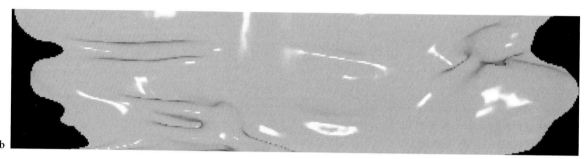

b

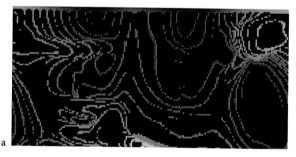

a

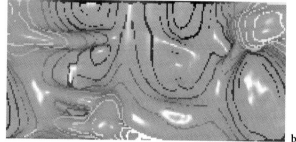

b

Fig. 18.14a, b. Image enhancement for the 3D local flattening approach. **a** Contour lines with colour coding indicating the depth. **b** Combination of the contour lines and shaded image

18.4
Conclusion

In both fibreoptic colonoscopy and CT colonography polyps behind colonic folds may be not seen on standard oral views due to the tortuous structure of the colon. Further endoscopic view visualises only a small part of the inner colonic surface. The display techniques of virtual dissection presented here avoid these problems and present the colonic surface in the same manner as on the pathologist's table. Theoretically, due to the view from "above" all polyps should be displayed and not be hidden by the colonic folds.

Navigation through the colon in oral and aboral directions is a time-consuming and labour-inten-

sive task. The two methods presented for obtaining a virtual dissection are mainly automated, operator interaction being required only for starting the segmentation procedure. If skeletonisation produces unwanted side branches of the central path, the central path and the segmented colon can be converted to the standards of the virtual reality modelling language (VRML) and a VRML editor used to prune the central path from unwanted side branches. All other steps are automated and need no operator interaction. A total time amount of about 2 h with an operator attendance of minutes seems acceptable. Therefore virtual dissection seems to be a promising display technique for CT colonography, especially if mass screening for polyp detection is considered. It cannot yet be decided whether

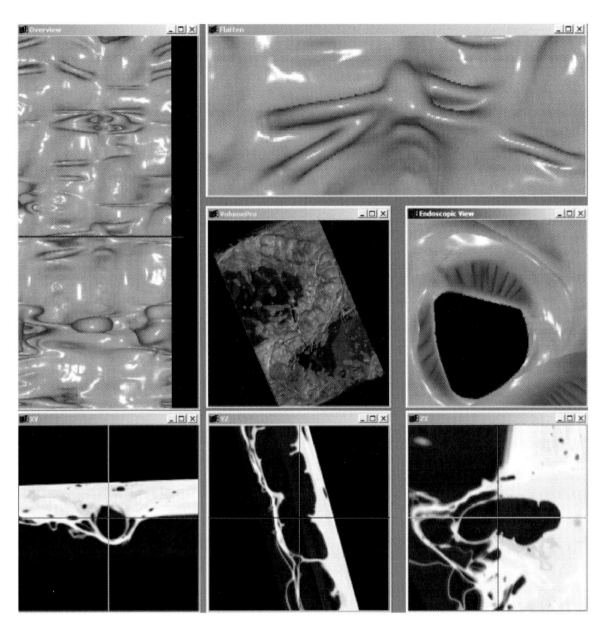

Fig. 18.15. Interactive application for evaluation of virtual dissection using the 3D local flattening approach. Seven different windows are shown on the computer screen. *Upper left corner*: virtual dissection of the colon using the 3D local flattening approach (constant angle sampling). The *red horizontal line* depicts the position of the virtual camera, which is used for anatomical cross-referencing on the other views. *Upper right corner*: magnified view from the left. *Middle row centre*: view from above. *Middle row right*: virtual endoscopic view. *Lower row*: axial CT slice and multiplanar reconstructions (coronal, sagittal) at the position of the virtual camera. Whenever the position of the virtual camera is moved upwards or downwards with the cursor keys all windows are updated automatically

the 2D flattening approach or the 3D local flattening approach will be the better choice for clinical routine. This has to be worked out in further, prospective clinical trials. An inherent disadvantage of virtual dissection is the deformation introduced by the individual steps of image processing. Therefore high-resolution source images are important, thus making it necessary to use MRDCT. A slice thickness of 1.0–1.5 mm with an overlap of 0.5–1.0 mm seems appropriate. A larger slice thickness will result in a lower resolution, higher deformation and therefore reduced image quality.

18.5
Further Work

18.5.1
Segmentation

A potential improvement of the colon segmentation procedure could be to use deformable models, which have received a lot of attention in the image analysis community in recent years. Deformable models were introduced by Kass et al. (1987). There are different variations of the active contours, but the basic approach behind all of them is this: in order to segment a region of interest (ROI) in the image, a contour is superimposed on this image and then deformed in order to fit the ROI. After a finite number of steps in which the contour moves and deforms in some way, depending on the particular active contour used, it settles to some position and shape which represents the ROI. The deformation of the active contour can be presented as an energy minimisation problem, where energy is defined as a function of the shape and position of the contour and the minimum of the energy term represents the optimal ROI. The energy consists of two terms: internal and external energy. The external energy connects shape with the underlying image. The internal energy is a function of the shape of the contour. Also, other energy terms can be introduced in order to enforce some specific behaviour on the active contour.

Active border is an extension of the active contour in 3D space. We can simplify the 3D model by assuming that the object of interest has tubular shape, meaning it can be represented by a set of 2D curves. Each curve interacts with neighbouring curves, but only force components in x and y directions are used, so the border nodes cannot move from one slice to another. This approach is used for segmentation of aortic aneurysm (Loncaric et al. 2000) but can be applied to other tubular structures such as the colon. An overview of the applications of the active contour paradigm to medical imagery can be found in McInerney and Terzopoulos (1996). Geometric deformable models have been proposed by Caselles et al. (1993) and Malladi et al. (1995). These deformable models overcome some of the difficulties of classical active contours. Their main advantage is that they easily represent complex structures and they can change topology (brake or merge) in a natural manner. The ability to represent complex shapes is useful in medical image segmentation because there are many different shapes to segment in the human body and pathological disorders can

produce particularly complex shapes (Subasic et al. 2001). These deformable models types are based on curve evolution theory and the level-set method (Osher and Sethian 1988). Here curves and surfaces are evolved using geometric measures (unit normal and curvature) instead of quantities dependent on parameters, which makes the geometric deformable model independent of parameterisation.

In geometric deformable models, evolving curves or surfaces are represented as a level set of higher-dimensional scalar function. This higher-dimension function is referred to as the level-set function. The level-set function is defined over the same domain as the image and its most common form is a signed distance function. Distances from an evolving curve or surface give values of the level-set function at each image point. Instead of evolving just a curve or a surface, the entire level-set function is evolved through time. This way, the level-set function always stays a smooth function even if its zero level set changes topology. The curve is evolved in its normal direction according to a speed function which determines the speed of evolution. This speed function is responsible for deformable model behaviour and is usually built from a constant speed term and a curvature-dependent speed term.

In order to segment images, the image influence has to be included in deformable model evolution. With geometric deformable models the image influence is included in the speed function as a multiplicative stopping term. The common stopping criterion is based on a gradient of the image data so that the deformable model stops at high gradient points.

References

Bartrolì AV, Wegenkittl R, König A (2001) Virtual colon flattening. In: Bartrolì AV (ed) VisSym '01 joint eurographics – IEEE TCVG symposium on visualisation (in press)
Blum H (1964) A transformation for extracting new descriptors of shape. Proceedings of the symposium on models for the perception of speech and visual form, pp 362–380
Byers T, Levin B, Rothenberger D (1997) American Cancer Society guidelines for screening and surveillance for early detection of colorectal polyps and cancer: update 1997. Cancer J Clin 47:154–160
Caselles V, Catte F, Coll T (1993) A geometric model for active contours. Numer Math 66:1–31
Gazelle G, McPhanon P, Schol F (2000) Screening for colorectal cancer. Radiology 215:327–335
Johnson C (1998) Virtual endoscopy: what's in a name? AJR 171:1201–1202
Johnson C (2000) CT colonography: the next colon screening examination? Radiology 216:331–341

Kass M, Witkin A, Terzopoulos D (1987) Snakes: active contour models. Int J Comput Vis 1:321–331

Kong T, Rosenfeld A (1989) Digital topology: introduction and survey. Comput Vis Graph Image Proc 48:357–393

Loncaric S, Kovacevic D, Sorantin E (2000) Semiautomatic active contour approach to segmentation of computed tomography volumes. SPIE Proc 3979:917–924

Malladi R, Sethian JA, Vemuri BC (1995) Shape modeling with front propagation. IEEE Trans PAMI 17:158–176

McInerney T, Terzopoulos D (1996) Deformable models in medical image analysis: a survey. Med Image Anal 1:91–108

Osher S, Sethian J (1988) Fronts propagating with curvature-dependent speed: algorithms based on Hamilton-Jacobi formulations. J Comput Physics 79:12–49

Palágyi K, Kuba A (1999) A parallel 3D 12-subiteration thinning algorithm. Graph Models Image Proc 61:199–221

Palágyi K, Sorantin E, Balogh E (2001) A sequential 3D thinning algorithm and its medical applications. Proceedings of the 17th international conference on information processing in medical imaging, IPMI 2001. Lecture notes in computer sciences. Springer, Berlin Heidelberg New York, pp 409–415

Saito T, Takahashi T (1990) Comprehensible rendering of 3-D shapes. SIGGRAPH '90 conference proceedings, annual conference series, pp 197–206

Subasic M, Loncaric S, Sorantin E (2001) 3-D deformable model segmentation of abdominal aortic aneurysm. SPIE Proc 4322 (in press)

Udupa JK, Samarasekera S (1996) Fuzzy connectedness and object definition: theory, algorithms, and applications in image segmentation. Graph Models Image Proc 58:246–261

Udupa JK, Odhner D, Samarasekera S (1994) 3DVIEWNIX: an open, transportable, multidimensional, multimodality, multiparametric imaging software system. SPIE Proc 2164:58–73

Udupa JK, Grossman RI, Nyúl LG (2000) Multiprotocol MR image segmentation in multiple sclerosis: experience with over 1000 studies. SPIE Proc 3979:1017–1027

Wang G, McFarland EG, Brown BP (1998) GI tract unraveling with curved cross-sections. IEEE Trans Med Imaging 17:318–322

Wang G, Dave SB, Brown BP (1999) Colon unraveling based on electrical field: recent progress and further work. SPIE Proc 3660:125–132

Winawer S, Fletcher R, Miller L (1997) Colorectal cancer screening: clinical guidelines and rationale. Gastroenterology 112:594–642

19 Liver

Riccardo Lencioni, Laura Crocetti, Emanuele Neri

CONTENTS

19.1
Introduction

Image processing is a very important tool to improve the quantity and quality of information given by ultrasound, computed tomography and magnetic resonance imaging of the liver. The liver is the largest organ in the body, has a very complex anatomy and can be affected by many different diseases, both diffuse and focal. Among diffuse diseases, cirrhosis has the highest prevalence and can be associated with portal hypertension and hepatocellular carcinoma (HCC) (Bartolozzi and Lencioni 1999). Cirrhotic patients are frequently candidates for orthotopic liver transplantation (OLT) and need an accurate evaluation of the liver itself and of its vascularization. Postprocessing with three-dimensional (3D) evaluation of surfaces, volumes and vessels is of crucial importance for surgical planning.

Many benign and malignant neoplasms, the latter being divided into primary and secondary tumours, can be located within the liver parenchyma. Diagnostic assessment of these neoplasms can be achieved by traditional examination techniques implemented by 3D reconstructions (Bartolozzi and Lencioni 1999). Malignant tumours can be treated with either surgery or interventional treatments (Bartolozzi and Lencioni 1999). Three-dimensional images allow a precise evaluation of the segmental location of the lesion, and of its relationship with vessels and surrounding organs. More information is also available with this technique about treatment outcome.

This chapter will deal with 3D image processing of the liver in the evaluation of patients who are candidates for surgery or interventional treatments.

19.2
Lobar and Segmental Anatomy of the Liver

Three-dimensional image processing has a crucial role in the pretreatment evaluation of patients who have to be placed on the active waiting list for transplantation or have to undergo surgery or other therapeutic procedures for hepatic neoplasm (Togo et al. 1998; Bartolozzi and Lencioni 1999). In all these patients conventional imaging implemented by 3D image processing is useful to assess hepatic morphology and vascular anatomy, to detect focal liver lesions, to calculate liver volume and to evaluate portal hypertension (Heath et al. 1995; van Leeuwen et al. 1995; Nghiem et al. 1999).

The surface anatomy of the liver can be shown by means of CT and MR shaded surface display (SSD), which allows the identification of the classical lobar anatomy of the liver (van Leeuwen et al. 1994a, b). A correlation between external landmarks (i.e. fissures) and internal landmarks (i.e. vessels) is possible, with an overview on anatomical variations, and the different course of internal and external landmarks. This information are very important for the surgeon because what he sees on the surface does not correspond to what he will find in the liver parenchyma.

R. Lencioni, MD
Diagnostic and Interventional Radiology, Department of Oncology, Transplants and Advanced Technologies in Medicine, University of Pisa, Via Roma 67, 56100 Pisa, Italy
L. Crocetti, MD
Diagnostic and Interventional Radiology, Department of Oncology, Transplants and Advanced Technologies in Medicine, University of Pisa, Via Roma 67, 56100 Pisa, Italy
E. Neri, MD
Diagnostic and Interventional Radiology, Department of Oncology, Transplants and Advanced Technologies in Medicine, University of Pisa, Via Roma 67, 56100 Pisa, Italy

The H-shaped indentations on the visceral faces of the liver divide it into four externally defined lobes: the right, left, quadrate and caudate lobes. The right-hand limb of the H is formed by the fossa for the gallbladder anteriorly and by a deep sulcus for the inferior vena cava posteriorly. The gallbladder fossa separates the anterior part of the externally defined right lobe from the quadrate lobe. The sulcus for the inferior vena cava separates the posterior portion of the right lobe from the caudate lobe. Between the gallbladder fossa and the sulcus for the inferior vena cava the right limb of the H is deficient where a caudate process connects the caudate lobe to the right lobe. The left limb of the H is formed by two deep fissures that contain true ligaments in their depths. Anteriorly it is formed by the deep fissure for the ligamentum teres, which separates the anterior part of the externally defined left lobe from the quadrate lobe. Posteriorly it is formed by the fissure for the ligamentum venosum, which separates the posterior part of the left lobe (FRIEDMAN and DACHMAN 1994).

Segmental anatomy is crucial in order to precisely localize a focal lesion, to evaluate the possibility of a resection, to determine the adequate technique for resection, and finally to estimate the ease or difficulty of a biopsy or any other percutaneous manoeuvre. Segmental anatomy is the basis of modern hepatic surgery (TOGO et al. 1998). Planes of resection in liver surgery and the correct positioning of devices for interventional treatment are largely determined by the precise position of tumour relative to the individual segmental anatomy. Consequently, localization of liver lesions and preoperative evaluation of resection planes requires consideration of the significant anatomical variations in the segmental anatomy of the liver (VAN LEEUWEN et al. 1995).

Each segment is supplied by a sheath containing branches of the hepatic artery and portal vein and a draining bile duct, which enters the middle of the segment. Venous drainage is via the hepatic vein, which tends to run between segmental divisions (HEALY and SCHROY 1953; COUINAUD 1957; GOLDSMITH and WOODBURNE 1957; HEALY 1970; MICHELS 1996; BISMUTH et al. 1988).

The left portal vein divides into three branches: lateral posterior, lateral anterior and medial. The lateral posterior branch feeds segment II, the lateral interior branch feeds segment III and the medial branch feeds segment IV.

The right portal vein divides into two branches: one anterior and one posterior. The anterior branch divides into a superior branch, for segment VIII, and an inferior branch, for segment V. Segment VIII is located between the middle hepatic vein (left), the right hepatic vein (right) and the inferior vena cava (superior and posterior). It lies over segment V. Segment V is located between the middle hepatic vein and the gallbladder fossa (left), the right hepatic vein (right) and the surface of the liver (inferior and anterior). It lies under segment VIII. Segment V does not reach the inferior vena cava. The posterior branch divides into a superior branch, for segment VII, and an inferior branch, for segment VI. Segment VII is located behind the right hepatic vein (right) and the inferior vena cava medial. It lies over segment VI, and is hidden by segment VIII when looking at the liver from the front. Segment VI is located behind the right hepatic vein and the surface of the liver (inferior and anterior). It lies under segment VII. Segment VI does not reach the inferior vena cava, but is usually located in front of the right kidney.

Segment I is not fed by a single portal vein, and drains through multiple short hepatic veins to the inferior vena cava. Segment I is located between the portal trunk (anterior), the inferior vena cava (posterior) and the liver surface (left), and is in complete continuity with segment VII on its right side.

Individualization of segment IX is a recent proposal from the major author on modern liver segmentation (COUINAUD 1998). This segment would be located in the right liver, in close relationship with the inferior vena cava. Segment IX is in close contact with the right aspect of the vena cava, rather symmetrical with segment I on the left side. Individualization of segment IX relies on the fact that many small portal branches arise from the portal arch. Branches arising from the left portal vein may feed some parts of segment IX. Also, like segment I, segment IX is drained by small hepatic veins entering either the caval axis directly, or the major hepatic veins. Segment IX and segment I together are the "dorsal sector", which is different from the right and left liver. Individualization of the dorsal sector may be important in understanding bleeding problems in resection or split liver transplantation.

Spiral CT allows the acquisition of consistent volumetric data of the entire liver during the peak of vascular enhancement. From these volumetric data, detailed 3D renderings can be created representing the intrahepatic portal branches, hepatic venous system and hepatic contour. By studying the portal branches from different angles and projections, in relation to the hepatic veins and hepatic contour, it is possible to assess the individual segmentation pattern of the liver in vivo and to represent it by means of surface rendering (VAN LEEUWEN et al. 1994a, b). When a resection is planned, it is of crucial importance for the surgeon to know were the avascular planes between the different portal territories are located. Because these avascular planes often are not discernible on the outside of the liver, it can be very helpful to the surgeon if the location of these planes is demonstrated preoperatively. Three-dimensional renderings are far closer to the surgical reality as perceived during liver resection than are transverse slices, and can help to plan a resection tailored to the individual segmental anatomy (VAN LEEUWEN et al. 1994a, b, 1995).

Cirrhotic changes within the liver in patients who are candidates for OLT or interventional treatment for HCC can be demonstrated by means of 3D CT and MR angiography: liver atrophy, nodularity, reduced size of the right hepatic lobe, and the enlargement of the left hepatic lobe or caudate lobe (SMITH et al. 1998).

The volume of the liver can be measured. The ability to measure liver volume before surgery can be useful in determining the extent and nature of hepatic resection. Accurate assessment of liver volume and an estimate of liver function may also allow prediction of post-operative liver failure in patients undergoing resection and can assist in embolization procedures, the planning of staged hepatic resection for bilobar disease and the selection of living related liver donors (GLOMBITZA et al. 1999; WIGMORE et al. 2001). A computer-based 3D virtual operation planning system may be available. The exact prediction of post-operative liver function can be provided by means of measures of the total and resected volume of liver parenchyma. Obviously also the correct loca-

tion of the tumour and of its relations with vessels can be established prior to liver resection (GLOMBITZA et al. 1999; WIGMORE et al. 2001).

Three-dimensional imaging can provide precise anatomical delineation of damaged areas after hepatic injuries, particularly in relation to major vessels. The 3D reconstruction can facilitate decisions regarding intraoperative, re-operative and non-operative management (GOODMAN et al. 1995).

19.3
Hepatic Vessels

Knowledge of hepatic vascular abnormalities prior to liver transplantation or liver resections can be crucial for the surgical planning. Three-dimensional CT and MR imaging evaluation, by means of maximum intensity projection (MIP), SSD and volume rendering projection, allow the visualization of many vascular findings. Volume rendering uses the entire spiral CT data set to create a 3D CT angiogram. The resultant 3D angiogram displays depth, surface relationships and relative CT attenuation values (KUSZYK et al. 1995; JOHNSON et al. 1996a, b).

The hepatic arterial supply can be categorized according to MICHELS' classification (MICHELS 1955) (Table 19.1) and diameters of the major vessels that supply the liver (coeliac axis, common hepatic artery, proper hepatic artery, replaced hepatic artery) can be measured. Classic hepatic arterial anatomy can be seen in 55% of patients, and the commonest arterial variant has been shown to be an aberrant right hepatic supply, which is seen in 13–18% of patients

Table 19.1. Normal variants of arterial supply to the liver: MICHELS' classification

Type I:	Conventional anatomy: proper HA arising from common HA and then giving rise to right and left HA as the sole supply of arterial blood to liver
Type II:	Replaced left HA arising from left gastric artery
Type III:	Replaced right HA arising from SMA
Type IV:	Both replaced right and left HA as described for types II and III
Type V:	Accessory left HA arising from left gastric artery
Type VI:	Accessory right HA arising from SMA
Type VII:	Accessory right HA arising from SMA and accessory left HA arising from left gastric artery
Type VIII:	Replaced right HA and accessory left HA or replaced left HA and accessory right HA
Type IX:	Entire hepatic trunk arising from SMA
Type X:	Entire hepatic trunk arising from left gastric artery

Major normal variants should be known as they may interfere with liver surgery. Liver resection and living related hepatic transplantation require an adequate evaluation of the precise anatomy of major vessels. The anatomy of the arterial supply to the liver can be categorized according to the standard classification system proposed by MICHELS (1955), who defined the 10 anatomical variations of the hepatic artery given above
HA hepatic artery; *SMA* superior mesenteric artery

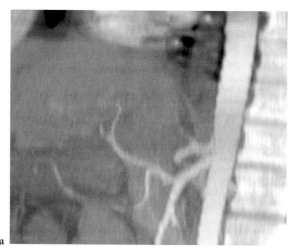

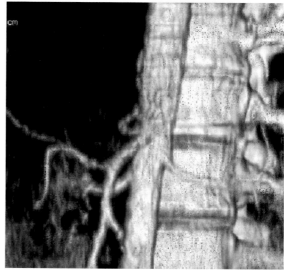

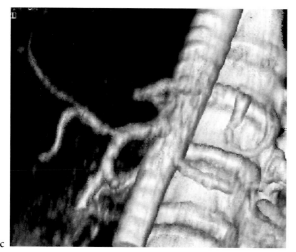

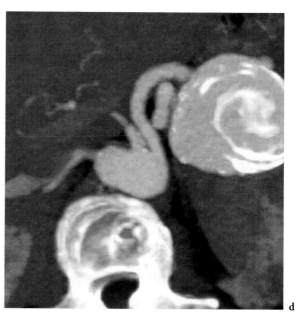

Fig. 19.1a–d. 3D CT angiography. Michels' type IX variant (entire hepatic trunk arising from the superior mesenteric artery) is well demonstrated on maximum intensity projection (MIP) (a) and volume rendered images (b, c). Hepatic artery arising from the aorta demonstrated on a MIP image (d); a splenic artery aneurysm can also be visualized

(COUINAUD 1986). Among various MICHELS' pattern, type IX anatomy can potentially change the surgical approach during liver transplantation. In this anatomical variant there is complete replacement of the hepatic trunk to the superior mesenteric artery. The aberrant course of this artery deep to the portal vein may necessitate altering the sequence of the vascular anastomoses so that the hepatic arterial reconstruction is performed prior to portal vein anastomoses (NGHIEM et al. 1999). 3D CT arteriography MIP, SSD and volume rendered images are equally useful for displaying the hepatic arterial anatomy (Fig. 19.1).

WINTER et al. (1995a) demonstrated that, in transplantation candidates, 3D CT arteriography was as accurate as angiography in the assessment of arterial anatomy. It was, of course, also safer, more convenient and more easily tolerated. Conventional CT plus 3D CT arteriography was therefore only 25% as expensive as the cost of conventional CT and conventional angiography (WINTER et al. 1995b; SMITH et al. 1998). Time-of-flight or phase contrast MR angiographic techniques are often adequate for the depiction of the portal vein but failed to yield reproducibly good-quality morphological images of the hepatic arterial blood supply and of the entire portal venous system. The phase contrast technique still allows functional studies, such as those of the measurement of portal venous blood flow (KOPKA et al. 1999). Contrast-enhanced MR angiography image quality is almost comparable to that of digital subtraction angiography (DSA) in terms of the MICHELS' classification. The entire arterial system of importance to the liver blood supply can be evaluated with high diagnostic confidence (KOPKA et al. 1999; LEE et al. 2000; GLOCKNER 2001). A recent approach is near-isotropic volumetric interpolated 3D MR imaging, which has the advantage of providing volumetric imaging of the entire liver with near-isotropic pixel size, thus offering the possibility of improved detection and characterization of small lesions (HAWIGHORST et al. 1999; ROFSKY et al. 1999; BLASBALG et al. 2000). Moreover, with the 3D sequence, the isotropic pixels allow for valuable angiographic reconstruction of the arterial data sets (LEE et al. 2000; GLOCKNER 2001; LAVELLE et al. 2001). Compared with spiral CT, MR eliminates exposure to ionizing radiation and uses contrast materials with favourable safety profiles compared with iodinated contrast materials (PRINCE et al. 1993; REIMER et al. 1999).

Anatomical variants can be found also in the portal and hepatic vein trees. A large right inferior hepatic vein, draining segment VI, is found in 15–20% of normal subjects. When a right inferior hepatic vein is present, the right hepatic vein is usually smaller, as it does not drain segment VI. In some cases the right hepatic vein is absent, or limited to a very small vessel, when a large inferior right hepatic vein is associated with a predominant middle hepatic vein. There is a balance in territories drained by each hepatic vein. For surgical purposes, evaluation of the approximate territory drained by each hepatic vein is interesting, especially in order to prevent intraoperative bleeding but also to preserve hepatic tissue. For example, an accessory inferior hepatic vein can allow preservation of the posteroinferior area of the right lobe despite transection of the right hepatic vein in partial hepatectomy (MAKUUCHI et al. 1987). The hepatic veins can be demonstrated with MR angiography, whereas this is almost impossible with DSA, and LEE et al. (2000) identified more inferior hepatic veins with 3D volumetric interpolated breath-hold MR images than did previously reported studies using CT and ultrasound methods (Fig. 19.2).

Portal vein variants occur in 20% of cases. In most instances, the portal bifurcation is located higher than usual, and may be strictly intrahepatic, which may represent a surgical problem when ligation of the right or left portal vein is required. The most usual abnormality is the left portal vein arising from the right portal vein or from the anterior branch of the right portal vein. Rarely, the right portal vein

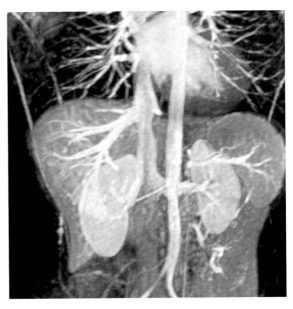

Fig. 19.2. MR angiography. MIP image of the right hepatic vein

arises from the intrahepatic left portal vein; usually, the anterior branch of the right portal vein arises from the segment IV branch of the left portal vein. The large number of variations in portal branching pattern determine the variation in segmental anatomy. Three-dimensional CT and contrast-enhanced MR angiography allow a precise evaluation of splenic, superior mesenteric and portal veins and of significant anatomical variation in the segmental anatomy of the liver (VAN LEEUWEN et al. 1994a,b; SOYER et al. 1996c; SADDIK et al. 1999; LEE et al. 2000; ITO et al. 2000) (Fig. 19.3). The evaluation of the portal venous system has been reported to be sufficient with time-of-flight and phase contrast techniques (KOPKA et al. 1999).

Not only the presence of vascular abnormality but also the evaluation of the diameter of the major vessels that supply the liver is of crucial importance during surgical planning of liver transplantation. Hepatic arterial reconstruction requires adequate inflow from the recipient artery. Inadequate inflow is commonly due to recipients having small-calibre vessels, which is often the case when there are multiple hepatic arteries with different origins. Moreover, the presence of coeliac axis stenosis (commonly due to impingement by the diaphragmatic crura) is important in liver transplantation candidates because the coeliac axis is the only source of arterial blood supply to the transplanted liver. Hepatocytes in fact are mostly supplied by the portal vein, while bile ducts

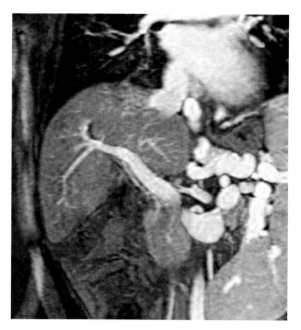

Fig. 19.3. MR angiography. MIP image of the portal vein

depend solely on arterial blood from the hepatic artery (NGHIEM et al. 1999).

Many patients who are candidates for OLT and interventional treatments for HCC have cirrhosis. It is very important to have an overview of the portal system of these patients, who are likely to have portal hypertension (OKUDA and BENHAMOU 1991).

Performance of a delayed acquisition during the portal phase of enhancement of a CT examination enables evaluation of the portal and variceal anatomy and of portosystemic shunts, without the need for an additional injection of contrast material. Three-dimensional reconstruction of portal-phase CT angiograms enhances the perception of the courses and anatomical relationship of varices and shunts, and the presence and extent of portal thrombosis (HENSELER et al. 2001). SSD can be very useful to display variceal anatomy during the portal phase and also 3D MR angiography can detect the presence and extent of collateral vessel pathways. Patients with portal hypertension benefit from the use of MR angiography, probably because of the increased contrast material sensitivity of the technique (SOYER et al. 1997; KOPKA et al. 1999). In particular, the region of the confluence of the portal vein can be evaluated with higher diagnostic confidence on MR angiograms than on DSA images, due to the inflow of unenhanced blood from the splenic vein (at splenoportography) or the superior mesenteric vein (at mesentericopor-

tography) (ONO et al. 1997; OKUMURA et al. 1999; KOPKA et al. 1999).

The demonstration of variceal anatomy provides important information to the surgeon or the interventional radiologist, anticipating difficult procedures in patient who often are already in a clinically tenuous condition. This knowledge is important not only for major operations such as liver transplantation but for more common procedures in which an unexpected varix can result in significant bleeding.

The most common and clinically important portosystemic shunt is through gastro-oesophageal varices, fed mainly by the left gastric vein. Bleeding from oesophageal varices is a major cause of death in patients with portal hypertension. It is very important to identify all the vessels shunting blood to the gastro-oesophageal varices to occlude them and thus prevent bleeding and, eventually, the significant steal of blood from the portal vein after transplantation (ONO et al. 1997; HENSELER et al. 2001) (Fig. 19.4).

Other collateral vessels include recanalized paraumbilical veins, which are of special clinical concern to the surgeon considering a large abdominal incision. Paraumbilical veins are small veins which runs in the falciform ligament, with the atrophied umbilical vein (ligamentum teres), and which may hypertrophy in the presence of elevated portal venous pressure. The recanalized paraumbilical vein originates from the left portal vein, courses along the falciform ligament, and usually extends towards the umbilicus,

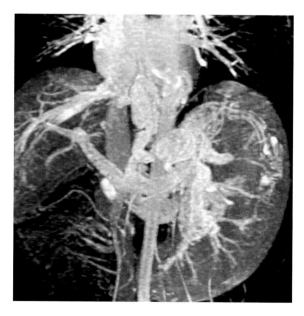

Fig. 19.4. MR angiography. MIP image showing gastro-oesophageal varices, fed by the left gastric vein

Liver

217

behind the anterior abdominal wall (Horton and Fishman 1998).

Collateral vessels originating from the splenic hilar region may communicate directly with the renal vein or travel a great distance before communicating with the systemic circulation (Fig. 19.5). Other retroperitoneal shunts which can be identified my means of CT a better visualized by 3D CT angiography are the iliolumbar, intercostal and phrenic veins shunts. These can be difficult to identify intra-operatively, and preoperative knowledge of their presence and course is valuable, since it is advantageous to ligate these varices to prevent steal of blood from the portal vein.

Intrahepatic collateral pathways can develop in cirrhotic patients with portal hypertension. Park et al. (1990) classified them into four types: type 1 when there is a vessel of large diameter which connects the right portal branch with the inferior vena cava; type 2 when there are one or more than one communications between portal vein and hepatic veins in one hepatic segment; type 3 when there is an aneurysmal shunt between the peripheral branches of the portal vein and hepatic veins; and type 4 where there are multiple communications between portal peripheral branches and hepatic vein branches in both hepatic lobes.

Patients with cirrhosis and portal hypertension are at increased risk for developing splenic artery aneurysms (Fig. 19.1). The major pathogenetic factor seems to be the high flow rate in the splenic artery, which causes dilatation, elongation and tortuosity of the main splenic artery in cirrhotic patients. The preoperative diagnosis of splenic artery aneurysms is crucial because this area is not routinely explored during transplantation surgery and the patient may be at higher risk for splenic artery aneurysm rupture in the post-transplant period. The decreased portal venous pressure and the increase in splenic arterial flow may cause the splenic artery aneurysms

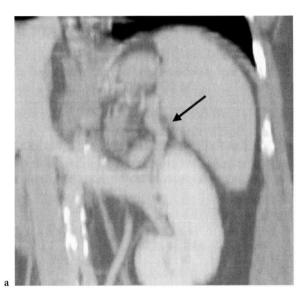

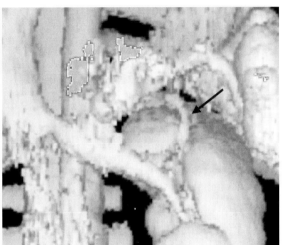

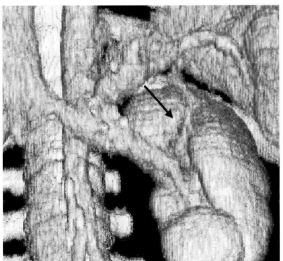

Fig. 19.5a–c. 3D CT angiography. Spleno-renal portosystemic shunt (*arrow*) demonstrated by MIP (**a**), surface shaded display (**b**) and volume rendering (**c**) techniques

to expand and rupture. 3D CT angiography provides a noninvasive means to evaluate the presence of splenic artery aneurysms, which have to be ligated before liver transplantation (NGHIEM et al. 1999).

Abnormalities of haemodynamics in the portal system or the presence of HCC may lead to portal thrombosis, the latter being a neoplastic thrombosis. Portal vein thrombosis seriously affects treatment choice in patients with HCC and was once considered a relative contraindication to OLT. Patients with complete portal thrombosis and multinodular or large HCC cannot undergo transcatheter arterial chemo-embolization and only palliative treatments can be performed. The use of increasingly sophisticated techniques to treat splanchnic venous thrombosis has eliminated the contraindication for OLT represented by portal thrombosis, but the knowledge of the extent of the thrombosis is crucial for planning a successful portal vein reconstruction. 3D CT angiograms and 3D MR imaging provide important information about the presence and extent of portal thrombosis, allowing appropriate treatment planning (SMITH et al. 1998; NGHIEM et al. 1999).

19.4
Liver Tumours

Three-dimensional rendering techniques provide a variety of methods for visualization of liver lesions in relation to the vessels and hepatic parenchyma, and can therefore provide important information to the surgeon and the interventional radiologist about the location of a lesion and its relations with surrounding vessels and organs (SOYER et al. 1991, 1996a). These techniques can also improve, as shown in recent studies, the morphological detection and characterization of benign and malignant lesions located in liver parenchyma (BENNETT et al. 1991; TAUPITZ et al. 1995; BJERNER et al. 1998).

HAWIGHORST et al. (1999) underlined that each hepatic lesion can be identified and characterized on the 3D gadolinium-enhanced MR angiographic images by analysing the spatial variations and evolution of contrast enhancement in each lesion. The functional information derived from this additional information at all three MR angiographic phases significantly improved lesion characterization of all lesions compared with the characterization using conventional sequences. A complete 3D volume set offers the opportunity to reformat hepatic lesions with multiple views. This allows liver anatomy and

vascular structures to be assessed with multiplanar reconstructions. Furthermore, MIP images improve the assessment of lesion volume. MIP and multiplanar reconstructions can also improve lesion delineation and potentially enable the detection of the feeding and draining vessels (BENNETT et al. 1991; BJERNER et al. 1998; HAWIGHORST et al. 1999; BLASBALG et al. 2000) (Fig. 19.6).

Gadolinium chelate-enhanced 3D spoiled GRE (gradient recalled echo) source images, for example, seem to be superior to MIP reformatted images for the assessment of morphological features of focal nodular hyperplasia (FNH). MIP reconstructed images are superior to the corresponding source imaging for showing the main branches of the hepatic artery, an arterial branch going to the FNH, and a small artery within the FNH radiating to peripheral areas. The combination of 3D spoiled GRE source images and MIP allows the analysis of the morphological, haemodynamic and angioarchitectural pattern of FNH (SOYER et al. 1996b).

Among the different 3D imaging techniques, UCHIDA et al. (1999) found that volume rendered 3D CT images during intravenous injection without the MIP technique produced 3D images of high quality with excellent visualization of tumours and their relationship to vital structures. The MIP technique, in fact, cannot simultaneously depict internal structures such as liver lesions and vessels. Volume rendering is conversely capable of depicting multi-object displays including the surface of the liver tumours and vessels. Different threshold values can be established to reconstruct separately the liver surface, tumour, portal vein and hepatic veins, and then the volume rendered image can be contracted with all four reconstructed objects simultaneously displayed (simultaneous display). This multi-object display gives stereotactic understanding of hepatic mass lesions and the technique has proved to be effective in the assessment of tumour invasion of the portal and intrahepatic venous structures. Volume rendered images can be displayed in colour following Hounsfield unit values (UCHIDA et al. 1999) (Fig. 19.6).

If in assessing liver anatomy and vasculature 3D ultrasound (US) has not yet gained an established role, its capability for guiding interventional procedures and for providing more accurate localization and size estimation of tumours has been demonstrated (DOWNEY et al. 1995, 2000; STATE et al. 1996; NELSON and PRETORIUS 1998; CESARANI et al. 1999). Volume measurements with 3D US are more accurate than measurements with conventional sonography and comparable to or even better than those made

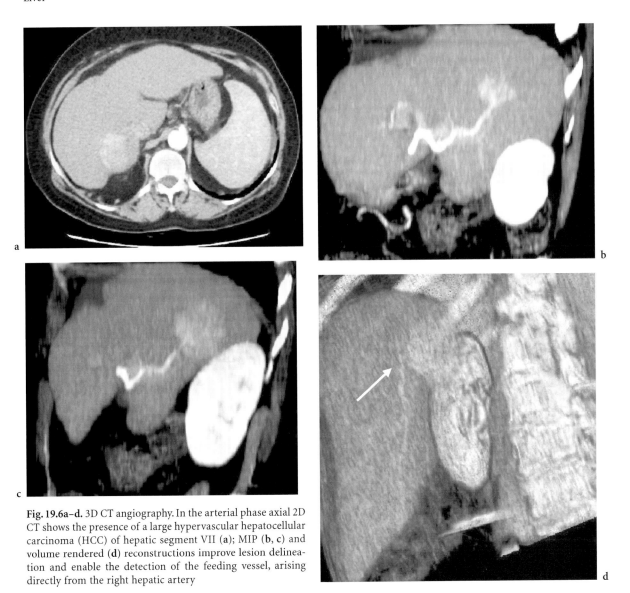

Fig. 19.6a–d. 3D CT angiography. In the arterial phase axial 2D CT shows the presence of a large hypervascular hepatocellular carcinoma (HCC) of hepatic segment VII (**a**); MIP (**b, c**) and volume rendered (**d**) reconstructions improve lesion delineation and enable the detection of the feeding vessel, arising directly from the right hepatic artery

using CT investigations (LIESS et al. 1994; WOLF et al. 1998; GILJA et al. 1999; LINNEY and DENG 1999). Moreover, changes in size can be more readily identified on serial studies and 3D US may be applied in conjunction with CT and MR imaging as an economical procedure for the follow-up of tumour disease (LIESS et al. 1994; WOLF et al. 1998; CESARANI et al. 1999).

Three-dimensional images can be reconstructed from a power US study, with or without administration of contrast medium, and visualized as a cine loop. The intratumoral blood flow of a focal liver lesion can thus be visualized, which can be useful for the differential diagnosis of hepatic tumours, especially HCC and FNH as these tumours have distinctly different intratumoral vascular structures (HIRAI et al. 1998; CAMPANI et al. 1998; CESARANI et al. 1999).

Three-dimensional reconstructions can also be useful in the follow-up of lesions after local therapies (percutaneous ethanol injection, trans-arterial chemo-embolization and radiofrequency thermal ablation). A comparison between the pre- and post-treatment imaging of the lesions is able to demonstrate the reduction in viable tumour tissue in the case of a successful treatment. The lesion can be isolated from the surrounding liver parenchyma and characterized by colour-coding and volume rendering. In this way, 3D imaging contributes to the precise estimation of tumour necrosis, and indicates whether or not the treatment has been successful (LENCIONI et al. 2000) (Fig. 19.7).

220

R. Lencioni et al.

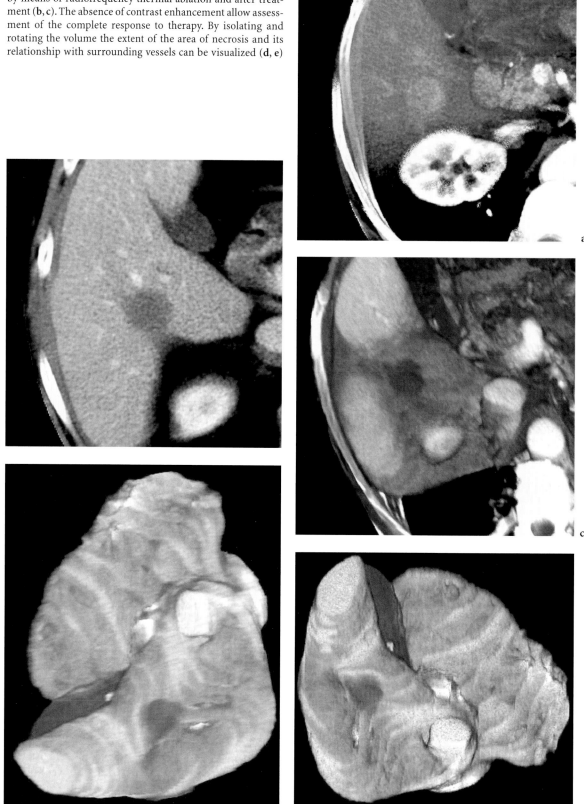

Fig. 19.7a–e. 3D CT angiography. Volume rendered reconstruction of a small HCC of hepatic segment VI before treatment (**a**) by means of radiofrequency thermal ablation and after treatment (**b, c**). The absence of contrast enhancement allow assessment of the complete response to therapy. By isolating and rotating the volume the extent of the area of necrosis and its relationship with surrounding vessels can be visualized (**d, e**)

References

Bartolozzi C, Lencioni R (1999) Liver malignancies. Springer, Berlin Heidelberg New York

Bennett WF, Bova JG, Petty L (1991) Preoperative 3D rendering of MR imaging in liver metastases. J Comput Assist Tomogr 15:979–984

Bismuth H, Castaing D, Garden OJ (1988) Segmental surgery of the liver. Surg Ann 20:291–310

Bjerner T, Johansson L, Haglund U (1998) 3D surface rendering of images from multiple MR pulse sequences in the pre-operative evaluation of hepatic lesions. Acta Radiol 39:698–700

Blasbalg R, Mitchell DG, Outwater EK (2000) Free MRA of the abdomen: postprocessing dynamic gadolinium-enhanced 3D axial images. Abdom Imaging 25:62–66

Campani R, Bottinelli O, Calliada F (1998) The latest in ultrasound: three dimensional imaging, part II. Eur J Radiol 27:S183–S187

Cesarani F, Isolato G, Capello S (1999) Tridimensional ultrasonography: first clinical experience with dedicated devices and review of the literature. Radiol Med 97:256–264

Couinaud C (1957) Le foie: études anatomiques et chirurgicales. Masson, Paris

Couinaud C (1986) Anatomie chirurgicale du foie: quelques aspects nouveaux. Chirurgie 112:337–342

Couinaud C (1998) The dorsal sector of the liver. Chirurgie 123:8–15

Downey DB, Chin JL, Fenster A (1995) Three-dimensional US-guided cryosurgery. Radiology 197:(P)539

Downey DB, Fenster A, Williams JC (2000) Clinical utility of three-dimensional US. Radiographics 20:559–571

Friedman AC, Dachman AH (1994) Radiology of the liver, biliary tract, and pancreas. Mosby, St Louis

Gilja OH, Hausken T, Bersted A (1999) Measurements of organ volume by ultrasonography. Proc Inst Mech Eng 213:247–259

Glockner JF (2001) Three-dimensional gadolinium enhanced MR angiography: applications for abdominal imaging. Radiographics 21:357–370

Glombitza G, Lamade W, Demiris AM (1999) Virtual planning of liver resections: image processing, visualization and volumetric evaluation. Int J Med Inf 53:225–237

Goldsmith NA, Woodburne RT (1957) The surgical anatomy pertaining to liver resection. Surg Gynecol Obstet 195:310–318

Goodman DA, Tiruchelvan V, Tabb DR (1995) 3D CT reconstruction in the surgical management of hepatic injuries. Ann R Coll Surg Engl 77:7–11

Hawighorst H, Schoenberg SO, Knopp MV (1999) Hepatic lesions: morphologic and functional characterization with multiphase breath-hold 3D gadolinium-enhanced MR angiography – initial results. Radiology 210:89–96

Healy JE (1970) Vascular anatomy of the liver. Ann NY Acad Sci 170:8–17

Healy JE, Schroy PC (1953) Anatomy of the biliary ducts within the human liver: analysis of prevailing pattern of branchings and major variations of the biliary ducts. Arch Surg 66:599–619

Heath DG, Soyer PA, Kuszyk BS (1995) Three-dimensional spiral CT during arterial portography: comparison of three rendering techniques. Radiographics 15:1001–1011

Henseler KP, Pozniak MA, Lee FT (2001) Three-dimensional CT angiography of spontaneous portosystemic shunts. Radiographics 21:691–704

Hirai T, Ohishi H, Yamada R (1998) Three-dimensional power Doppler sonography of tumor vascularity. Radiat Med 16:353–357

Horton KM, Fishman EK (1998) Paraumbilical vein in the cirrhotic patient: imaging with 3D CT angiography. Abdom Imaging 23:404–408

Ito K, Blasbalg R, Hussain SM (2000) Portal vein and its tributaries: evaluation with thin section three-dimensional contrast-enhanced dynamic fat-suppressed MR imaging. Radiology 215:381–386

Johnson PT, Heath DG, Bliss DF (1996a) Three dimensional CT: real-time interactive volume rendering. AJR 167:581–583

Johnson PT, Heath DG, Kuszyk BS (1996b) CT angiography with volume-rendering: advantages and applications in splanchnic vascular imaging. Radiology 200:564–568

Kopka L, Rodenwaldt J, Vosshenrich R (1999) Hepatic blood supply: comparison of optimized dual phase contrast-enhanced three-dimensional MR angiography and digital subtraction angiography. Radiology 211:51–58

Kuszyk BS, Heath DG, Ney DR (1995) CT angiography with volume rendering: image findings. AJR 165:445–448

Lavelle MT, Lee VS, Rofsky NM (2001) Dynamic contrast-enhanced three-dimensional MR imaging of liver parenchyma: source images and angiographic reconstructions to define hepatic arterial anatomy. Radiology 218:389–394

Lee VS, Lavelle MT, Rofsky NM (2000) Hepatic MR imaging with a dynamic contrast-enhanced isotropic volumetric interpolated breath-hold examination: feasibility, reproducibility, and technical quality. Radiology 215:365–372

Lencioni RA, Neri E, Caramella D (2000) Radiofrequency thermal ablation of liver malignancies: assessment of treatment outcome by volume-rendered spiral CT. Radiology 217:228

Liess H, Roth C, Umgelter A (1994) Improvements in volumetric quantification of circumscribed hepatic lesions by three-dimensional sonography. Z Gastroenterol 32:488–492

Linney AD, Deng J (1999) Three-dimensional morphometry in ultrasound. Proc Inst Mech Eng 213:235–245

Makuuchi M, Hasegawa H, Yamazaki S (1987) Four new hepatectomy procedures for resection of the right hepatic vein and preservation of the inferior right hepatic vein. Surg Gynecol Obstet 164:68–72

Michels N (1955) Blood supply and anatomy of the upper abdominal organs with a descriptive atlas. Lippincott, Philadelphia

Michels N (1996) Newer anatomy of the liver and its variant blood supply and collateral circulation. Am J Surg 112:337–347

Nelson TR, Pretorius DH (1998) Three-dimensional ultrasound imaging. Ultrasound Med Biol 24:1243–1270

Nghiem HV, Dimas CT, Mc Vicar JP (1999) Impact of double helical CT and three-dimensional CT arteriography on surgical planning for hepatic transplantation. Abdom Imaging 24:278–284

Okuda K, Benhamou JP (1991) Portal hypertension: clinical and physiological aspects. Springer, Berlin Heidelberg New York

Okumura A, Watanabe Y, Dohke M (1999) Contrast-enhanced three-dimensional MR portography. Radiographics 19:973–987

Ono N, Toyonaga A, Nishimura H (1997) Evaluation of magnetic resonance angiography on portosystemic collaterals in cirrhotic patients. Am J Gastroenterol 92:1515–1519

Park JH, Cha SH, Han JK (1990) Intrahepatic portosystemic venous shunt. AJR 155:527–528

Prince MR, Yucel EK, Kaufman JA (1993) Dynamic gadolinium-enhanced three-dimensional abdominal arteriography. J Magn Reson Imaging 3:877–881

Reimer P, Allkemper T, Matuszewski L (1999) Contrast-enhanced 3D-MRA of the upper abdomen with a bolus-injectable SPIO (SH U 555 A). J Magn Reson Imaging 10:65–71

Rofsky NM, Lee VS, Laub G (1999) Abdominal MR imaging with a volumetric interpolated breath-hold examination. Radiology 212:876–884

Saddik D, Frazer C, Robins P (1999) Gadolinium-enhanced three-dimensional MR portal venography. AJR 19:973–987

Smith PA, Klein AS, Heath DG (1998) Dual-phase spiral CT angiography with volumetric 3D rendering for preoperative liver transplant evaluation: preliminary observations. J Comput Assist Tomogr 22:868–874

Soyer P, Roche A, Gad M (1991) Preoperative segmental localization of hepatic metastases: utility of three-dimensional CT during arterial portography. Radiology 180:653–658

Soyer P, de Givry SC, Gueye C (1996a) Detection of focal hepatic lesions with MR imaging: prospective comparison of T2-weighted fast spin-echo with and without fat suppression, T2-weighted breath-hold fast spin-echo, and gadolinium chelate enhanced 3D gradient-recalled imaging. AJR 166:1115–1121

Soyer P, Dufresne AC, Somveille E (1996b) Focal nodular hyperplasia of the liver: assessment of hemodynamic and angioarchitectural patterns with gadolinium chelate-enhanced 3D spoiled gradient-recalled MRI and maximum intensity projection reformatted images. J Comput Assist Tomogr 20:898–904

Soyer P, Heath D, Bluemke DA (1996c) Three-dimensional helical CT of intrahepatic venous structures: comparison of three rendering techniques. J Comput Assist Tomogr 20:122–127

Soyer P, Dufresne AC, Somveille E (1997) MR imaging of the liver: effect of portal hypertension on hepatic parenchymal enhancement using a gadolinium chelate. J Magn Reson Imaging 7:142–146

State A, Livingston MA, Garrett WF (1996) Technologies for augmented reality systems: realizing ultrasound-guided needle biopsies. Proceedings of SIGGRAPH '96. Comput Graph 13:439–446

Taupitz M, Speidel A, Hamm B (1995) T2-weighted breath-hold MR imaging of the liver at 1.5 T: results with a three-dimensional steady-state free precession sequence in 87 patients. Radiology 194:439–446

Togo S, Shimada H, Kanemura E (1998) Usefulness of three-dimensional computed tomography for anatomic liver resection: sub-subsegmentectomy. Surgery 123:73–78

Uchida M, Ishibashi M, Abe T (1999) Three-dimensional imaging of liver tumors using helical CT during intravenous injection of contrast medium. J Comput Assist Tomogr 23:435–440

van Leeuwen MS, Fernandez MA, van Es HW (1994a) Variations in venous and segmental anatomy of the liver: two- and three-dimensional MR imaging in healthy volunteers. AJR 162:1337–1345

van Leeuwen MS, Noordzij J, Fernandez MA (1994b) Portal venous segmental anatomy of the right hemiliver: observations based on three-dimensional spiral CT renderings. AJR 163:1395–1404

van Leeuwen MS, Noordzij J, Hennipman A (1995) Planning for liver surgery using three dimensional imaging techniques. Eur J Cancer 31:1212–1215

Wigmore SJ, Redhead DN, Yan XJ (2001) Virtual hepatic resection using three-dimensional reconstruction of helical computed tomography angioportograms. Ann Surg 233:221–226

Winter TC Jr, Freeny PC, Nghiem HV (1995a) Hepatic arterial anatomy in transplantation candidates: evaluation with three-dimensional CT arteriography. Radiology 195:363–370

Winter TC Jr, Nghiem HV, Freeny PC (1995b) Hepatic arterial anatomy: demonstration of normal supply and vascular variants with three-dimensional CT angiography. Radiographics 15:771–780

Wolf GK, Lang H, Prokop M (1998) Volume measurements of localized hepatic lesions using three-dimensional sonography in comparison with three-dimensional computed tomography. Eur J Med Res 23:157–164

20 Biliary Tract

Piero Boraschi, Simone Lodovigi, Giuditta Campori, Roberto Gigoni, Emanuele Neri

CONTENTS

20.1
Introduction

The advent of endoscopic biliary surgery and the recent introduction of magnetic resonance cholangiopancreatography (MRCP) (Morimoto et al. 1992; Hall-Craggs et al. 1993; Ishizaki et al. 1993; Guibaud et al. 1994; Takehara et al. 1994; Macaulay et al. 1995; Barish et al. 1995; Reinhold et al. 1995; Reinhold and Bret 1996; Soto et al. 1995a, b; Becker et al. 1997; Boraschi et al. 1999a, b) have renewed an interest in the techniques of pancreatobiliary tract imaging.

Among the imaging techniques currently advocated for evaluating the biliary tree, sonography and computed tomography are most frequently used in the initial non invasive approach in patients with symptoms and signs referable to the pancreaticobiliary system. In many instances, particularly in cases of malignant bile duct obstruction, sonography and CT provide the necessary information for planning further treatment.

However, although these modalities are sensitive in the detection of biliary obstruction, direct cholangiography, including endoscopic retrograde cholangiopancreatography (ERCP) and, to a lesser extent, percutaneous transhepatic cholangiography (PTC), remain the reference standard for visualizing the presence and level of the biliary obstruction, as well as suggesting its etiology. Significant advantages of ERCP include the unparalleled resolution obtained with this procedure and the ability to perform therapeutic measures at the time of initial diagnosis. Nevertheless, ERCP is operator-dependent and is limited by considerable morbidity (1–7%) and mortality (0.2–1%). Complications, including pancreatitis, sepsis, hemobilia, and bowel perforation, can be life-threatening and delay or even diminish the chance of managing the primary disease. Consequently, a safe and highly accurate diagnostic procedure is needed to replace diagnostic ERCP, or to be performed in patients in whom ERCP is unsuccessful or incomplete.

The situation has changed since the advent of MRCP, which was introduced in 1991 by Wallner et al. This technique is an absolutely non invasive imaging modality, requires no injection of contrast material, combines the benefits of projection and cross-sectional imaging techniques, and provides an overview of the entire biliary and pancreatic ductal system by means of data acquisition and image reconstruction rendered in the coronal plane in a conventional cholangiography fashion. A major challenge of MRCP is to achieve an accuracy comparable to that of ERCP for the most frequent clinical indications requiring direct opacification of the pancreaticobiliary system.

20.2
MR Cholangiopancreatography

MRCP has become a reliable non invasive diagnostic method of investigating the biliary tree and the pancreatic ductal system. Technical improvements in imaging sequences (half-Fourier rapid acquisition

P. Boraschi, MD, R. Gigoni, MD
2nd Department of Radiology, Pisa University Hospital, Via Paradisa 2, 56124, Pisa, Italy
S. Lodovigi, MD, G. Campori, MD, E. Neri, MD
Diagnostic and Interventional Radiology, Department of Oncology, Transplants and Advanced Technologies in Medicine, University of Pisa, Via Roma 67, 56100 Pisa, Italy

with relaxation enhancement) and use of phased-array coils allow high-quality imaging comparable to that available with ERCP. This technique has shown high diagnostic potential, and has been effectively introduced into clinical practice for the evaluation of many pancreaticobiliary diseases (REINHOLD et al. 1995; BECKER et al. 1997).

A comparable diagnostic accuracy with respect to ERCP in the diagnosis of choledocholithiasis is reported by various authors for MRCP (GUIBAUD et al. 1994; BORASCHI et al. 1999b). MRCP may help in establishing the diagnosis of malignant obstruction and is useful in evaluating those patients in whom ERCP was unsuccessful or incomplete. MRCP also plays a crucial role in evaluating post-surgical biliary tract alterations and can demonstrate a variety of congenital anomalies of the biliary tract (aberrant ducts, choledochal cysts, Caroli disease, pancreas divisum). In addition, intentional or incidental imaging of the gallbladder with MRCP can be used to identify calculi or help determine the presence and extent of neoplastic disease.

The MRCP technique is based on heavily T2-weighted images obtained with different pulse sequences. As a result, stationary fluids, including bile and pancreatic secretions, have a high signal intensity while solid organs have a low signal intensity. This combination of imaging characteristics means that MRCP provides optimal contrast between the hyperintense signal of bile and the hypointense signal of the background.

T2-weighted gradient echo sequences with the steady-state free precession (SSFP) technique were initially used by WALLNER, MORIMOTO, HALL-CRAGGS and ISHIZAKI (WALLNER et al. 1991; MORIMOTO et al. 1992; HALL-CRAGGS et al. 1993; ISHIZAKI et al. 1993). Subsequently, other investigators have utilized two-dimensional (2D) and three-dimensional (3D) heavily T2-weighted fast spin echo sequences for MRCP (TAKEHARA et al. 1994; BARISH et al. 1995; REINHOLD et al. 1995; SOTO et al. 1995a, b; REINHOLD and BRET 1996; BORASCHI et al. 1999a,b). In a study comparing 2D fast spin echo and 3D SSFP pulse sequences, REINHOLD et al. (1995) have demonstrated that fast spin-echo sequences are significantly better for the visualization of both biliary tree and pancreatic ducts. More recent studies have described the clinical usefulness of MRCP performed with a new heavily T2-weighted sequence, the half-Fourier rapid acquisition relaxation enhancement (RARE) sequence, with or without image reconstruction for the evaluation of the pancreaticobiliary system; this new technique has a very fast acquisition time and

shows slow-flowing fluids such as bile and urine as being very bright (REGAN et al. 1996b; MIYAZAKI et al. 1996).

20.3
Image Processing Techniques

Biliary tract examinations using rapid 3D volumetric techniques can be performed with helical CT and MRCP. Integration between volumetric acquisition and 3D surface and volume rendering techniques permits the study of the biliary tract in a non invasive way. Knowledge of segmental anatomy and intersegmental biliary connections is an essential prerequisite to the effective management of patients with complex bile duct anatomy (e.g., congenital abnormalities, bilio-enteric anastomoses). Three-dimensional imaging techniques are also useful for an accurate anatomical assessment before surgery.

Preliminary studies on 3D reconstructions of the biliary system have been carried out by some investigators with surface and volume rendering of CT cholangiography data sets for preoperative evaluation before laparoscopic cholecystectomy (KINAMI et al. 1999). Three-dimensional CT cholangiography (KLEIN et al. 1993; ZEMAN et al. 1995; FLEISCHMANN et al. 1996; FURUKAWA et al. 1997; PRASSOPOULOS et al. 1998; RAPTOPOULOS et al. 1998; KINAMI et al. 1999; SAJJAD et al. 1999) has been reported as a 3D shaded surface display image of the biliary tract obtained by using helical CT after intravenous administration of biliary contrast medium (meglumine iotroxate). This technique can also be performed by means of a percutaneous transhepatic cholangio-drainage tube. Slice thickness of 3 mm with a pitch up to 1.7 in a single breath-hold acquisition is considered essential for an optimal scanning protocol. A 3D helical CT study of the biliary tract without cholangiographic contrast material has been proposed by ZEMAN et al. (1995).

CT techniques are especially useful when MR imaging is unavailable or contraindicated, or when the quality of MRCP images is suboptimal (CT cholangiography, in fact, has a better spatial resolution, hence its clearer depiction of small ducts), but to date the use of radiation, low availability of biliary contrast media and possible adverse reactions to iodinated contrast agents have all had a negative impact on the large-scale diffusion of CT techniques. Optimization of CT cholangiography using multi-row helical scanners should improve the potentialities of this technique (NINO-MURCIA et al. 2001). Multi-row CT captures four helical scans in a single 0.5 s gantry rotation and this increase in speed allows routine use of a very thin collimation with higher-quality 3D reformations.

The diagnostic approach to pancreaticobiliary tract pathology has undergone a major change because of the recent introduction of MRCP. This is a new non invasive imaging technique for the visualization of the biliary and pancreatic ducts with images similar to those obtained with ERCP, PTC or even CT cholangiography, but with no contrast agent injection. One of its advantages is the possibility of processing its data sets to generate 3D reconstructions, which can be obtained with both external and endoluminal points of view of the organ anatomy.

The maximum intensity projection (MIP), shaded surface display (SSD), the real time volume rendering, and the multiplanar volume reconstruction (MPVR) algorithms provide external views of the pancreaticobiliary tract. Endoluminal points of view can be obtained with virtual endoscopy.

20.3.1
Maximum Intensity Projection and Shaded Surface Display

With the SSD algorithm a threshold value in the Hounsfield density/intensity scale is set so that only tissues with voxel values equal or superior to the threshold are rendered. Then a virtual light source creates light and shading effects simulating a 3D perspective. The result resembles a cast, as only external overlapping surfaces can be appreciated, while all the information beyond this interface is lost.

In the MIP algorithm a beam of parallel rays is projected through a 3D matrix of interpolated data to create an image where any pixel is assigned the maximum value encountered by the ray along its axis with no information loss. Alternatively, an analog algorithm can assign the minimum value to the pixels generating a minimum intensity projection (MinIP) image (Raptopoulos et al. 1998).

MIP and SSD provide a global map of the pancreaticobiliary tree anatomy that can be helpful in the interpretation of 2D MRCP images (particularly postsurgical anatomy, anatomical variants of the pancreaticobiliary ductal system and large biliary neoplasms).

In fact, in patients with cholangiocarcinomas and bilio-enteric anastomoses, 3D reconstructed images are helpful in identifying the infiltration of the common bile duct and intrahepatic ducts and in assessing post-surgical anatomy of the biliary system correctly.

However, various authors have stressed the limitations of such algorithms in the depiction of small intraductal pathology, and particularly in the detection of small calculi in the common bile duct (Boraschi et al. 1996, 1999b; Chan et al. 1996; Regan et al. 1996a; Reinhold and Bret 1996). Therefore, meticulous review of 2D coronal and also axial images is extremely important to allow the identification of small endoluminal pathologies. If fluid completely surrounds the intraluminal filling defect, the latter is missed on the reconstructed MIP and SSD images because it is obscured by the higher signal intensity of surrounding bile (Fig. 20.1).

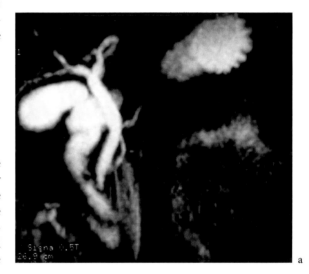

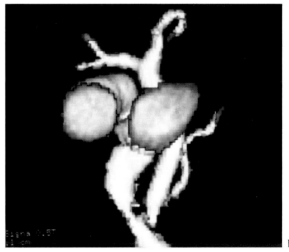

Fig. 20.1a,b. In this patient with a small calculus at the level of the distal tract of the common bile duct, both maximum intensity projection (MIP) (a) and surface shaded display (SSD) (b) reconstructions fail to reveal the stone

20.3.2
Volume Rendering

Volume rendering is the latest development for 3D visualization of the anatomy of the pancreaticobiliary tree (WIELOPOLSKI et al. 1999; NERI et al. 2000; KONDO et al. 2001). This method allows the simultaneous display of different anatomical structures imaged within a single volume. It provides an image created by simulated rays of light, arising from a virtual source (i.e., the eye of the user looking through the computer display), traversing the imaging volume that has been attenuated by its contents, and assigns certain characteristics, such as opacity, color, light and shininess, to specific voxel values. Volume rendering has the advantage of providing a clear roadmap of the entire biliary tree, but its real role in demonstrating pathological changes deserves further clinical evaluation. We have identified possible applications of this method in the follow-up of patients who have undergone bilio-enteric anastomoses (Fig. 20.2) (BORASCHI et al. 2000). Recently,

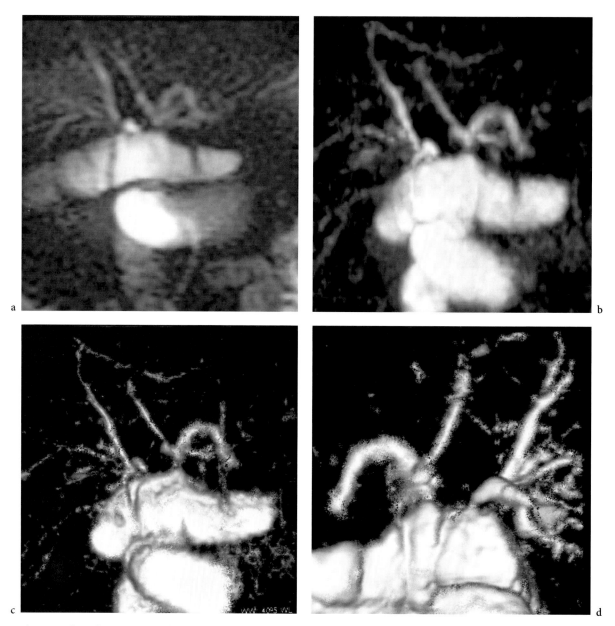

Fig. 20.2a–d. In this woman, single-shot fast spin echo acquisition (**a**) and frontal view MIP (**b**) show the presence of a double bilio-enteric anastomosis. Anterior (**c**) and posterior (**d**) views of MR volume rendering clearly show the right and left hepatic ducts that are anastomosed with the jejunal loop. No complication is present in this case

furthermore, the volume rendering technique has also been proposed for evaluating choledocholithiasis as an alternative to MIP reconstructions of MR cholangiography (KONDO et al. 2001).

20.3.3
MR and CT Virtual Cholangioscopy

Virtual endoscopy (VE) permits intraluminal structures within the body to be visualized from inside in three dimensions. With either CT or MR imaging data sets, the approach has been successfully applied in the investigation of the colon, vessels, bronchial tree, middle and inner ear, cerebrospinal fluid spaces, urinary tract and biliary tract (WOOD et al. 1998).

The exploration of the biliary tract with fiberoptic cholangioscopy is a relatively new and well-established procedure that has found interesting applications in the diagnostic approach to and therapeutic management of biliary stones, in the differential diagnosis between benign and malignant lesions, and in the staging of ductal malignancies (PICUS 1995; ROSSI et al. 1996).

The technique is operator-dependent, expensive, time-consuming, but most of all invasive and affected by many complications related to the use of the cholangioscope, such as hemorrhage into the biliary ducts (with a percentage ranging between 4.1% and 12%), laceration of the bile duct (2%), bacteremia, vagal reactions, nausea, fever and diarrhea. Moreover, the large number of failed acquisitions has to be taken into consideration (PICUS 1995; ROSSI et al. 1996).

Virtual simulation of fiberoptic endoscopy can be obtained with a new software tool based on surface or volume rendering techniques, called virtual cholangioscopy when specifically applied to the study of the biliary system (BORASCHI et al. 1997; NERI et al. 1997a, b, 1999a–c; DUBNO et al. 1998; PRASSOPOULOS et al. 1998). Endoluminal views of the pancreatic and bile ducts can be obtained by rendering CT or MR data sets.

Virtual CT cholangiopancreatoscopy (NERI et al. 1997a; PRASSOPOULOS et al. 1998) is a relatively new technique which permits the exploration of the common bile duct (CBD) and the pancreatic duct (PD) from an endoluminal point of view. The application of the VE surface algorithm to helical CT data sets with proper setting of the thresholds allows the rendering of the interface pixels only, that is to say those pixels on the border between endoluminal fluid (bile, pancreatic secretions) and surrounding soft tissue (CBD/PD wall). CT acquisition parameters are 120 kVp, 220–260 mA, 3 mm collimation, pitch 1.3–1.7 in a single breath-hold coverage, with reconstruction intervals of 1–1.5 mm.

The use of MR data sets for VE was first reported by DAVIS et al. (1996) in the study of the aorta and its branches with MR angiography. Due to the high signal intensity of the blood generated with this acquisition technique, the voxels representing the aorta correspond to the brightest gray level. In this approach the voxels of the vascular structures can easily be segmented to be used for VE.

Since MRCP images have comparable characteristics to the images provided by MR angiography, segmentation and generation of endoscopic views is potentially feasible (BORASCHI et al. 1997; NERI et al. 1997b, 1999b,c; DUBNO et al. 1998). Segmentation of MRCP data sets has been made feasible by the high contrast difference between the bile ducts (brightest voxels) and the surrounding tissue (darkest voxels). Therefore MR VE has clearly shown internal views of the biliary tract, although in some cases (i.e., normal subjects with no bile duct dilatation) the signal intensity is not sufficient to provide the necessary number of voxels for segmentation.

Navigation sequences can be simulated through the common bile duct, hepatic duct (HD), left (LHD) and right (RHD) hepatic ducts and intrahepatic branches, pancreatic duct, cystic duct (CD) and gallbladder. All these anatomical details appear as tubular structures, with a smooth internal surface. The confluence between intrahepatic branches, LHD and RHD, PD and CBD, CD and CBD can also be represented. In all cases the CD and PD are the most difficult structures to be visualized from the inside because of their small caliber.

The endoluminal patterns of pathological findings showed by MRCP images were depicted in a recent study by our group (NERI et al. 1999c). Three types of endoluminal pattern were identified: endoluminal "polyp-like" mass, luminal stenosis and luminal occlusion. "Hole artefacts" through the internal wall were also observed and interpreted as errors of segmentation, due to incorrect threshold selection (Fig. 20.3).

According to our data, biliary stones were depicted mainly as polyp-like endoluminal masses (85% of cases) (Fig. 20.4). Thus, it is supposed that the polyp-like pattern is their most probable appearance inside the lumen; but in a few cases, when the stones produced an important degree of

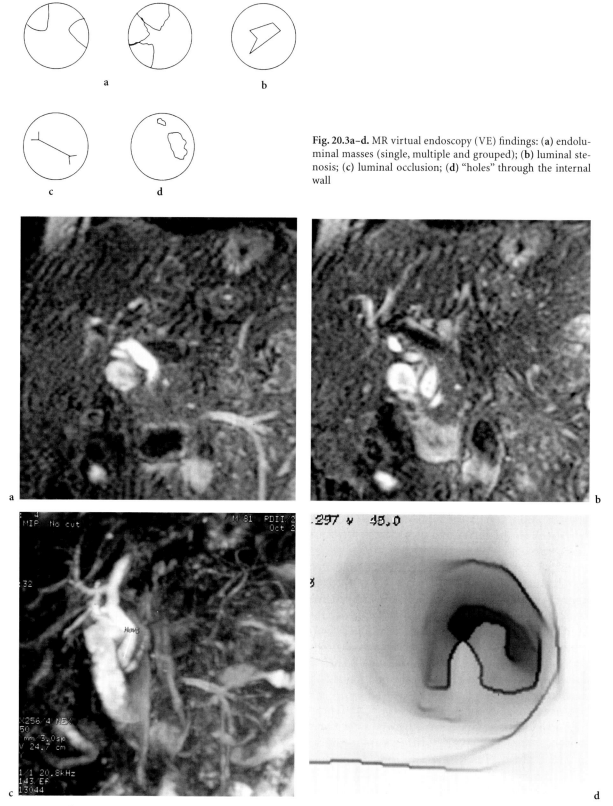

Fig. 20.3a–d. MR virtual endoscopy (VE) findings: (a) endoluminal masses (single, multiple and grouped); (b) luminal stenosis; (c) luminal occlusion; (d) "holes" through the internal wall

Fig. 20.4a–d. On coronal fast spin-echo T2-weighted images (a, b) of this 81-year-old man we suspected the presence of microcalculi at the distal portion of the common bile duct. Rendering from the inside these data sets, the MR VE view can be simulated in the cephalocaudal direction looking toward the ampulla (c). Two polyp-like masses can be observed in the internal wall (d)

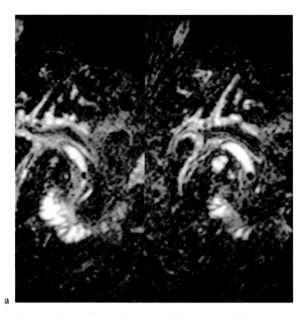
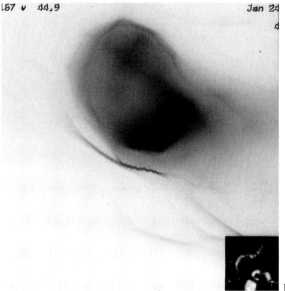

Fig. 20.5a,b. In this patient MR cholangiograms (**a**) reveal a stone in the CBD, causing a biliary obstruction. The MR VE view (**b**), simulated to look toward the ampulla, shows the luminal stenosis pattern of the CBD from the inside. A residual lumen is evident

stenosis of the lumen, they were identified as luminal stenosis (10%) (Fig. 20.5) and occlusion (5%). In these cases, the polyp-like morphology of the stone was not recognized because the lumen did not provide sufficient voxels for virtual navigation.

In the remaining cases, the pathological conditions of the bile ducts were variably interpreted as stenoses or occlusions (Fig 20.6), but the morphology of the endoluminal changes was never detected by the observers. This means that MR VE does not show the cause of luminal involvement but only provides information about the effects of this involvement (high sensitivity, low specificity). Luminal stenosis and occlusion patterns were equally represented in patients with inflammatory ampullary stenosis, whereas endoluminal occlusion was the most common finding observed in cholangiocarcinoma and pancreatic tumors.

In order to evaluate the applications of MR cholangioscopy in a clinical setting, we set out to establish whether MRCP, together with VE, could improve the non invasive detection of common bile duct stones (NERI et al. 1999c). VE is particularly helpful in detecting small CBD stones (<5 mm across). When applied to MRCP as a complementary technique it improves the detection of CBD calculi; on its own it can not provide any useful information though, as it never allows characterization of incidental lesions.

This limitation can be overcome by the use of cursors that allow observers to point at the surface of interest and obtain, interactively, in real time, the corresponding multiplanar MR images or 3D reconstructions crossing through the indicated point. In this way each abnormal finding can be characterized with the T2 signal of the lesion. This novel combined approach permits lesions to be identified more easily using VE and then characterized on the basis of standard MR signal characteristics, allowing in this case CBD stones (signal void) to be precisely identified.

20.4
Conclusion

In most cases 3D imaging does not add quantitative information to MRCP, but the main advantage with respect to cross-sectional anatomy is represented by a different rendering of data, more familiar to the human eye.

Constant integration between 2D source images and 3D reconstructions, with both external and endoluminal points of view, represents an added value to the diagnostic potentialities of MRCP in the evaluation of biliary tract diseases.

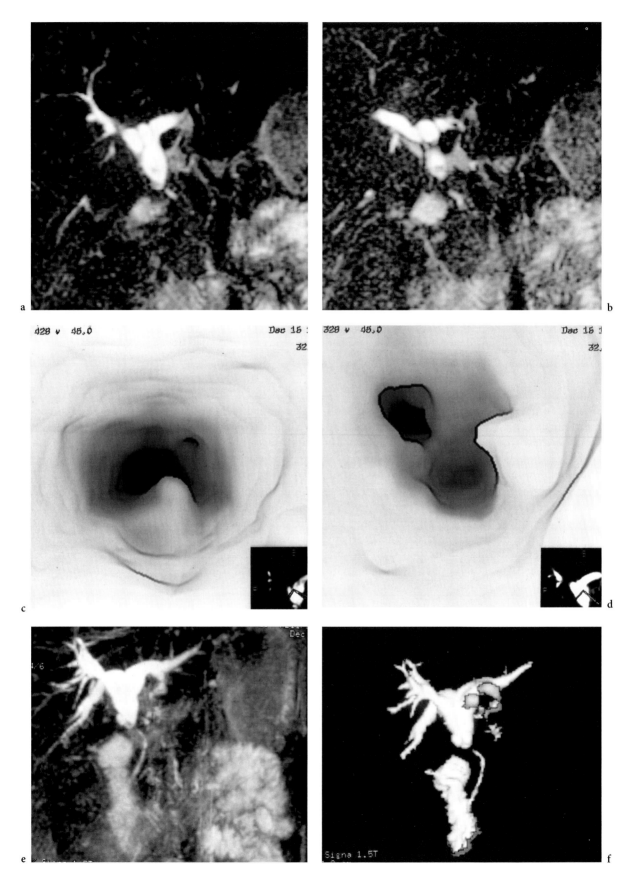

Fig. 20.6a–f. In this young woman, coronal MR cholangiograms (**a, b**) obtained 7 months after orthotopic liver transplantation, demonstrate an anastomotic stricture, with a small filling defect in the dilated pre-anastomotic biliary tract. The MR VE views (**c, d**), simulated in the cephalocaudal direction to look toward the biliary anastomosis, confirm the presence of a small calculus and show the endoluminal occlusion pattern and the lumen of the residual cystic duct. Both MIP (**e**), and SSD (**f**) reconstructions fail to reveal a stone

References

Barish MA, Yucel EK, Soto JA (1995) MR cholangiopancreatography: efficacy of three-dimensional turbo spin-echo technique. AJR 165:295–300

Becker CD, Grossholz M, Mentha G (1997) MR cholangiopancreatography: technique, potential indications and diagnostic features of benign, postoperative and malignant conditions. Eur Radiol 7:865–874

Boraschi P, Braccini G, Geloni M (1996) MR cholangiopancreatography: two-dimensional fast spin-echo imaging versus 3D MIP reconstructions. Radiology 201:S501

Boraschi P, Neri E, Caramella D (1997) MR cholangioscopy. 15th EuroPACS annual meeting Pisa (Italy), 25–27 Sept 1997, pp 75–78

Boraschi P, Braccini G, Gigoni R (1999a) MR cholangiopancreatography: value of axial and coronal fast spin-echo fat-suppressed T2-weighted sequences. Eur J Radiol 32:171–181

Boraschi P, Neri E, Braccini G (1999b) Choledocolithiasis: diagnostic accuracy of MR cholangiopancreatography. Three-year experience. Magn Reson Imaging 17:1245–1253

Boraschi P, Neri E, Gigoni R (2000) MR volume-rendering of bilio-enteric anastomoses. Radiology 217:S667

Chan Y, Chan ACW, Lam WWM (1996) Choledocholithiasis: comparison of MR cholangiography and endoscopic retrograde cholangiography. Radiology 200:85–89

Davis CP, Ladd ME, Romanowski BJ (1996) Human aorta: preliminary results with virtual endoscopy based on three-dimensional MR imaging data sets. Radiology 199:37–40

Dubno B, Debatin JF, Luboldt W (1998) Virtual MR cholangiography. AJR 171:1547–1550

Fleischmann D, Ringl H, Schofl R (1996) Three-dimensional spiral CT cholangiography in patients with suspected obstructive biliary disease: comparison with endoscopic retrograde cholangiography. Radiology 198:861–868

Furukawa H, Sano K, Kosuge T (1997) Analysis of biliary drainage in the caudate lobe of the liver: comparison of three-dimensional CT cholangiography and rotating cine cholangiography. Radiology 204:113–117

Guibaud L, Bret PM, Reinhold C (1994) Diagnosis of choledocholithiasis: value of MR cholangiography. AJR 163:847–850

Hall-Craggs MA, Allen CM, Owens CM (1993) MR cholangiography: clinical evaluation in 40 cases. Radiology 189:423–427

Ishizaki Y, Wakayama T, Okada Y (1993) Magnetic resonance cholangiography for evaluation of obstructive jaundice. Am J Gastroenterol 88:2072–2077

Kinami S, Yao T, Kurachi M (1999) Clinical evaluation of 3D-CT cholangiography for preoperative examination in laparoscopic cholecystectomy. J Gastroenterol 34:111–118

Klein HM, Wein B, Truong S (1993) Computed tomographic cholangiography using spiral CT scanning and 3D image processing. Br J Radiol 66:762–767

Kondo H, Kanematsu M, Stiratori Y (2001) MR cholangiography with volume rendering: receiver operating characteristics curve analysis in patients with choledocholithiasis. AJR 176:1183–1189

Macaulay SE, Schulte SJ, Sekijma JH (1995) Evaluation of a non-breath-hold MR cholangiography technique. Radiology 196:227–232

Miyazaki T, Yamashita Y, Tsuchigame T (1996) MR cholangiopancreatography using HASTE (half-Fourier acquisition single-shot turbo spin-echo) sequences. AJR 166:1297–1303

Morimoto K, Shimoi M, Shirakawa T (1992) Biliary obstruction: evaluation with three-dimensional MR cholangiography. Radiology 183:578–580

Neri E, Caramella D, Bartolozzi C (1997a) Spiral CT, three-dimensional reconstructions and virtual endoscopy of the biliary tract. Eur Radiol 7[Suppl 1]:311

Neri E, Boraschi P, Braccini G (1997b) Virtual endoscopy (VE) of the pancreaticobiliary tract with perspective surface rendering on MRCP data sets. Radiology 205:689

Neri E, Boraschi P, Braccini G (1999a) MR virtual endoscopy of the pancreaticobiliary tract: a feasible technique? Abdom Imaging 24:289–291

Neri E, Boraschi P, Braccini G (1999b) MR virtual endoscopy of the pancreaticobiliary tract. Magn Reson Imaging 17:59–67

Neri E, Caramella D, Boraschi P (1999c) Magnetic resonance virtual endoscopy of the common bile duct stones. Surg Endosc 13:632–633

Neri E, Boraschi P, Caramella D (2000) Real-time volume rendering of MRCP: clinical applications. MAGMA 10:35–42

Nino-Murcia M, Jeffrey RB, Beaulieu CF (2001) Multidetector CT of the pancreas and bile duct system: value of curved planar reformations. AJR 176:689–693

Picus D (1995) Percutaneous biliary endoscopy. J Vasc Interv Radiol 6:303–310

Prassopoulos P, Raptopoulos V, Chuttani R (1998) Development of virtual CT cholangiopancreatoscopy. Radiology 209:570–574

Raptopoulos V, Prassopoulos P, Chuttani R (1998) Multiplanar CT pancreatography and distal cholangiography with minimum intensity projections. Radiology 207:317–324

Regan F, Fradin J, Khazan R (1996a) Choledocholithiasis: evaluation with MR cholangiography. AJR 167:1441–1445

Regan F, Smith D, Khazan R (1996b) MR cholangiography in biliary obstruction using half-Fourier acquisition. J Comput Assist Tomogr 20:627–632

Reinhold C, Bret PM (1996) Current status of MR cholangiopancreatography. AJR 166:1285–1295

Reinhold C, Guibaud L, Genin G (1995) MR cholangio-pancreatography: comparison between two-dimensional fast spin-echo and three-dimensional gradient-echo pulse sequences. J Magn Reson Imaging 4:379–384

Rossi P, Bezzi M, Fiocca F (1996) Percutaneous cholangioscopy. Semin Interv Radiol 13:185–193

Sajjad Z, Oxtoby J, West D (1999) Biliary imaging by spiral CT cholangiography – a retrospective analysis. Br J Radiol 72:149–152

Soto JA, Barish MA, Yucel EK (1995a) MR cholangiopancreatography: findings on 3D fast spin-echo imaging. AJR 165:1397–1401

Soto JA, Barish MA, Yucel EK (1995b) Pancreatic duct: MR cholangiopancreatography with a three-dimensional fast spin-echo technique. Radiology 196:459–464

Takehara Y, Ichijo K, Tooyama N (1994) Breath-hold MR cholangiopancreatography with a long-echo-train fast spin-echo sequence and a surface coil in chronic pancreatitis. Radiology 192:73–78

Wielopolski PA, Gaa J, Wielopolski DR (1999) Breath-hold MR cholangiopancreatography with three-dimensional, segmented, echo-planar imaging and volume rendering. Radiology 210:247–252

Wallner BK, Schumacher KA, Weidenmaier W (1991) Dilated biliary tract: evaluation with MR cholangiography with a T2-weighted contrast-enhanced fast sequence. Radiology 181:805–808

Wood BJ, O'Malley ME, Hahn PF (1998) Virtual endoscopy of the gastrointestinal system outside the colon. AJR 171:1367–1372

Zeman RK, Berman PM, Silverman PM (1995) Biliary tract: three-dimensional helical CT without cholangiographic contrast material. Radiology 196:865–867

21 Upper Urinary Tract

Emanuele Neri, Piero Boraschi, Simone Lodovigi, Giuditta Campori

CONTENTS

21.1
3D Imaging of the Kidneys
and Upper Urinary Tract: CT and MR

Recent improvements in image processing and three-dimensional (3D) visualization increased the potential of current imaging techniques for the study of the kidneys and upper urinary tract. In this case spiral computed tomography and magnetic resonance imaging have become crucial techniques for an accurate evaluation of anatomy and pathology. The ideal imaging method should combine the evaluation of kidney parenchyma and urinary tract. However, to date the competition between CT and MR is still going on: whereas spiral CT is still the preferred technique for the study of parenchyma, MR is gaining a role in the study of the urinary tract. The examination of kidney and urinary tract requires specific protocols for dedicated imaging of this anatomical region.

The study of parenchyma can be optimally performed with single- and multislice CT (Fishman 2000; Lee et al. 2001). The scanning protocol should be a triphasic one (Roy 2000). As for other examinations in which 3D reconstructions are integrated, no oral contrast agent should be administered, to avoid artefacts. The single-slice scanning protocol includes a collimation of 3 or 5 mm, variable pitch and a reconstruction interval of 1–2.5 mm. With multislice technology the acquisition can be performed with the collimation reduced to 1 mm, exploiting the possibility of scanning 4 rows per rotation. For example, if we study the kidneys with single-slice CT with 3 mm collimation and pitch 2 (6 mm/s), in 25 s the volume covered will be 150 mm; using a fixed matrix multislice CT with collimation 1.25 mm and pitch 6 (15 mm/s), in 25 s the volume covered will be 375 mm. The advantages of multidetector technology can therefore be summarized as follows: large volume coverage in a short time frame, thin collimations, optimal use of contrast and less patient cooperation needed (Fishman 2000).

In a triphasic study the initial phase is unenhanced; this allows localization of the kidneys and eventual suspected masses, and reveals incidental calcifications (or calculi) and even fatty lesions. After administration of intravenous contrast medium (130–180 ml at a rate of 3–5 ml/s) an arterial phase is obtained (subject to calculation of the delay time to maximum vascular enhancement). This phase combines the enhancement of the renal arterial vasculature and cortical parenchyma, generally obtained after 30 s from injection. Then a nephrographic phase is obtained, about 90–100 s from injection, with the same parameters as the baseline scan. This provides information about the whole renal parenchyma and incidental focal lesions. A fourth, additional, delayed acquisition (about 5 min after injection) captures the contrast within the collecting system, the ureters and the bladder in a urographic fashion (Zeman 1996).

However, the study of the upper urinary tract that has been proposed with MR urography (MRU) provides a projectional roadmap of the entire urinary tract. Two methods have been proposed on the basis of unenhanced and gadolinium-enhanced studies. The unenhanced study is based on the acquisition of so-

E. Neri, MD, S. Lodovigi, MD; G. Campori, MD
Diagnostic and Interventional Radiology, Department of Oncology, Transplants, and Advanced Technologies in Medicine, University of Pisa, Via Roma 67, 56100, Pisa, Italy
P. Boraschi, MD
2nd Department of Radiology, Pisa University Hospital, Via Paradisa 2, 56124, Pisa, Italy

called water images using heavily T2-weighted turbo spin echo or half-Fourier acquisition single-shot turbo spin echo sequences and other variations of these techniques. These approaches do not require contrast medium administration and are feasible in patients with urinary tract obstruction (Roy 1994; Rothpearl 1995; O'Malley 1997; Louca 1999; Catalano 1999). The gadolinium-enhanced study, performed using T1-weighted gradient echo sequences provides morphological and functional information about the urinary tract (Nolte-Ernsting 1998, 1999).

MRU is performed with a non-breath-hold, fat-suppressed, respiratory-triggered two-dimensional heavily T2-weighted fast spin echo sequence in the coronal plane. Imaging parameters are as follows: TR range/TE, 7000–18,000/253; echo train length, 32; section thickness, 3 mm with no interslice gap. Acquisition time ranges from 5 min to 7 min.

21.2
3D Image Processing Techniques

The state-of-the-art 3D imaging of the kidney and upper urinary tract is represented by spiral CT and in particular by multislice technology: this captures four helical scans in a minimum single 0.5 s gantry rotation with an increase in speed that allows routine use of very thin collimation and higher-quality 3D reconstructions (McTavish 2000).

Integration between volumetric acquisition and 3D surface and volume rendering techniques permits the study of the upper urinary tract in a non invasive manner.

Some investigators have carried out preliminary studies on 3D reconstructions of the collecting system with surface rendering of MRU data sets (Nolte-Ernsting 1999; Neri et al. 2000). Experiences with 3D volume rendered CT of the kidney for evaluating renal tumors (Coll 1999), potential kidney donors (Dachman et al. 1998) and congenital urinary tract anomalies (Farres et al. 1998) have also been reported, which aimed to provide an accurate anatomical assessment before surgery.

Three-dimensional reconstructions can be obtained with both external and endoluminal points of view of the organ anatomy. The maximum intensity projection (MIP), shaded surface display (SSD), volume rendering and multiplanar volume reconstruction (MPVR) algorithms provide external views of the kidney and upper urinary tract. Endoluminal points of view of the upper urinary tract can be obtained with virtual endoscopy (VE) by using either MRU or the nephrographic phase of spiral CT.

21.3
Role of 3D Imaging in the Study of Pathological Findings

Non-vascular renal pathology is well studied using spiral CT and/or MR. Postprocessing techniques can offer added value in solving anatomical dilemmas. Current potential applications of 3D imaging include the non invasive study of congenital anomalies, preoperative evaluation in kidney donors, detection of lithiasis and preoperative planning of surgery for neoplasms.

21.3.1
Congenital Anomalies/Kidney Donors

The importance of accurate knowledge of the renal anatomy, especially in a kidney to be transplanted, is of fundamental relevance in the preoperative assessment of these patients. Also the presence of supplementary arteries may have therapeutic implications in hypertensive patients. For this, CT angiography has maintained an essential role in the preoperative diagnostic investigation. Native axial images remain the best way to examine kidney dimensions, morphology and parenchyma condition before and after contrast enhancement and to detect arterial and venous anomalies (accessory arteries and/or veins, early branching) or infrequent congenital ureteral anomalies (uretero-pelvic junction obstruction, double ureteral district). Two-dimensional (multiplanar reconstructions/coronal planes with MIP) and 3D (SSD, volume rendering) techniques rarely add information that may result in a different therapeutic approach, but help to provide a different point of view on patient anatomy, which shunts the mental reconstruction of a 3D model from axial images – an immediacy much sought after by surgeons (Fig. 21.1).

Fig. 21.1a–f. Multislice CT study of the kidneys. a Volume rendering (panoramic view) of the abdominal aorta, coeliac trunk, superior mesenteric artery, renal arteries and both kidneys. b Volume rendering of the left renal artery shows the entire path of the vessel in great detail, even at the level of the renal hilum. Slight contrast enhancement occurs even in the renal calices (*arrows*) and pelvis (*p*). c Maximum intensity projection of the same kidney (posterior view) which demonstrates, in a later phase of the study, the morphology of the upper urinary tract. (*s*) superior calices, (*m*) median calices, (*i*) inferior calices, ▶ ▶

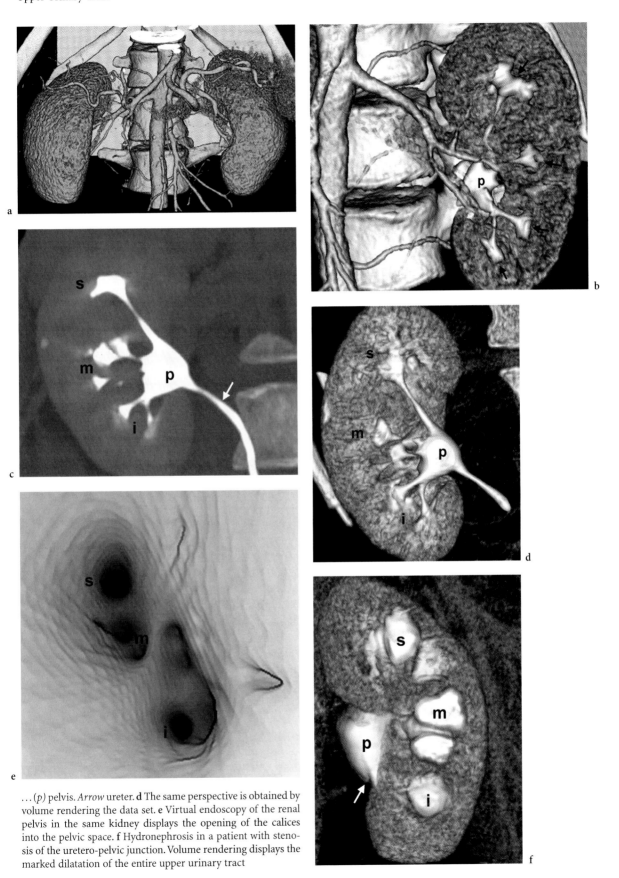

... (*p*) pelvis. *Arrow* ureter. **d** The same perspective is obtained by volume rendering the data set. **e** Virtual endoscopy of the renal pelvis in the same kidney displays the opening of the calices into the pelvic space. **f** Hydronephrosis in a patient with stenosis of the uretero-pelvic junction. Volume rendering displays the marked dilatation of the entire upper urinary tract

21.3.2
Lithiasis

Spiral CT is progressively gaining a role in the management of patients with suspect lithiasis of the urinary tract. A single scan of the entire abdomen performed in a single breath-hold, at high-resolution, allows the depiction of calcifications in the urinary tract. In difficult cases where the position of calcification cannot be precisely defined, the use of intravenous contrast helps in delineating the entire urinary map and allows calculi located in the renal pelvis to be distinguished from calcified plaques of the arterial system. If surgery of lithiasis is planned, the spiral CT study should include the evaluation of the renal parenchyma and renal arteries, as during surgery the presence of accessory renal arteries, as well as malformations of the kidneys, represents a further difficult problem.

In studying the renal arteries volume rendering is suggested as the ideal method. As mentioned elsewhere in this book the classic MIP provides a projectional roadmap of the arterial system but is limited by its poor perception of depth and relationships with contiguous anatomical structures. This limitation can be overcome by volume rendering, which displays in the same image the branches of the renal artery in the renal hilum, the urinary tract and the parenchyma. Since volume rendering is fast in generating 3D displays, it could be suitable even in emergency conditions (renal colic).

21.3.3
Neoplasms

Three-dimensional volume rendering applied to tri-phasic spiral CT also represents a useful tool for delineating kidney neoplasms (position, extent) and global anatomy (relationship with adjacent vascular structures and collecting system) before surgery, with an eye to saving the maximum amount of renal parenchyma (nephron-sparing surgery) and minimizing complications such as ischemic injury or intraoperative bleeding (COLL 1999), (Fig. 21.2). This technique allows the depiction of complex renal anatomy in a single non invasive examination with the possibility, in selected cases, of avoiding preoperative angiography (FISHMAN 2000).

21.4
Virtual Endoscopy of the Upper Urinary Tract

The simulation of a fibreoptic perspective can be obtained through dedicate software which reconstructs CT/MR images in three dimensions by creating surface or volume rendered endoscopic images. The dilatation of the urinary tract is a prerequisite for generating virtual endoscopy of MRU data sets, since the dilatation of the ureter or renal pelvis increases the availability of bright image pixels and, consequently, the voxels that VE can use to reconstruct the lumen in three dimensions and to create the virtual space for endoscopic navigation. In CT acquisition an adequate filling of the upper urinary tract by contrast medium is obtained even in normal subjects (Fig. 21.1). The feasibility of virtual endoscopy with MRU has been proposed both with and without gadolinium (NOLTE-ERNSTING 1999; NERI et al. 2000).

Previous experiences in the application of VE to MR data sets concerned the study of vessels, biliary tract, colon and cerebral ventricles. Our series included 26 patients with neoplastic lesions ($n=9$) located in the renal pelvis, calices and/or ureter, calculi ($n=8$) located in the ureter, pelvi-ureteric junction stenoses ($n=4$), postoperative fibrotic strictures ($n=3$) and extrinsic compressions ($n=2$) located in the lumbar tract of the ureter. MRU was done with a non-breath-hold, fat-suppressed, respiratory-triggered, two-dimensional, heavily T2-weighted fast spin echo sequence in the coronal plane.

VE views were displayed in a combined fashion with MR source images and VE findings could be correlated with the coronal views. VE of the renal pelvis and calices was feasible in all cases at the side of urinary obstruction. VE of the ureter, from the pelvi-ureteric junction to the site of obstruction, was obtained with acceptable quality when its caliber was at least 5 mm. The contralateral side could be partially explored in 11 cases (43%), and navigation was feasible in the calices, renal pelvis and proximal tract of the ureter. The dilatation of the urinary tract was a prerequisite for generating endoscopic views and the majority of pathological patterns were described as occlusion of the lumen.

Neoplastic lesions appeared as endoluminal masses and VE demonstrated the endoluminal appearance of the lesions, their morphology, position with respect to calices, and extent.

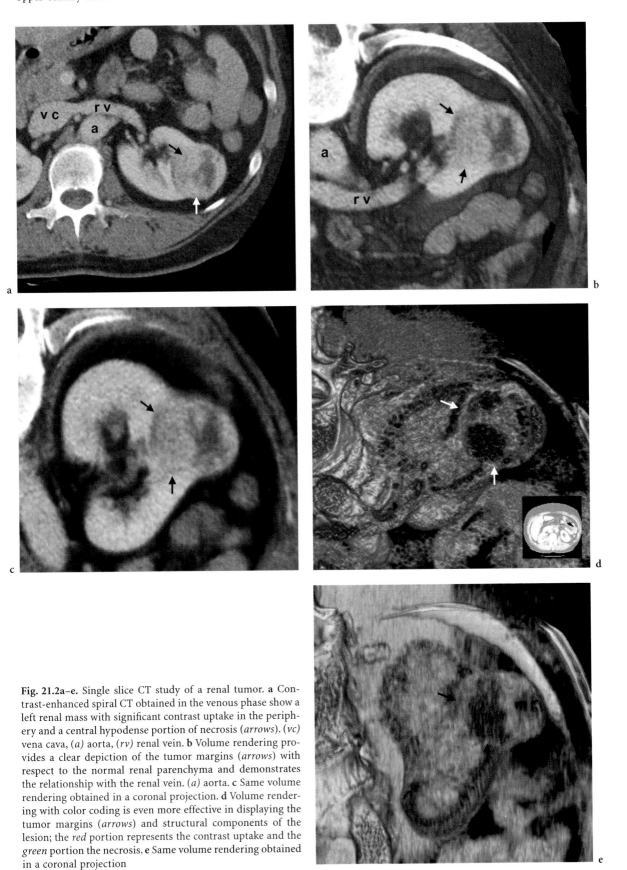

Fig. 21.2a–e. Single slice CT study of a renal tumor. **a** Contrast-enhanced spiral CT obtained in the venous phase show a left renal mass with significant contrast uptake in the periphery and a central hypodense portion of necrosis (*arrows*). (*vc*) vena cava, (*a*) aorta, (*rv*) renal vein. **b** Volume rendering provides a clear depiction of the tumor margins (*arrows*) with respect to the normal renal parenchyma and demonstrates the relationship with the renal vein. (*a*) aorta. **c** Same volume rendering obtained in a coronal projection. **d** Volume rendering with color coding is even more effective in displaying the tumor margins (*arrows*) and structural components of the lesion; the *red* portion represents the contrast uptake and the *green* portion the necrosis. **e** Same volume rendering obtained in a coronal projection

References

Catalano C (1999) MR pyelography and conventional MR imaging in urinary tract obstruction. Acta Radiol 40:198–202

Coll DM (1999) Three-dimensional volume rendered computerized tomography for preoperative evaluation and intraoperative treatment of patients undergoing nephron sparing surgery. J Urol 161:1097–1102

Dachman AH, Newmark GM, Mitchell MT (1998) Helical CT examination of potential kidney donors. AJR 171:193–200

Farres MT, Pedron P, Gattegno B (1998) Helical CT of the ureteropelvic junction obstruction: accuracy in detection of crossing vessels. J Comput Assist Tomogr 22:300–303

Fishman EK (2000) Multidetector CT with 3D angiography: applications in the evaluation of renal pathology. Radiology 217:S633

Lee CT, Hilton S, Russo P (2001) Renal mass within a horseshoe kidney: preoperative evaluation with three-dimensional helical computed tomography. Urology 57:168

Louca G (1999) MR urography in the diagnosis of urinary tract obstruction. Eur Urol 35:102–108

McTavish JD (2000) Multidetector CT urography: analysis of techniques and comparison with IVU. Radiology 217:S225

Neri E, Boraschi P, Braccini G (2000) MR virtual endoscopy of the upper urinary tract. AJR 1775:1696–1702

Nolte-Ernsting CC (1998) Gadolinium-enhanced excretory MR urography after low-dose diuretic injection: comparison with conventional excretory urography. Radiology 209:147–157

Nolte-Ernsting CC (1999) MR virtual ureterorenoscopy of the upper urinary tract. Rofo Fortschr Geb Rontgenstr Neuen Bildgeb Verfahr 170:550–556

O'Malley ME (1997) MR urography: evaluation of a three-dimensional fast spin-echo technique in patients with hydronephrosis. AJR 168:387–392

Rothpearl A (1995) MR urography: technique and application. Radiology 194:125–130

Roy C (1994) Evaluation of RARE-MR urography in the assessment of ureterohydronephrosis. J Comput Assist Tomogr 18:601–608

Roy C (2000) Helical CT of urinary tract: clinical applications. J Radiol 81[Suppl 9]:1071–1081

Zeman RK (1996) Helical CT of renal masses: the value of delayed scans. AJR 167:771–776

22 Lower Urinary Tract

CONTENTS

22.1
Introduction

Bladder cancer is one of the most common malignancies of the urinary tract. Carcinoma of the urinary bladder accounts for 7% of all malignant tumors in men and 4% in women (Parker 1997). More than 50,000 new cases of bladder cancer are diagnosed in the United States each year with the majority in men older than 60 years (Carson 1979; Lynch and Cohen 1995; Parker 1997). Ninety-five percent of these tumors are transitional cell carcinomas, with the rest being comprised of a mixture of squamous cell carcinoma, adenosquamous cell carcinoma and the rare sarcoma. Seventy percent of transitional cell carcinomas of the bladder are superficial, papillary tumors (Rife 1979; Messing 1995). Only 5% of patients with such tumors will die of their disease within 5 years following diagnosis, although 50% will develop another bladder tumor, usually of the same low-grade superficial type (Prout 1992). Many of these patients undergo surveillance cystoscopy at 3–6 month intervals. The remaining 30% of bladder tumors are invasive. These patients are treated using

A.G. Schreyer, MD
Department of Radiology, University Hospital Regensburg, Franz-Josef-Strauss Allee 11, 93053 Regensburg, Germany

surgery, chemotherapy or a combination of the two.

Given the excellent prognosis, especially of non-invasive bladder cancer, early diagnosis is a prerequisite for successful therapy. Microscopic hematuria, usually detected by standard urine analysis or a urine dipstick, is indicative of a bladder cancer in less than 5% of cases (Woolhandler 1989). After identifying hematuria the diagnostic investigation usually includes urine cytology, intravenous urography to assess the kidneys and ureters, and cystoscopy to detect bladder masses.

In conventional fiberoptic cystoscopy the patient is placed in the lithotomy position and an endoscope is passed through the urethra into the bladder under local or general anesthesia. The urologist can manipulate the endoscope in order to visualize the inner surface of the bladder wall. Once a tumor is identified, the endoscope may be used to obtain a tissue specimen for biopsy or to guide therapy, such as excision or fulguration. Conventional cystoscopy is reported to have 87% sensitivity in the detection of bladder tumors. However, using a rigid cystoscope limits the evaluation at the bladder neck, structures within diverticula and deeply trabeculated portions of the bladder wall (Rife 1979). Also, because only the inner surface of the bladder is visualized, extension of tumor into or through the wall cannot be discerned without biopsy. In addition to the discomfort induced during the procedure, there is a 5–10% rate of urinary tract infection following cystoscopy.

Having a noninvasive or at least minimally invasive screening test for patients with hematuria would be a great benefit, especially because only 5% of this group really suffers from bladder cancer. Additionally a replacement for surveillance cystoscopy in those patients with a history of superficial bladder cancer would be beneficial.

Virtual endoscopy is a new imaging approach in radiology that is able to visualize a volumetric sectional data set such as is obtained by CT or MR within one comprehensive three-dimensional (3D) model (Fig. 22.1). Using certain mathematical algorithms the distortion of an optical lens as in a real endoscope

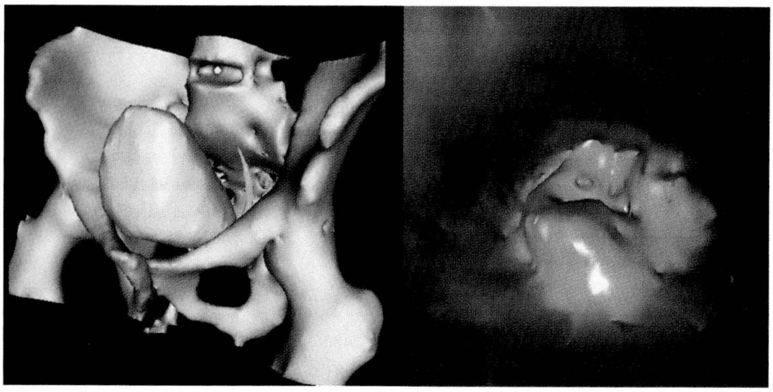

Fig. 22.1. *Left*: exterior view of a 3D reconstructed bladder. *Right*: a urinary bladder tumor depicted using the "virtual endoscopy" view. [Images by Andreas G. Schreyer, MD created at the SPL (Surgical Planning Lab), Brigham and Women's Hospital, Harvard Medical School, Boston, Mass., USA, using "Slicer" software (www.slicer.org)]

can be simulated. A frequently discussed and used application of this new visualization technique is so-called virtual colonoscopy, first described in 1996 by Vining.

The urinary bladder seems to be a more or less perfect hollow organ for virtual endoscopic applications. Its geometry embodies a smooth ellipse within the pelvis. It is surrounded by fatty tissue which gives a good contrast for CT and MR imaging. Additionally because of the fixation within the pelvis it is barely affected by breathing artefacts. Because of its short distension along the body axis even high-resolution CT imaging with minimal slice thickness is feasible.

Several studies are addressing virtual cystoscopy for different clinical applications, most of which are using CT scanning for data acquisition. Scanning strategies for virtual cystoscopy are described in the following section.

22.2
Imaging Strategies for 3D Reconstruction of the Lower Urinary Tract

22.2.1
CT Imaging

Volumetric imaging is a prerequisite for 3D reconstruction and therefore virtual endoscopy. Most studies on virtual cystoscopy are applying spiral CT for data acquisition. The urinary bladder has to be scanned using single breath-hold technique because of possible motion artefacts. A 10–12 F Foley catheter is inserted transurethrally into the bladder. After the urine has been drained 300–550 ml of room air (Narumi 1996; Fenlon 1997; Sommer 1997) or CO_2 (Song 2001) is instilled into the urinary bladder. Currently there are no studies concerning the impact on patient comfort of air versus CO_2 for urinary bladder filling. Given the preliminary results from virtual colonoscopy, CO_2 could be more comfortable for patients because of the physiological absorption of the gas after the examination. On the other hand special equipment has to be used in the scanner room which increases scanning time and costs.

A scout image is necessary to check for adequate bladder distension and filling. Scanning in the supine and prone positions appears to be obligatory for satisfactory visualization of the complete inner bladder surface; up to 19% of tumors can be missed if just one position is used. In most cases a second application of an additional 100 ml CO_2 between the prone and supine imaging is necessary (Song 2001).

Using a single-slice spiral CT imaging is performed with a collimation of 3 mm and a pitch of 1 or slightly larger if necessary. Most studies have used reconstruction intervals ranging from 0.6 mm to 2 mm. However, a 1 mm reconstruction interval seems to be sufficient to achieve a fair isotropic voxel resolution for 3D imaging. Parameters of 120–220 mA with 110–120 kV are used for scanning. The overall scan time is approximately 30 min including the placement of the urinary catheter.

Another application of CT-based virtual cystoscopy is the visualization of a reconstructed lower urinary tract. Stenzl (1998) used a 10 F Foley catheter inserted transurethrally or transrectally to empty the reservoir, and then instilled a saline and iodine contrast mixture until a first sensation of a full pouch. Usually 250–400 ml of contrast/saline mix is necessary. In this particular study electronic beam CT was used, but any spiral CT with collimation, pitch and reconstruction intervals like those mentioned above should be sufficient.

Urinary bladder CT scanning without any catheterization represents a completely different approach (Merkle 1998). After an unenhanced bladder scan, an arterial-phase image is acquired 50 s after the start of an injection of approximately 150 ml non-ionic contrast medium at an injection rate of 3 ml/s. After 30 min a third scan of the contrast-filled bladder is performed. Patients are not allowed to void during the 30 min waiting time. The advantage of this method is that there is no need for transurethral catheterization, which has some known side effects such as infection. On the other hand there are certain side effects of intravenously applied non-ionic contrast media, and the high cost of the contrast media is another disadvantage. Nevertheless this seems to be a interesting approach which needs to be examined in further clinical studies.

Regarding the most common preparation and scanning approach of a voided and air-filled urinary bladder, in our experience another problem is that of urine entering the bladder during the scan. To make the inner bladder surface discernible from urine that entered during scanning we applied some drops of iodine contrast medium after draining the bladder and before the instillation of air (SCHREYER 2000). This resulted in a high contrast between the air and inner bladder surface and an enhanced urine signal (Fig. 22.2) which can easily be removed electronically. This approach is quite similar to so called fecal tagging and electronic cleansing in virtual colonoscopy, where the high-contrast feces that have been marked with barium are removed electronically after image acquisition.

22.2.2
MR Imaging

Currently there are no major studies applying MR imaging to virtual cystoscopy. Basically MR imaging would be well suited for examining the bladder because of its superior contrast resolution and its ability to obtain images in multiple planes. Additionally the T1 and T2 relaxation is useful to differentiate particular pathologies. On T1-weighted sequences bladder tumors have a relatively low signal intensity compared with perivesical fat, but a higher signal than urine within the bladder. On T2-weighted sequences, tumor has a higher signal than the bladder wall but a lower signal than either urine or the perivesical fat. Consequently T1-weighted images are best suited for demonstrating extravesical tumor spread whereas T2-weighted sequences are best for demonstrating spread of tumor into adjacent organs such as the prostate, seminal vesicles and cervix. The accuracy of staging bladder cancer using dynamic con-

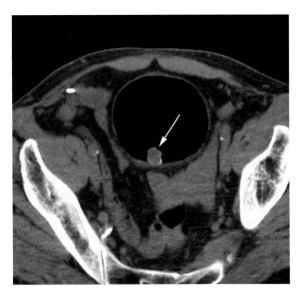

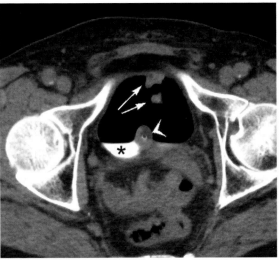

Fig. 22.2. CT scan of a bladder cancer on different slices (*arrows* tumor, *arrowhead* balloon on catheter, *asterisk* contrast medium mixed with urine which entered during scan). [Images by Andreas G. Schreyer, MD created at the SPL (Surgical Planning Lab), Brigham and Women's Hospital, Harvard Medical School, Boston, Mass., USA, using "Slicer" software (www.slicer.org)]

trast-enhanced MR imaging has been shown to be superior to that of both CT and conventional MR imaging (TANIMOTO 1992).

Using MR imaging it would be possible to scan the urinary bladder sufficiently for virtual cystoscopy without catheterization. Ultrafast heavily T2-weighted sequences such as the HASTE sequence could depict the urine-filled bladder without any contrast. For T1-weighted images gadopentetate dimeglumine (e.g. Magnevist, Schering, Berlin, Germany) given intravenously would be useful. After waiting several minutes the bladder concentrates the contrast medium, which would result in a positive contrasted bladder lumen suitable for virtual cystoscopy.

For 3D visualization and MR-based virtual cystoscopy a T1-weighted 3D FLASH (fast low angle shot) sequence as used in MR angiography would be appropriate because of its isotropic voxel dimensions and the ability to scan the entire volume within one breath-hold.

MR-based virtual cystoscopy could be a fascinating application which has yet to be evaluated in clinical trials. Especially because there is no radiation, there is huge potential for the technique as a screening and follow-up tool in bladder imaging.

22.2.3
3D Reconstruction Techniques

For 3D visualization of sectional image data there are basically two different reconstruction techniques: so-called volume rendering, which represents a volume visualization method, and surface rendering, which only visualizes the computed virtual surface of the segmented structure. Both techniques will be briefly explained, including their advantages and disadvantages for 3D urinary bladder visualization.

22.2.3.1
Volume Rendering

Volume rendering represents a quite new 3D visualization technique which demands dedicated powerful computer workstations with huge internal RAM (random accessible memory) capacities. All sectional image data have to be loaded into the computer memory. All voxels of the sectional data are visualized three-dimensionally by computing the whole data set in real time. Based on the density value of each voxel, a voxel is represented by applying certain default or user-created histograms. These histograms assess each voxel as being a certain shade of color, opacity and reflectivity on the basis of voxel density. Using this technique there is barely a need for major time-consuming manual postprocessing. Three-dimensional visualization can be done in real time. This reconstruction approach requires sectional images with high contrast differences of the desired structure relative to the background. The contrast of an air- or contrast-medium-filled urinary bladder should be sufficient for this technique. There is no need for manual segmentation of the hollow

organ, which reduces reconstruction time and user faults. In contrast to the surface rendering technique the whole image data set is used. On the other hand a quantitative analysis of the 3D model is barely possible. Additionally it requires quite powerful and expensive dedicated computer hardware.

For virtual cystoscopy volume rendering seems to be superior and more practicable than surface rendering (FENLON 1997). Volume rendered images provide a more "fluoroscopic" appearance compared with the flat opaque surface of reconstructions created with surface shaded display. Although there are no studies comparing the two modes for virtual cystoscopy, volume rendering should be the preferred technique because of the negligible postprocessing and the more accurate representation of lesion morphology and tissue composition.

22.2.3.2
Surface Rendering

Shaded surface rendering represents a different reconstruction approach. All two-dimensional (2D) images have to be segmented before creating a 3D model. Segmentation means a 2D definition or outlining of the desired structure on each slice of the data set. Segmentation can be done manually by outlining the shape of each structure (Fig. 22.3). Semiautomatic segmentation is the most commonly used approach. One semiautomatic method is intensity-based segmentation, i.e., each structure within a defined intensity threshold is outlined automatically. In CT imaging bony structures, which have a fairly high intensity, can be segmented by this method very easily. Another helpful tool for semiautomatic segmentation is a connectivity algorithm: each voxel within a certain intensity threshold which has a defined connectivity to its neighboring voxel is automatically segmented. Using this approach many connected slices of the data stack can be segmented in one step. After semiautomatic segmentation some slices of the data set have to be fine tuned manually, because of the presence of similar-intensity structures on sectional images. After segmentation has been done a computer algorithm connects each point of the outlined structure on all slices of the data stack. Using dedicated visualization pipelines, a wire frame model representing the surface of the segmented data is created. The wire frame model can be covered by a virtual surface. Assigning colors, reflective properties and virtual light sources to the surface creates an impression of a 3D model.

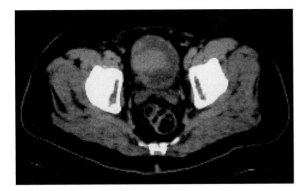

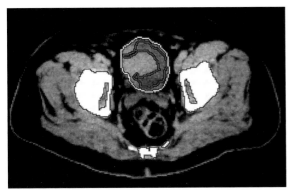

Fig. 22.3. Segmentation for surface rendering requires an intensity-based outlining of the desired structures (here a huge bladder cancer within the bladder lumen). [Images by Andreas G. Schreyer, MD created at the SPL (Surgical Planning Lab), Brigham and Women's Hospital, Harvard Medical School, Boston, Mass., USA, using "Slicer" software (www.slicer.org)]

Because of the segmentation process the anatomy of the reconstructed models is very detailed. Even quantitative analysis such as precise measurement of diameters can be done on segmented data. The drawback of this method is the time-consuming segmentation. Additionally only approximately 10% of all sectional image data are used for the final 3D reconstruction (JOHNSON 1996).

22.2.3.3
Virtual Endoscopy

Virtual endoscopy uses 3D dimensional rendering algorithms such as the volume rendering or surface rendering methods described above. Virtual endoscopy uses perspective rendering with optical simulation of a real endoscopic lens. Basically perspective rendering causes objects to grow larger as the observer approaches. Even the angle of the lens and the size of the virtual camera can be altered. Employing these capacities even particular endoscopes from

certain manufacturers can be simulated. There are several commercially available software packages for virtual endoscopy. The user interface of the software allows the data to be inspected in three different ways: an exterior view provides general orientation, the virtual endoscopic view allows inspection of the interior bladder walls, and the cross-sectional images allow the assessment of the morphology below the surface. Cross-referencing between the 2D and 3D images is provided by a simple mouse interaction. The direction of movement through the preferred structure is based on such cross-references. For tubular structures such as the colon, automated path calculation algorithms are useful. In virtual cystoscopy free navigation within this ellipsoid hollow organ is sufficient. The motion should be calculated and executed in real time. Conceptually, the "virtual endoscope" is attached to the mouse pointer by a virtual "rubber band". Wherever the pointer moves, the virtual camera moves as well. Applying this technique, a comprehensive 3D dimensional visualization of the urinary bladder including simulated endoscopic view is feasible (Figs. 22.1, 22.4, 22.5).

Transverse and virtual views are complementary in lesion detection and characterization. SONG (2001) and colleagues found that some lesions of less than 5 mm were identified only on the virtual views.

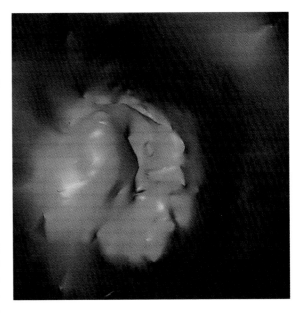

Fig. 22.4. Bladder cancer visualized by virtual cystoscopy. [Image by Andreas G. Schreyer, MD created at the SPL (Surgical Planning Lab), Brigham and Women's Hospital, Harvard Medical School, Boston, Mass., USA, using "Slicer" software (www.slicer.org)]

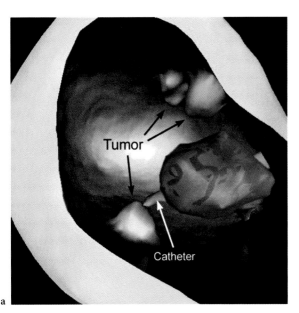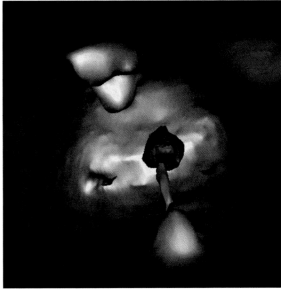

a   b

Fig. 22.5a, b. Virtual cystoscopy of the tumors depicted in Fig. 22.2. [Images by Andreas G. Schreyer, MD created at the SPL (Surgical Planning Lab), Brigham and Women's Hospital, Harvard Medical School, Boston, Mass., USA, using "Slicer" software (www.slicer.org)]

22.3
Clinical Applications

Having a minimally invasive radiological method for the diagnostic investigation of microscopic hematuria identified by standard urine analysis would be very appealing. Less than 5% of microscopic hematuria is indicative for bladder cancer (WOOLHANDLER 1989), so there is a need for a sensitive minimally invasive diagnostic method.

Conventional cystoscopy remains the standard technique of exploring bladder abnormalities. There are, however, certain limitations. The method is invasive, expensive and time-consuming. Sedation is frequently required and iatrogenic injury of the urethra and bladder may occur. Urinary sepsis can develop in 5–10% of patients. Moreover, because of the limited flexibility of fiberoptic cystoscopes particular regions of the bladder mucosa, such as the bladder neck, are recognized as potential blind spots. Bladder diverticula are not accessible for uncomplicated inspection.

Bladder tumors can be identified radiologically by intravenous pyelography, contrast-enhanced cystography, ultrasound, MR imaging or contrast-enhanced CT. Applying 3D reconstruction techniques and virtual endoscopy could add some additional value to these methods. Sectional imaging and virtual endoscopy should be considered complementary in urinary bladder diagnosis. One study has shown that particularly small lesions, which were not even seen retrospectively on sectional images, can only be diagnosed using virtual endoscopy (SONG 2001). NARUMI (1996) detected 77% of lesions smaller than 10 mm. SONG (2001) had a detection rate of 60% for lesions smaller than 5 mm with an overall detection rate of 90% compared with conventional cystoscopy. All available studies are based on small skewed patient groups. Nevertheless the method seems to be capable of detecting tumors bigger than 5 mm with a sensitivity of more than 80%.

A shortcoming of virtual cystoscopy is the fact that subtle color changes of the mucosa indicating inflammation or malignancy can not be seen. Also, flat lesions smaller than 5 mm are difficult to visualize and a histological evaluation based on sectional radiological imaging is not possible. There exist different techniques to overcome these problems by adding more sectional image information to the 3D reconstructed inner surface. One approach could be color coding of wall thickness in virtual endoscopy (SCHREYER 2000). This algorithm can be indicative of subtle thickness changes of hollow organs, which is a sign of inflammation or malignant tumors (Fig. 22.6).

Besides screening tests for bladder cancer there is a major need for follow-up examinations after treatment. In particular, patients with low-grade disease will develop another bladder cancer of the same low-

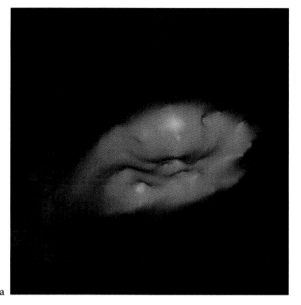 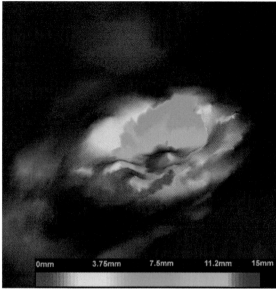

a   b

Fig. 22.6a, b. Flat tumor depicted by virtual cystoscopy. (**a**) An algorithm which basically color-codes the wall thickness of the bladder indicating the tumor (**b**). [Images by Andreas G. Schreyer, MD created at the SPL (Surgical Planning Lab), Brigham and Women's Hospital, Harvard Medical School, Boston, Mass., USA, using "Slicer" software (www.slicer.org)]

grade type after therapy (PROUT 1992). Surveillance cystoscopy at 3–6 month intervals is essential in these patients. Additionally virtual cystoscopy could be an interesting tool for monitoring the treatment response in patients with nonresectable tumors. Because this technique is based on sectional imaging even extravesical metastases or the infiltration of surrounding organs can be diagnosed.

Another indication for virtual cystoscopy is patients with urethral stricture or marked prostate hypertrophy, because catheters for air instillation are smaller than endoscopes.

22.4
Conclusion

Although the clinical value of CT- and MR-based virtual cystoscopy has not yet been established, it may have several potential roles. It could be used as a diagnostic examination for patients with obstacles to conventional cystoscopy such as urethral stricture or warfarin therapy. It could be beneficial to integrate it into the imaging algorithm for evaluation of hematuria. Certainly it is a useful tool for monitoring treatment response in patients with known unresectable bladder cancer and to follow-up patients with treated low-grade cancer. Furthermore it is a fascinating tool

with growing fields of application with improved CT and MR imaging. However, it has to be improved and evaluated in larger prospective studies in a general population.

References

Carson CC (1979) Clinical importance of microhematuria. JAMA 241:149–150
Fenlon HM (1997) Virtual cystoscopy: early clinical experience. Radiology 205:272–275
Johnson PT (1996) Three-dimensional CT: real-time interactive volume rendering. AJR 167:581–583
Lynch CF, Cohen MB (1995) Urinary system. Cancer 75 [Suppl 1]:316–329
Merkle EM (1998) Virtual cystoscopy based on helical CT scan datasets: perspectives and limitations. Br J Radiol 71:262–267
Messing EM (1995). Comparison of bladder cancer outcome in men undergoing hematuria home screening versus those with standard clinical presentations. Urology 45:387–396
Narumi Y (1996) The bladder and bladder tumors: imaging with three-dimensional display of helical CT data. AJR 167:1134–1135
Parker SL (1997). Cancer statistics. CA Cancer J Clin 47:5–27
Prout GR (1992) Treated history of noninvasive grade 1 transitional cell carcinoma. J Urol 148:1413–1419
Rife CC (1979). Urine cytology of transitional cell neoplasms. Urol Clin North Am 6:599–612
Schreyer AG (2000) Virtual CT cystoscopy: color mapping of bladder wall thickness. Invest Radiol 35:331–334

Sommer FG (1997) Volume rendering of CT data: applications to the genitourinary tract. AJR 168:1223–1226

Song JH (2001). Bladder tumor detection at virtual cystoscopy. Radiology 218:95–100

Stenzl A (1998) 3-Dimensional computerized tomography and virtual reality endoscopy of the reconstructed lower urinary tract. J Urol 159:741–746

Tanimoto A (1992) Bladder tumor staging: comparison of conventional and gadolinium-enhanced dynamic MR imaging and CT. Radiology 185:741–747

Vining DJ (1996) Virtual endoscopy: is it reality? Radiology 200:30–31

Woolhandler S (1989) Dipstick urinalysis screening of asymptomatic adults for urinary tract disorders. JAMA 262:1214–1219

23 Musculoskeletal System

ANNE COTTEN, SANDRINE IOCHUM, ALAIN BLUM MOYSE

CONTENTS

23.1
Introduction

Musculoskeletal applications of three-dimensional (3D) imaging were among the first to be developed and remain its most common clinical application , as this noninvasive method offers a unique tool to characterize the bone morphology and to understand the architecture and kinematics of normal and pathologic joints in vivo. Indeed, accurate evaluation of complex anatomy or complex spatial relationships between the lesions and adjacent anatomic structures plays a major role in clinical applications of 3D imaging, as it represents a dramatic improvement over the use of planar cross-sectional imaging alone. This imaging has been shown to have an impact on diagnosis and surgical management in a number of skeletal applications including trauma, malformations and tumors. Moreover, 3D images frequently integrate hundreds of sections in a form that is often easier to interpret than the sections themselves (CALHOUN et al. 1999).

Three-dimensional imaging has been developed from images obtained with multiple modalities, but computed tomography and magnetic resonance imaging represent the most common data sets in the musculoskeletal applications of 3D imaging.

23.2
3D CT and MR Imaging

Three-dimensional medical images of CT and MR data sets can be generated with a variety of computer algorithms. The three most commonly used techniques are shaded surface display (SSD), maximum intensity projection (MIP) and, more recently, 3D volume rendering (CALHOUN et al. 1999).

23.2.1
Computer Algorithms

23.2.1.1
Shaded Surface Display

SSD is a process in which apparent surfaces are determined within the volume of data and an image representing the derived surfaces is displayed (CALHOUN et al. 1999). Because this process reduces the original data volume down to a compact surface model, surface rendering algorithms can operate very rapidly, with flexibility in image rendering (KUSZYK et al. 1996). In general, surface rendered images have the clearest volume depth cues of all 3D images, producing skeletal images that appear more three-dimensional than those created using volume rendering (CALHOUN et al. 1999). Applications in surgical planning take advantage of this capability that allows surface models to be interactively repositioned and manipulated.

However, their clinical utility in skeletal pathology is compromised by an inability to show subcortical detail (CALHOUN et al. 1999) (Fig. 23.1). Indeed, surface rendering depicts only the bone surface. Most of the available data is not incorporated into the 3D

A. COTTEN, MD
Service de Radiologie Ostéo-Articulaire, Hôpital R. Salengro – CHRU de Lille, Boulevard du Pr. J. Leclercq, 59037 Lille Cédex, France
S. IOCHUM, MD, A. BLUM MOYSE, MD
Service de Radiologie, Hôpital Central, 29, avenue Maréchal de Lattre de Tassigny, 54035 Nancy Cédex, France

a 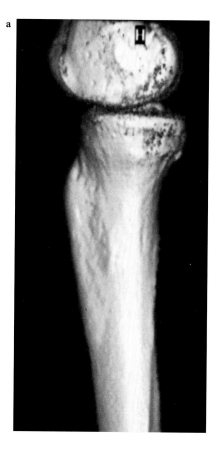 b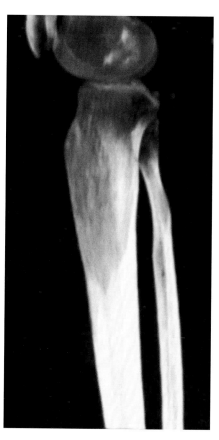

Fig. 23.1a, b. Paget's disease. **a** Shaded surface display (SSD) demonstrates only the enlargement of the tibial tuberosity. **b** Volume rendering clearly underlines the characteristic tibial advancing wedge-shaped radiolucent edge

image. In cases where the pathology of interest is subcortical or obscured by overlying bone, surface rendering does not display the lesion. Another drawback is poor image fidelity. Surface rendering simplifies the data into a binary form, classifying each pixel as either 100% bone or 0% bone. This finite voxel size in medical data produces many voxels that are only fractionally composed of bone, and classifying them as all or none introduces stair-step artefacts into the image (DREBIN et al. 1989; WANG and VANNIER 1994). By varying the threshold minimally, a fracture gap can open or close, bony processes lengthen and shorten, and "holes" in the cortex are created and fused (KUSZYK et al. 1996). The last drawback is that surface rendering is not adequate for the visualization of structures that do not have naturally well differentiated surfaces (CALHOUN et al. 1999).

23.2.1.2
Maximum Intensity Projection

MIP is the simplest of all 3D rendering techniques. In MIP, the intensity assigned to a pixel in the rendition is simply the maximum scene intensity encountered along the projection line. It is most effective when

the objects of interest are the brightest in the scene and have a simple 3D morphology and a minimal gradation of intensity values. One limitation of this technique that must be taken into account to interpret the rendered images properly is that MIP images misrepresents anatomic spatial relationships because the planar projected data do not take spatial location into account (CALHOUN et al. 1999). The anterior anatomic structures cannot be differentiated from the posterior ones.

The sliding thin slab maximum intensity projection (STS-MIP) and multiplanar volume reconstruction (MPVR) represent alternatives to MIP in which the volume is restricted to a thin slab that is only a few voxel widths in depth (NAPEL et al. 1993). Preprocessing is no longer required and the resulting images have a high contrast resolution.

Contrast material enhanced CT angiography and MR angiography are ideal applications for MIP (UDUPA 1999) (Fig. 23.2). They both offer more rapid examination than conventional angiography and a lower or no radiation dose. In addition, the 3D nature of the acquired data makes them amenable to postprocessing and reprojection from any angle (NAPEL et al. 1992).

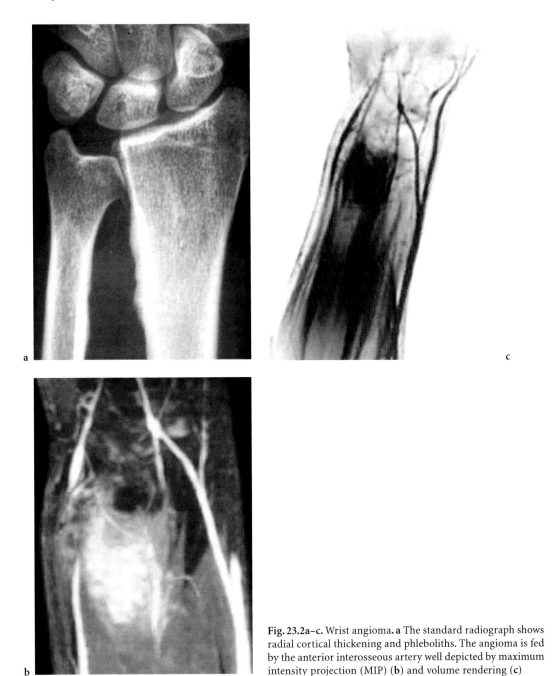

Fig. 23.2a–c. Wrist angioma. a The standard radiograph shows radial cortical thickening and phleboliths. The angioma is fed by the anterior interosseous artery well depicted by maximum intensity projection (MIP) (b) and volume rendering (c)

Another application of MIP for the diagnosis of craniostenosis and fracture of the calvaria has recently been reported (MEDINA 2000).

23.2.1.3
Volume Rendering

Unlike surface rendering, volume rendering uses a percentage classification that provides a realistic depiction of voxels that are only fractionally composed of

bone (KUSZYK et al. 1996) (Fig. 23.1). Moreover, the algorithm incorporates all the data contained in the volume into the displayed image, leading to greater fidelity in the data. This algorithm has the advantage of showing multiple overlying and internal features with a displayed intensity related to the amount of bone encountered along a line extending through the volume. The main drawback associated with volume rendering is the difficulty in appreciating 3D relationships in very transparent volume rendered images.

Three volume rendering techniques (unshaded bone, shaded bone and shaded opaque bone) can help reveal both surface and internal detail and can be used for a better understanding of the volume rendered images:

- The unshaded bone algorithm creates images that appear similar to plain radiographs. The lack of surface shading and enhancement makes these images the simplest, most artefact-free of the three volume rendering techniques. For some authors (Kuszyk et al. 1996), the ability to depict multiple overlying structures with few artefacts has made this algorithm the most useful volume rendering technique for most skeletal applications. Video loop rotation greatly enhances 3D understanding when viewing these images.
- The shaded bone algorithm incorporates surface shading and enhancement at interfaces of tissues with different CT numbers. This can be useful for accentuating lytic or sclerotic lesions, or clearly defining the medullary canal. However, this technique increases computer rendering time and can serve as a source of artefact which can make these images difficult to interpret. Kuszyk et al. (1996) have found the shaded bone to be the least helpful of the three volume rendering algorithms.
- The opaque bone algorithm may be useful in applications in which detail and 3D understanding are of importance. Indeed, opacity dramatically improves 3D anatomic relationships with a degree of clarity similar to that of surface rendering. In the extreme case where the opacity is 100%, no internal detail is visible and the resulting image is effectively a surface model (Kuszyk et al. 1996). However, the decreased transparency in these images can make it more difficult to appreciate multiple overlying structures and subcortical lesions.

Color can be used for differentiation between anatomic structures of different densities. For example, it may be helpful in displaying the tendons. However, it must be determined whether the use of color provides additional information.

As volume rendering is now possible on inexpensive desktop computers, it seems to be the most valuable algorithm for most skeletal applications as it has the advantages of both MIP (good contrast and good differentiation between tissues) and SSD (precise location of the lesion in the space). Moreover, with this algorithm it is easy to delete some tissues, to highlight others, to isolate bones or to present them with their adjacent soft tissues or vessels.

23.2.2 Clinical Applications

23.2.2.1 Trauma

The first applications of 3D imaging were in the evaluation of skeletal fractures and planning for orthopedic surgery. Indeed, a precise classification and an optimal understanding of fractures are the basis of conservative treatment or adequate surgery. Three-dimensional images are particularly useful for planning surgery, especially in determining the surgical approach and screw placement. This is especially the case for acetabular fractures, where 3D evaluation is of the utmost importance for precise definition of the direction and magnitude of displacement of the bone. The hip joint space and its relationship to the fracture must be accurately analyzed. In selected cases, the femur can be disarticulated from the acetabulum. Preoperative planning of fractures in anatomically complex areas such as the scapula, the spine, the foot and the wrist can also be improved by 3D imaging.

Fractures analysis is frequently based on the axial sections as well as on multiplanar reconstructions (MPRs) and 3D surface shaded rendering. However, although MPR allows precise quantification of the displacement of the fragments, it does not display a global and comprehensible view of the lesions. This explains why surgeons usually prefer 3D images for surgical planning (Pretorius and Fishman 1999a). Three-dimensional surface shaded rendering greatly facilitates the evaluation of complex fractures, but can fail to recognize minimally displaced fractures and lesions beneath the bony surface. Moreover, the images can demonstrate stair-step artefacts.

Volume rendering has been found highly superior to shaded surface rendering for the accurate demonstration of subtle fractures, particularly those oriented in the axial plane (Pretorius and Fishman 1999b) (Fig. 23.3). It also clearly demonstrates complex injuries and complicated spatial information about the relative positions of fracture fragments. The use of intravenously administered contrast material allows simultaneous evaluation of osseous and vascular structures within the affected area. Associated vascular injuries can be identified or excluded. Moreover, reconstructions can be optimized to achieve high spatial or density resolution. Finally the images do not demonstrate stair-step artefacts.

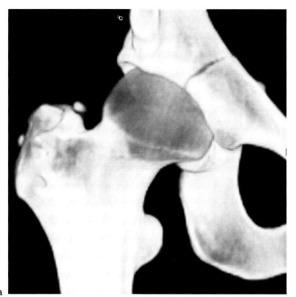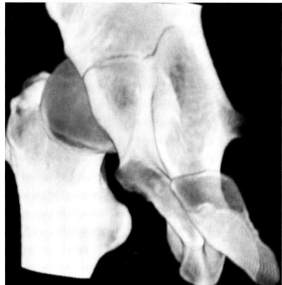

a   b

Fig. 23.3a, b. Acetabulum fracture. Volume rendering allows the clear and precise visualization of this nondisplaced fracture. It provides an accurate depiction of the extent of the fracture line

23.2.2.2
Malformations and Complex Osteoarticular Relationships

Three-dimensional images represent an efficient and comprehensive way to understand preoperatively the complexity of anatomic and pathologic relationships in the case of bone and joint malformations. For example, 3D CT can be a useful tool in the assessment of patients with congenital scoliosis, in that the 3D images provide easier comprehension of the anomalous segments and their relationship with other vertebrae. Indeed, the complex 3D nature of the vertebral malformations makes their characterization by planar cross-sectional imaging methods difficult. Even if curved sagittal reconstructions can be helpful for the analysis of the relationship between the spine and the cord, MPR images do not display the global morphology of the anomalous segments and their interrelationships in an easily perceived manner. BUSH and KALEN (1999) have reported that, in four of their 12 cases of congenital scoliosis, 3D CT was markedly superior to CT with MPR in displaying the pathology, in that the pathology revealed by the 3D images was difficult to comprehend on both axial CT sections and the reformatted images, even in retrospect.

Three-dimensional display of CT data is also extremely valuable for planning reorientation osteotomies for the treatment of residual dysplasia of the hip. Three-dimensional reconstructions also greatly facilitate the diagnosis of rare pathologies such as snapping scapula (MOZES et al. 1999), related to mechanical impingement between the scapula and the rib cage, by demonstrating the bony component of this entity. Three-dimensional CT has also been found helpful in delineating Sprengel deformity in detail, and in planning scapuloplasty (CHO et al. 2000).

23.2.2.3
Tumors

Three-dimensional imaging is also valuable in the evaluation of tumor extent and helps confirm the initial decision regarding tumor resectability and preoperative planning for the most appropriate type of tumor resection. Both CT and MR imaging can provide precise vascular cartography (Figs. 23.2, 23.4). However, CT volume rendering is the only 3D modality that allows, on the same image, clear visibility of the tumoral bone, soft tissue and vessels. Two or three CT acquisitions must be performed. The first must be obtained at the peak of the contrast bolus in the artery and the second at the venous time. Sometimes it may be interesting to perform a third acquisition at a distance from the first contrast administration, and consequently to wait for the enhancement of the tumor. A second intravenous administration of contrast medium can then be performed to reveal the precise relationship between the enhanced tumor and the adjacent vessels (BLUM and REGENT 1995).

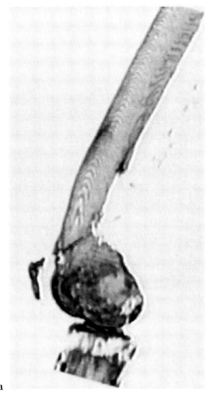
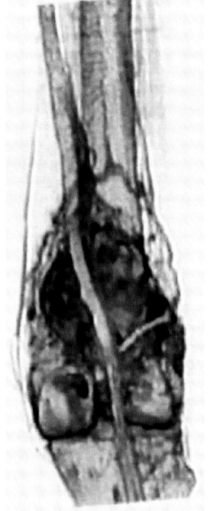

Fig. 23.4a, b. Osteosarcoma of the distal femur in Paget's disease with supracondylar fracture. **a** Volume rendering allows reconstruction of the bony structures alone with depiction of supracondylar fracture and posterior osteolysis. **b** It also allows simultaneous visualization of bone, tumor and vessels

23.2.2.4
Control of Orthopedic Hardware

Postoperative review of patients with orthopedic hardware can be effectively accomplished by 3D volume rendering as this technique eliminates the vast majority of streak artefact (Fig. 23.5) and clearly delineates the relationship between hardware, bones and bone fragments (CALHOUN et al. 1999; PRETORIUS and FISHMAN 1999b).

23.2.2.5
Functional Anatomy of the Musculoskeletal System

Three-dimensional reconstructions of CT and MR images can delineate precisely the spatial relationship between bones and musculotendinous structures and produce a good 3D visual presentation of biodynamic events of human joints. Rotational motion of a shoulder, knee flexion, and other complex musculoskeletal motions can be assessed, as well as the effect of muscle dysfunction and its relevance to the mechanics of joints (TOTTERMAN et al. 1998). This method is of great interest because many biomechanical studies are based on dramatically simplified anatomic models.

Assessment of the dynamic compression of the subclavian artery when it crosses one of the tunnels of the thoracic outlet has been performed with both CT and MR imaging (Fig. 23.6). With CT, the arterial compression seems better depicted with volume rendered reconstructions than with the 3D shaded surface images and with sagittal reformations (REMY-JARDIN et al. 2000). With MR imaging, MIP or volume rendering can be performed.

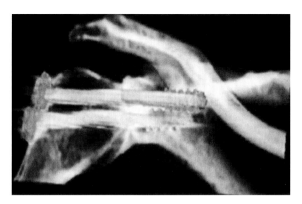

Fig. 23.5. Surgical procedure on the shoulder. Volume rendering attenuates metal artefacts

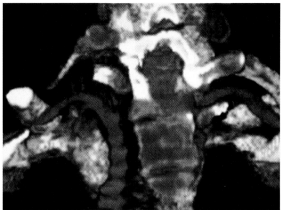

a

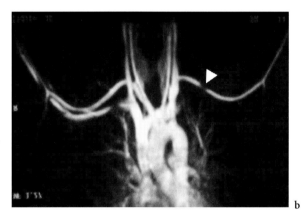

b

Fig. 23.6a, b. Thoracic outlet syndrome .Thoracic outlet syndrome in two different patients explored with CT (**a**) and MR imaging (**b**). The *arrowhead* points to subclavian artery compression in the costoclavicular space. A right cervical rib can also be seen

23.2.2.6
Cartilage

The emergence of new therapeutic concepts for treating cartilage disorders explains the increasing demand for accurate and objective evaluation of cartilage morphology in vivo (HYHLIK-DURR et al. 2000), especially with MR imaging due to its noninvasive nature. Because sectional images cannot be identically reproduced in longitudinal studies, 3D reconstruction postprocessing methods have been developed to quantify cartilage morphology (volume and thickness) independent of the respective section position and orientation (HYHLIK-DURR et al. 2000). Several studies suggest the interest of quantitative MR-based cartilage morphometry as a tool to diagnose, stage and follow cartilage loss in the knee.

Sequences must be optimized to achieve a high spatial resolution and a fast acquisition time. As sequences must allow analysis of the cartilage with high contrast to the surrounding tissue, thin sliced 3D spoiled gradient echo sequences with spectral fat suppression (ECKSTEIN et al. 1998) or with selective water excitation (HYHLIK-DURR et al. 2000) are usually performed. The water excitation protocol allows the water-bound protons in the cartilage to be excited selectively and directly. Therefore, no prepulse is required as in conventional fat-suppressed imaging protocols.

Segmentation of the cartilage is then performed semiautomatically on a section by section basis by using a gray value oriented region-growing algorithm. An isotropic voxel size can be obtained with a shape-based interpolation method, and the cartilage is reconstructed in three dimensions with an opti-

mized surface reconstructing algorithm (ECKSTEIN et al. 1998; HYHLIK-DURR et al. 2000). The cartilage volume is then computed from these reconstructions. The cartilage thickness can be determined by using a 3D minimal distance algorithm (LÖSCH et al. 1997; ECKSTEIN et al. 1998).

23.2.2.7
Navigation in Diagnosis and Therapy

Software systems simulating surgery and image-guided navigation for surgery and other therapeutic interventions have grown in importance in recent years. Key elements in image navigation systems are preoperative 3D imaging, a graphical display and interactive input devices. CT and MR imaging are commonplace today and 3D images are useful in complex interventions. Osteotomy and setting of pedicle screws in orthopedic surgery profit greatly from the high targeting precision of this technique (Laine et al. 2000). The term computer-aided surgery is now mainly used for intraoperative navigation within the body combining a 3D digitizer with preoperative CT/MR imaging.

Other navigation systems may also use intraoperative acquisition of images (Woodard et al. 2001; Haberland et al. 2000). These systems are consequently able to reflect the intraoperative changes.

23.3
3D Ultrasound

Three-dimensional ultrasound (3D US) is in the early stages of clinical assessment but seems to offer several advantages over conventional US, including 3D US image reconstruction with a single pass of the US beam, virtually unlimited viewing perspectives, and repeatable evaluation of anatomic structures and diseases entities (Downey et al. 2000). Image acquisition must be performed very cautiously, as unplanned transducer movement or involuntary patient motion (e.g., cardiac motion, respiratory motion) may produce artefacts severely degrading the quality of the images.

Three-dimensional US data acquisition systems can be tracked freehand systems (in which devices are attached to the transducer), untracked freehand systems (in which the images are digitized as the operator moves the transducer with a smooth, steady motion), mechanical assemblies (in which the transducer is propelled or rotated mechanically) or two-dimensional arrays (in which a square-faced or circular-faced transducer obtains true 3D data from an array of detectors) (Downey et al. 2000). Three-dimensional reconstruction techniques use a 3D surface model or a voxel-based volume model. Three different rendering modes can be selected: surface rendering for photorealistic images of objects, transparent rendering as either a maximum mode to enhance hyperechoic structures (e.g., bones) a minimum mode to accentuate hypoechoic structures (e.g., blood vessels and cysts) or color mode rendering for spatial reconstructions of volumes including Doppler or angiographic information (Brandl et al. 1999). MPR can also be performed.

23.3.1
Clinical Applications

If 3D US seems promising in fetal, gynecologic, prostate, breast and power Doppler imaging, the clinical applications of this technique in musculoskeletal diseases are still uncertain. Leotta and Martin (2000) have reported a technique for measuring the thickness of the rotator cuff from the 3D compound volumes. To the best of our knowledge, only two papers have reported the usefulness of 3D US in the assessment of the rotator cuff lesions. For these authors, 3D US appears to facilitate diagnosis of partial-thickness rotator cuff tears both in patients and in artificial rotator cuff lesions of cadaveric shoulder joints (Wallny et al. 2000). However, further studies are required to confirm these results. Indeed if this modality may appear to be a powerful adjunctive tool to 2D US in providing a more comprehensive visualization of lesions, it must be determined whether the use of 3D US provides additional information and has an effect on patient management.

Three-dimensional high-resolution US has also proved to be useful for in vitro assessment of cartilage remodeling of rat patella in osteoarthritis (Lefebvre et al. 1998). Another application of 3D US could be in performing biopsy. Indeed, it has been suggested that 3D US can help facilitate needle localization and guidance during biopsy.

Finally, although it may appear time-consuming to measure the volume of lesions using 3D US, this technique of volume calculation allowing images of multiple areas to be obtained simultaneously in uniform conditions must be assessed, as it may have valuable applications in tumors and in the assessment of synovial disorders.

References

Blum A, Regent D (1995) Scanner hélicoïdal. Principes et modalités pratiques d'utilisation. Collection d'Imagerie Radiologique. Masson, Paris
Brandl H, Gritzky A, Haizinger M (1999) 3D ultrasound: a dedicated system. Eur Radiol 9:S331–S333
Bush CH, Kalen V (1999) Three-dimensional computed tomography in the assessment of congenital scoliosis. Skeletal Radiol 28:632–637

Calhoun PS, Kuszyk BS, Heath DG, et al (1999) Three-dimensional volume rendering of spiral CT data: theory and method. Radiographics 19:745–764

Cho TJ, Choi IH, Chung CY, et al (2000) The Sprengel deformity: morphometric analysis using 3D CT and its clinical relevance. J Bone Joint Surg Br 82:711–718

Downey DB, Fenster A, Williams JC (2000) Clinical utility of three-dimensional US. Radiographics 20:559–571

Drebin RA, Magid D, Robertson DD, et al (1989) Fidelity of three-dimensional CT imaging for detecting fractures gaps. J Comput Assist Tomogr 13:487–489

Eckstein F, Tieschky M, Faber SC, et al (1998) Effect of physical exercise on cartilage volume and thickness in vivo: MR imaging study. Radiology 207:243–248

Haberland N, Ebmeier K, Grunewald JP, et al (2000) Incorporation of intraoperative computerized tomography in a newly developed spinal navigation technique. Comput Aided Surg 5:18–27

Hyhlik-Dürr A, Faber S, Burgkart R, et al (2000) Precision of tibial cartilage morphometry with a coronal water-excitation MR sequence. Eur Radiol 10:297–300

Kuszyk BS, Heath DG, Bliss DF, et al (1996) Skeletal 3-D CT: advantages of volume rendering over surface rendering. Skeletal Radiol 25:207–214

Laine T, Lund T, Ylikoski M, et al (2000) Accuracy of pedicle screw insertion with and without computer assistance: a randomised controlled clinical study in 100 consecutive patients. Eur Spine J 9:235–240

Lefebvre F, Graillat N, Cherin E, et al (1998) Automatic three-dimensional reconstruction and characterization of articular cartilage from high-resolution ultrasound acquisitions. Ultrasound Med Biol 24:1369–1381

Leotta DF, Martin RW (2000) Three-dimensional spatial compounding of ultrasound scans with weighting by incidence angle. Ultrason Imaging 22:1–19

Lösch A, Eckstein F, Haubner M, et al (1997) A non-invasive technique for 3-dimensional assessment of articular cartilage thickness based on MRI. I. Development of a computational method. Magn Reson Imaging 15:785–804

Medina LS (2000) Three-dimensional CT maximum intensity projections of the calvaria: a new approach for diagnosis of craniosynostosis and fractures. AJNR Am J Neuroradiol 21:1951–1954

Mozes G, Bickels J, Ovadia D, et al (1999) The use of three-dimensional computed tomography in evaluating snapping scapula syndrome. Orthopedics 22:1029–1033

Napel S, Marks MP, Rubin GD, et al (1992) CT angiography of spiral CT and maximum intensity projection. Radiology 185:607–610

Napel S, Rubin GD, Jeffrey RB, et al (1993) STS-MIP: a new reconstruction technique for CT of the chest. J Comput Assist Tomogr 17:832–838

Pretorius ES, Fishman EK (1999a) Spiral CT and three-dimensional CT of musculoskeletal pathology. Radiol Clin North Am 37:953–974

Pretorius ES, Fishman EK (1999b) Volume-rendered three-dimensional spiral CT: musculoskeletal applications. Radiographics 19:1143–1160

Remy-Jardin M, Remy J, Masson P, et al (2000) CT angiography of thoracic outlet syndrome: evaluation of imaging protocols for the detection of arterial stenosis. J Comput Assist Tomogr 24:349–361

Totterman S, Tamez-Pena J, Kwok E, et al (1998) 3D visual presentation of shoulder joint motion. Stud Health Technol Inform 50:27–33

Udupa JK (1999) Three-dimensional visualization and analysis methodologies: a current perspective. Radiographics 19:783–806

Wallny TA, Theuerkauf I, Schild RL, et al (2000) The three-dimensional ultrasound evaluation of the rotator cuff an experimental study. Eur J Ultrasound 11:135–141

Wang GE, Vannier MW (1994) Stair-step artifacts in three-dimensional helical CT: an experimental study. Radiology 191:79–83

Woodard EJ, Leon SP, Moriarty TM, et al (2001) Initial experience with intraoperative magnetic resonance imaging in spine surgery. Spine 26:410–417

Special Topics

24 Analysis of Functional Images

Alan Jackson and Neil A. Thacker

CONTENTS

24.1 Introduction

The advances in MR image acquisition have led to the increasing use of parametric or calculated images, which are designed to display physiological features of tissues rather than simply anatomical structure. Many of these rely on the analysis of changes in signal intensity that occur over time in response to some physiological stimulus. In this chapter we will review the basic concepts of the three commonest types of functional imaging: blood oxygen level dependent (BOLD) imaging, dynamic susceptibility contrast-enhanced imaging of perfusion (DSC-MR) and imaging of endothelial permeability.

24.2 Blood Oxygen Level Dependent Imaging

Blood oxygen level dependent imaging, was first described in 1991 and resulted from the observation

A. Jackson, MD, N.A. Thacker, PhD
Imaging Science and Biomedical Engineering, The Medical School, University of Manchester, Oxford Road, Manchester, M13 9PT, UK

that areas of neuronal activation within the brain show changes in signal intensity on T2-weighted images. From that simple observation has grown one of the most commonly used tools for studying the human brain. The worldwide growth of BOLD imaging has been startling, reflecting the advantages of a technique which allows safe non invasive imaging of brain activation, can be repeated as often as needed and allows simple correlation with high-quality anatomical images. The BOLD technique can be performed on most conventional scanners and allows the production of high-resolution functional maps within a few minutes. These features allow studies of activation patterns in individuals and the design of complex cognitive paradigms using inter- and intra-subject comparisons. The subject has been the topic of many thousands of publications and this chapter will only provide the reader with an overview of the basic technique. For those requiring a more detailed understanding readers are directed to the excellent book on the subject edited by Moonen and Bandettini (2000).

Brain activation is a complex process involving a variety of physiological responses designed to mediate inter-neuronal transmission. Generically, incoming action potentials activate synaptic release of a neurotransmitter that will cross the synaptic cleft causing activation or inhibition of a neurone or of a secondary synapse acting on a neurone. The passage of the action potential and the synaptic activity create a local metabolic demand, which requires increased glucose utilisation and oxygen delivery. Synaptic uptake of glucose increases and it is the local synaptic activity that appears to govern acute changes in local glucose utilisation. However, the metabolic processes associated with activation are more complex and non-oxidative metabolism of glucose takes place in neurones resulting in the production of lactate, which undergoes further oxidative metabolism within glial cells. One of the physiological responses to neuronal activation is an increase in local capillary blood flow, which is produced by an increased flow rate of blood through the capillary network. This increase is larger than would be expected if the change were proportional to the increase in local oxygen demand and has been described as "uncoupled". The reasons for this uncoupling remain unclear; however, it has recently been suggested that the increase in flow is needed to increase the rate of deoxyhaemoglobin washout and thereby increase the local intra-capillary oxygen tension and the oxygen gradient between the blood and tissues. This flow-related maintenance of oxygen extraction would explain the disproportionate increase in blood flow and would indicate a tight, but non-linear, coupling between blood flow and metabolism.

The increase in local blood flow and the consequent decrease in deoxyhaemoglobin concentration is central to the BOLD imaging technique. The oxygenated haemoglobin iron atom is diamagnetic; the bulk magnetic susceptibility effect (BMS) is zero. Deoxyhaemoglobin is paramagnetic so that the BMS is related to the local concentration of deoxyhaemoglobin. The increase in blood flow associated with cerebral activation causes a decrease in local deoxyhaemoglobin concentration and the BMS increases causing a local increase in signal intensity. It is this increase in signal intensity that forms the basis of the BOLD technique. The level of this signal change in modern MR scanners is still quite small and of the same order as the noise in the data (a few per cent). The most common way of extracting this signal has thus been to produce repeated changes in the regional blood flow to produce a temporal integration of signal to boost statistical power. The most common technique requires a relatively restricted "on-off" block paradigm in order to generate data sets during known functional activity/inactivity (Fig. 24.1). This experimental approach uses alternating periods of activation and rest or differing forms of activation to produce local variations in cerebral activation with time, whose time course can be approximated from the task or stimulus schedule. In the block paradigm the on period is designed to last long enough for the maximal local change in blood flow and therefore in signal to occur in order to maximise the differences between the on and off states. The maximum rate that can be achieved is determined by the haemodynamic response function, which typically shows a delay of approximately 6 s from the onset of the activation to the maximal signal change. This mechanism fundamentally limits the temporal resolution of BOLD experiments independently of the level of noise in the scanner.

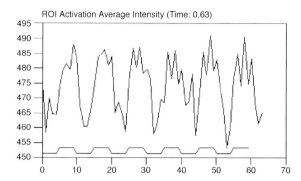

Fig. 24.1. Signal response to a visual paradigm in the primary visual cortex. The subject was stimulated using an alternating checkerboard during the on periods indicated along the bottom of the graph. Note the delay in the signal rise after the onset of the stimulus and the variation in signal intensity due to noise in the imaging process

24.2.1
Analysis of BOLD Data

Unfortunately, BOLD is not the only physical mechanism which can lead to a signal change in functional magnetic resonance imaging (fMR) experiments. There are also blood flow oxygen level dependent (b-FOLD), oxygen CSF oxygen level dependent (COLD), CSF flow oxygen level dependent (c-FOLD) and motion oxygen level dependent (MOLD) signal mechanisms (HAJNAL et al. 1997). Because of these multiple signal mechanisms much care has to be taken during data analysis to ensure that the observed signal is genuinely due to BOLD.

The magnitude of the b-FOLD contribution will depend on the choice of imaging sequence, so that it can be the predominant source of signal change. Some image acquisition sequences dramatically reduce or even eliminate this flow-related component (Fig. 24.2). The b-FOLD signal can be considered as complementary to the BOLD signal as an alternative indicator of functional activation and has the advantage of increasing signal-to-noise ratio within the data. However, the flow response has a less specific spatial location since it will occur in vessels distal to the activation site so that the increase in sensitivity may be gained at the expense of spatial accuracy. The CSF-related signal is not expected to correlate with the stimulus paradigm due to the much shorter time scales. Of the various other ways that signal can be generated in a BOLD activation experiment, c-FOLD and COLD can be removed by anatomical masking of CSF areas.

Therefore, the main problem with ensuring valid signal from a BOLD analysis is in controlling the

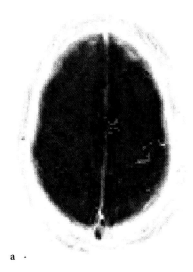 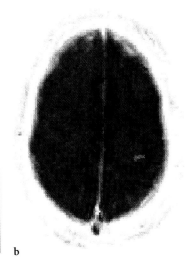

a ·   b

Fig. 24.2a, b. Functional images from a motor paradigm involving movement of the thumb. a Data acquired using single-shot gradient echo EPI which is sensitive to flow effects. b Data acquired using multi-shot 3D segmented EPI with echo shifting which is insensitive to flow effects. Note the difference in apparent area of activation in b due to the loss of signal from draining veins

effects of motion, which can be considerable during the course of an extended experiment and often correlate directly with the paradigm task. The importance of motion correction in fMR has been widely recognised in the literature (HAJNAL et al. 1997; THACKER et al. 1999). Many of the stages of BOLD data analysis are geared towards minimising or eliminating this effect, the aim being to pre process the data in order to obtain the data that would have been acquired had the subject remained perfectly motionless throughout the study. The solution to this problem involves the use of a co-registration procedure, the alignment in three dimensions of two volume data sets by automatic means which was described in Chap. 8. The success of the co-registration step can be visually assessed by production of a simple scattergram of correlation against edge strength in the image. These plots will show increasing correlation values in areas of high edge strength if stimulus-correlated motion is a significant contributor to apparent areas of activation (Figs. 24.3, 24.4). The processing strategy involves four basic steps:

- Co-registration of all the image volumes to the first image to determine the transformation between the volumes.
- Reslicing of all the image volumes which demonstrate movement using an appropriate interpolation function (preferably sinc).
- Analysis of the signal changes with time in each voxel for correlation with the timing of the "on-off" paradigm (some pre processing may be needed prior to this stage to eliminate scanner artefacts such as receive coil heterogeneity).
- Translation of the high correlation results into a standardised coordinate system such as the Talairach system.

These standardised activation maps can then be fused with anatomical information or used for intra- or inter-subject comparisons (Figs. 24.5, 24.6).

There seems to be a standard approach emerging to the problem in clinical environments making use of software available on the Internet, such as the Automatic Image Registration package (AIR) (JIANG 1995; WOODS et al. 1993, 1998a,b), which assumes a rigid body motion. Depending on the details of the data acquisition, a rigid body assumption may be considered a little naive. In some cases slices of image data may undergo different amounts of motion and in other cases the data may suffer from motion blurring. These processes could leave residual motion artefacts in the data which bias subsequent interpretation. Many groups now routinely make use of rigid body co-registration and it has been proven that the effects caused by motion are reduced to an acceptable level in the subsequent fMR analysis (THACKER et al. 1999). Following the co-registration and reslicing stage it is appropriate to perform pixel by pixel analysis on the signal intensity changes which have occurred over the time course of the experiment.

There have been many approaches to the analysis of fMR images proposed in the literature. Considered from a statistical point of view these techniques can be grouped as either non-parametric or parametric. It is generally accepted that whilst non-parametric techniques are initially more robust, parametric techniques will ultimately have better discrimination once the analytical models have been refined. We will therefore concentrate on these approaches here. For parametric approaches, analysis can be basically decomposed into two stages: the application of a voxel by voxel time-dependent analysis, followed by a regional analysis of clusters (FRISTON et al. 1996;

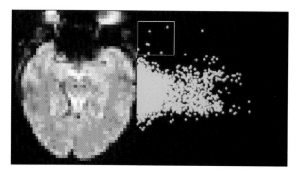

Fig. 24.3. Functional experiment using visual activation. The areas of activation can be seen in regions of low edge strength on the corresponding scattergram

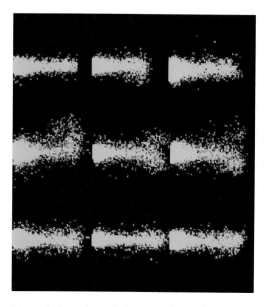

Fig. 24.4. Plots of correlation score (*vertical axis*) against edge strength (*horizontal axis*). The top row represents three slices from a subject at rest with no movement or stimulus. The m*iddle row* is from three slices in a subject performing a simple motor paradigm. Note the spread of high correlation values at high edge strength due to stimulus-correlated motion. The b*ottom row* is the same data after co-registration

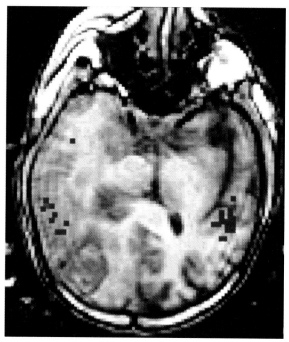

Fig. 24.5. Functional experiment showing the relationship between the primary auditory cortex and right-sided glioma

LANGE 1996). The first of these is designed as a significance test, the hypothesis being that the data seen in the image can be accounted for entirely by random noise fluctuations. The voxel-based null hypothesis test is generally implemented as a correlation measure (see Box 24.1). The details of this vary in the literature, but all successful measures have the same fundamental statistical origin, which is effectively that some measure of correlation C is normalised by its expected variance var(C) in order to produce a measure which can be treated like a t-test or Z-score (LANGE 1996). The subsequent thresholding

of this measure, to detect significant signals, invariably assumes a Gaussian distribution for this test statistic and must generally take into account temporal correlations in the image formation process (VAN GELDEREN et al. 1995). The specific choice of correlation measure varies depending on the authors. Some have suggested using a set of sinusoidal correlation functions and computing the effective "power" of the data (BULLMORE et al. 1996). There seem to be two main justifications for this approach. The first is that although the stimulus in the experiment is invariably a simple "on" or "off" task (i.e. a "box car" function of known period), we do not know the true shape or phase of the signal. Such a Fourier approach to analysis thus gives a method of estimating signal content which is independent of phase or specific details of the shape of the response curve. The second justification is simply that such an approach delivers measures which are completely independent of phase. A simpler analysis than a Fourier decomposition involves correlation with a "box car" function (BAUDENDISTEL et al. 1995), which can be shifted as necessary in order to locate the maximum phase response. Though this second technique does not take variability of shape into account there may be some merit in restricting the freedom of the response function to something resembling the initial stimulus. As we do

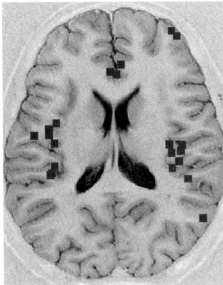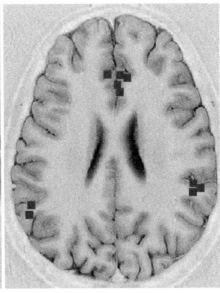

Fig. 24.6. Mapping of cortical areas activated in response to a painful rectal stimulus

not know the true shape of the signal we are looking for, it would be difficult to know which of these two approaches is superior. However, in general the "box car" approach will be more specific as it requires not only a signal, but a signal with a particular shape. One model, which has been justified empirically, is a convolution of the stimulus function with the Poisson distribution. This can be generalised to the gamma variate, which is also a popular choice for perfusion analysis (BENNER et al. 1997). Another simple variant is to construct pooled estimates of signal from off and on periods and then to apply a simple t-test (SADATO et al. 1996). Simple algebra can show that this is statistically equivalent to correlation with a "box car" function. Clearly such an approach does not take correct account of either temporal correlations or the specific shape of the response curve. Finally, some authors have suggested correlation measures which cannot be directly interpreted as a t-test. The measure used both in BANDETTINI et al. (1993) and PRESCIUTTI et al. (1997) in particular is a measure which occurs in the commonly used STIMULATE software. Though this has intuitive properties (it is normalised between –1 and 1) it cannot be reliably thresholded in order to identify true signal as the measure has different statistical scaling for each experimental design. In BRAMMER et al. (1997) the test statistic is defined as a power-quotient which is the power of the sought frequencies divided by a normalisation factor other than the expected variance. This particular form of measure is only monotonically related to the standard form described above.

However, before this measure is used it is renormalised using a Monte Carlo technique to re-impose the standard statistical interpretation. A similar step would also be necessary with the measure in BANDETTINI et al. (1993) and PRESCIUTTI et al. (1997) before it could be used in earnest. In doing so this would be reverting to the previous measures.

24.2.2
Interpretation of Activity Maps

The interpretation of activation maps from fMR experiments must be performed carefully and the user must be aware of the assumptions underlying the analysis. Firstly there is an assumption that the signal change will be sited over the active region. In fact the site of maximum signal change can be affected by local blood volume and blood flow related signal, and these will be greatly affected by the choice of scanning technique. In some data sets this will limit the spatial resolution of the approach to millimetres; however, careful choice of scanning technique and the use of high field systems can allow the detection of fMR changes with considerable accuracy. Secondly, the use of a correlation analysis to identify regions of activation assumes a close relationship between activational change and paradigm. Such an analysis will measure local changes correctly, but if the brain is continually active the correlation with the paradigm may be small. Thus we have to be particularly careful when interpreting BOLD responses: absence of evidence is not evidence of absence. We cannot say that regions which do not correlate with the stimulus were not active and BOLD correlations should not be equated directly to brain activity. Finally, the location of cortical activations must be carefully considered, particularly when conducting inter-patient studies, since cortical areas do not demonstrate a true one-to-one spatial correspondence in simple stereotactic coordinate spaces, and therefore anatomically identical areas of activation in different subjects may occur in different spatial locations within the coordinate system.

24.3
Dynamic Susceptibility Contrast-Enhanced Imaging

There are two commonly used methods for measuring cerebral blood flow using MR. Arterial spin labelling magnetically labels the water in the blood entering the sample to provide an endogenous tracer of flow. Although it is highly attractive this technique is not yet sufficiently robust for routine clinical use (CALAMANTE et al. 1999). Dynamic susceptibility contrast-enhanced MR imaging uses rapid measurements of MR signal change following the injection of a bolus of a paramagnetic MR contrast agent (ROSEN et al. 1991a,b; BOXERMAN et al. 1997; CALAMANTE et al. 1999). The signal loss resulting from passage of the contrast agent bolus on T2-weighted images can be used to calculate estimates of cerebral blood volume (CBV), mean transit time (MTT) and cerebral blood flow (CBF). DSC-MR is simple to perform in a clinical environment and is now the MR perfusion technique most commonly used in clinical studies (SORENSEN and REIMER 2000).

The use of first-pass bolus studies to measure cerebral perfusion is fundamentally attractive. The use of contrast injection produces controllable decreases in signal intensity, whilst basing the analysis purely on first-pass data imposes a short image acquisition which can easily be incorporated into existing clinical imaging protocols. First-pass bolus kinetics are also well documented and highly generic, so that any successful technique can be used with a range of imaging technologies including both MR and CT.

24.3.1
Collecting DSC-MR Data

MR imaging of bolus passage is a relatively straightforward process. The imaging technique must collect a time course series of T2-weighted images of the area of interest with sufficient temporal resolution to allow accurate analysis and without significant slice-to-slice movement. The typical imaging strategy is to collect data using a fast imaging technique such as single- or multi-shot echo planar imaging (EPI) to produce a temporal resolution of approximately 2 s. During this 2 s acquisition window it is usually possible to acquire in the region of 5–15 slices at a resolution of 128×128 dependent on the scanner specifications. The imaging sequence can be a gradient echo sequence which will maximise T2 weighting or alternatively a spin echo approach can be used which will minimise the signal contribution from large vessels. Many authors prefer the latter approach since it produces signal changes which predominantly reflect the passage of contrast through the capillary bed.

The patient should be comfortably positioned with adequate cushioning to reduce movement and light restraining straps should be used in the same way as for normal MR imaging. This level of restraint, combined with the relatively short acquisition times, usually result in data with no significant movement, so that data co-registration is seldom required. A series of at least 5 precontrast images should be collected prior to the passage of the bolus and many centres will collect for up to 1 min to provide a large number of precontrast images to improve the estimation of the signal intensity baseline during analysis.

The contrast agent is administered by intravenous injection and the injection technique must be carefully standardised. A standard contrast dose (0.1 mmol/kg) is adequate in most cases although some centres use double this dose in order to improve the signal-to-noise ratio. The use of an automated pressure injector is recommended and should be programmed to deliver the contrast over approximately 4 s followed by a saline flush of at least 25 ml/s delivered at the same rate. A careful manual injection technique can produce acceptable and reproducible results. The injection should be given through a large cannula, preferably introduced into a large antecubital vein; the cannula should be at least 18G for manual injection to reduce the resistance of the injection system. Manual injection should be given at an even rate over a 4 s period and should be immediately followed by a chaser of the same amount of normal saline given at the same rate to ensure immediate washout of contrast from the arm veins.

24.3.2
Analysis of DSC-MR Data

24.3.2.1
Basic Theory

One of the main aims of DSC-MR is the production of quantified images of blood flow. In theory this is a relatively straightforward process. However, in practice a number of major problems exist which have considerably restricted the clinical use of the technique. These are discussed separately in the next section.

The conventional approach to modelling the perfusion measurement process relies upon three key assumptions:

- that the change in contrast concentration can be derived from the observed signal changes,
- that the regional CBV can be derived by integration of the contrast density profile,
- that the MTT can be derived from measurements of the shape and width of the contrast bolus.

If these assumption are true then it is possible to calculate tissue perfusion from the time-varying MR signal following contrast administration. The DSC-MR technique uses the area under the contrast concentration curve as an estimate of blood volume within the pixel (CBV) and the width of the contrast bolus as an estimate of the mean transit time (MTT). The blood flow can then be calculated using the central volume theorem:

$$CBF = CBV/MTT$$

The initial calculation of local contrast concentration can be performed using the observed signal change by calculation of the T2 rate changes ($\Delta R2$) using the relationship

$$\Delta R2 = -\ln[S(t)/S(0)]/TE$$

where $S(0)$ is the baseline signal intensity, $S(t)$ is the pixel intensity at time t and TE is the echo time. This allows transformation of signal intensity time course data to contrast concentration time course data (Fig. 24.7). The CBV will be proportional to the cumulative integral of the concentration time course curve shown in Fig. 24.7 and is calculated analytically as:

$$rCBV = \int_{t_0}^{t_e} \Delta R2(t)dt$$

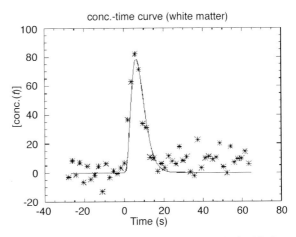

Fig. 24.7. Variation in $\Delta R2$ (contrast concentration) with time in a voxel of grey matter following injection of contrast. The data points are fitted using a gamma variant to produce the theoretical data shown as a *continuous line*

where t_0 is the time of first arrival of contrast and t_e is the time at which $\Delta R2$ returns to baseline values. The MTT is then estimated as the width of the curve at half the maximum height and these values can be used to calculate parametric maps of CBV, MTT and CBF (CBV/MTT).

In addition to these flow-related parameters it is possible to produce maps based on the time the contrast takes to arrive in the voxel using the time of arrival (t_0) or, more commonly the time to peak concentration (TTP). These parameters are unique to bolus tracking techniques (Fig. 24.8).

24.3.2.2
Problems with DSC-MR

Unfortunately this deceptively simple approach to the measurement of CBF is subject to major errors arising from a number of sources. These errors have led to several modifications of the analysis approach in an attempt to produce more accurate quantitative estimates of blood flow. We will discuss four main problems with the technique:

Contrast Recirculation. Analysis of the contrast bolus passage assumes that the bolus passes through the voxel and that the concentration of contrast then returns to zero. In fact the contrast recirculates through the body, and a second recirculation peak is commonly seen following the first. As the contrast circulates the bolus disperses and widens so that the second peak is lower and broader than the second,

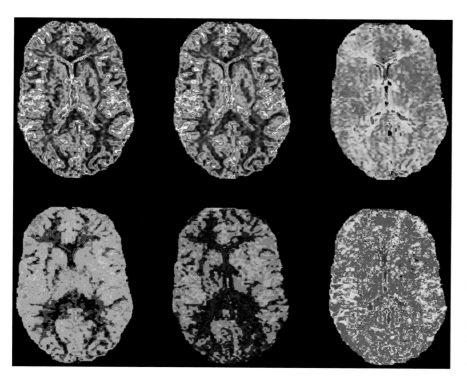

Fig. 24.8. Maps of *r*CBV (*top left*), *r*CBF (*top centre*), MTT (*top right*), *t0* (*bottom left*), TTP (*bottom centre*) and standard fitting error (*bottom right*) in one of the authors

and by the time of the third recirculation the intravascular contrast has mixed evenly throughout the blood volume causing a small constant baseline elevation in contrast concentration (Fig. 24.7). Measurement of CBV is therefore subject to errors due to the presence of both first-pass and recirculating contrast in the vessels during the later part of the bolus passage. In addition the identification of the end of the bolus passage is complicated by the second recirculation of the bolus.

One way in which this can be approached is by using a γ variate curve-fitting technique to produce a mathematical description of the contrast concentration changes from the early part of the bolus passage. The use of curve fitting smoothes the data, effectively reducing noise and eliminating the contamination of the first-pass bolus due to contrast agent recirculation (BELLIVEAU et al. 1989; ROSEN et al. 1990; BENNER et al. 1997; BOXERMAN et al. 1997). The γ variate function is shown in Box 24.2 and Fig. 24.7.

Contrast Leakage and Tissue Enhancement. The analysis of contrast bolus studies assumes that the signal change observed results entirely from contrast within the blood vessels. However, leakage of contrast into the interstitial space will cause signal changes, principally by relaxivity mechanisms (Fig. 24.9). Susceptibility-based imaging methods offer the opportunity to separate these relaxivity- and susceptibility-based

effects and to produce images in which the effect of contrast leakage is eliminated or minimised. In theory, the use of a true intravascular contrast medium, or a contrast with negligible relaxivity effects, such as iron oxide, would allow pure susceptibility measurements. In fact, the restrictions of standard contrast media force us to use methods to separate as far as possible the susceptibility and relaxivity effects. The use of techniques with reduced T1 sensitivity, such as low flip angle gradient echo based sequences, has become a common technique (ARONEN et al. 1994; KUHL et al. 1997a; MAEDA et al. 1997). This technique effectively removes relaxivity effects, although some workers have still observed residual effects in rapidly enhancing tumours (MAEDA et al. 1997). The major problem with this method is the loss of signal-to-noise ratio produced by the reduction in flip angle. However, this can be partially compensated by increased contrast doses (ARONEN et al. 1994). Another approach to reducing T1 sensitivity is to use a dual echo technique in which the T1-weighted first echo is used to correct the predominantly T2-weighted second echo (MIYATI et al. 1997). This method is a simple and effective way to remove relaxivity effects. Unfortunately, the requirement for two echoes places considerable demands on the sampling time and inevitably restricts the number of samples, and therefore slices, which can be obtained. In addition, the use of a cal-

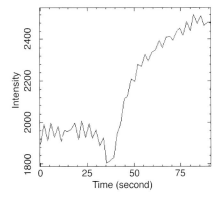
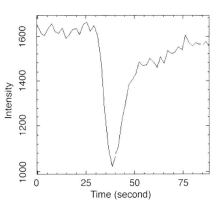

Fig. 24.9. Signal change in an enhancing meningioma without (*left*) and with (*right*) pre-enhancement. Note the rise in signal due to the relaxivity effects in the left graph. Following pre-enhancement the signal fails to return to the base-line due to delayed outflow of contrast from the abnormal tumour vasculature

culated parameter of this type derived from single pixels in noisy data sets produces a mathematical coupling effect on background noise which adversely affects the signal-to-noise ratio.

The use of pre-enhancement techniques is based on the signal changes that occur in response to changing concentrations of contrast medium. The change in signal intensity resulting from T1 shortening is bi-exponential, so that for any given sequence there exists a plateau phase during which signal intensity remains relatively constant (Fig. 24.10). The position and length of this plateau phase will vary with the sequence. The effect of this response curve is that pre-enhancement of tumours will reduce the relaxivity-based signal intensity responses to subsequent contrast doses. The major problem with this approach is that the efficiency of the technique is dependent on the interstitial contrast concentration at the time of the bolus passage. Since tumours show differing contrast diffusion rates (BULLOCK et al. 1991; GOWLAND et al. 1992), this concentration cannot be accurately predicted although it can be measured. Elimination of T1 shine-through requires an interstitial contrast concentration (Gd-DTPA-BMA) greater that 0.4 mmol/l and this figure will differ slightly depending on the relaxivity of the contrast. Another problem with pre-enhancement techniques is the residual contrast effects seen in sequential dynamic susceptibility contrast experiments (LEVIN et al. 1995). The use of sequential injections demonstrates a change in the signal response curve so that it no longer conforms to a γ variate pattern and demonstrates elevation of $\Delta R2$ during the re-circulation phase. The cause of these effects is unclear, although they do not appear to result from relaxivity changes (LEVIN et al. 1995; KUHL et al. 1997b). The effect of these changes is that analysis of the perfusion data using standard γ variate fitting techniques becomes less accurate and may result in

significant levels of fitting error (LEVIN et al. 1995; KUHL et al. 1997b).

Each of these methods has specific advantages and disadvantages. The choice of technique must be made by considering the requirements of the individual study. Dual-echo methods will reliably eliminate relaxivity effects but suffer from poor signal-to-noise ratio and limited sampling volume. Low flip angle methods provide reliable elimination of relaxivity effects as long as TR (repetition time) times are adequate. These methods are fast but also suffer from poor signal-to-noise ratios in normal tissue. Pre-enhancement techniques allow the use of sequences which are sensitive to relaxivity changes and consequently provide good signal-to-noise ratio. However, the effect of pre-enhancement on T1 shine-through will be highly dependent on tumour contrast concentration, which will vary from tumour to tumour. In addition, pre-enhancement causes residual bolus effects, which affect the dynamics of signal change during subsequent bolus passage in normal tissue.

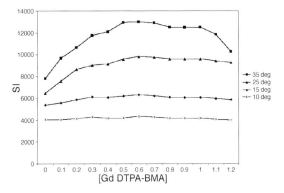

Fig. 24.10. The effect of gradient echo flip angle on enhancement characteristics of contrast medium at different concentrations

Statistical Stability. The production of parametric images derived from mathematical calculations performed on each voxel raises additional problems since the accuracy of the estimates and therefore the potential errors will vary from voxel to voxel. In particular the use of a γ variant curve-fitting technique may obscure variations in the quality of the original data leading to generation of parametric images (derived by fitting to data) in which noise is the dominant, or only, cause of variation (Fig. 24.11). Previous studies have shown that the accuracy of the calculated CBV is decreased if the signal-to-noise ratio in the temporal data is poor, or if the signal drop induced by bolus passage is small (Boxerman et al. 1992, 1997; Robson and Gore 1994).

In clinical practice it is clearly impossible to assess the accuracy with which parametric variables reflect the true underlying changes in concentration of contrast agent since these are, by definition unknown. It

is possible, however, to measure the signal-to-noise ratio and the magnitude of the signal drop and to derive a simple parameter that reflects the quantified uncertainty in the estimated perfusion parameters. If the changes in contrast concentration truly conform to a γ variate function, then the root mean fitting error between the calculated γ variate and the time course data provides an estimate of the uncertainty reflecting the signal-to-noise ratio in the temporal domain. In fact, as we have described above, the accuracy with which the γ variate function will reflect the underlying changes in gadolinium concentration will also be affected by the magnitude of the signal drop induced by bolus passage of contrast agent. Thus a very large signal drop will obviate the effect of high background noise in the images. Given the scale similarity of γ variate curves, it is appropriate to scale the measurement of root mean fitting error with the area under the fitted curve to allow for variations in MSD (mean standard deviation) (Box 24.2). This scaled fitting error (SFE) measurement scales approximately linearly with the errors in the estimation of MTT and CBV and provides an important index of the reliability of individual parametric maps (Li and Zhu 1998). Since the SFE can be used to generate a parametric map of error (Figs. 24.8, 24.12) this can be used to control the inclusion of erroneous measurements of MTT or CBV in regions for analysis.

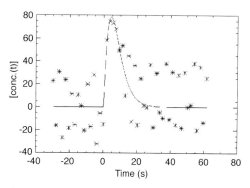

Fig. 24.11. An apparently successful γ variate fit in extremely noisy data from a poorly perfused area of oedematous white matter adjacent to a tumour

Bolus Dispersion and the Measurement of Absolute CBF. The use of the central volume theorem to calculate values for CBF assumes that the technique can produce quantitative measurements of CBV and MTT. In fact the use of the area under the curve

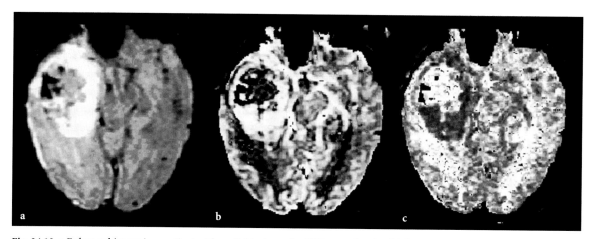

Fig. 24.12. a Enhanced image in a patient with a glioblastoma. **b** *r*CBV map showing high CBV in the enhancing portion of the tumour. **c** SFE map showing low errors in the enhancing areas of the tumour but higher errors in the normal white matter and in the central necrotic area of the tumour

to estimate CBV results in relative measures which allow comparison of CBV between tissues rather than producing an absolute measurement. These relative measures can be calibrated in a number of ways by use of standard tissue values such as grey or white matter or by measurement of CBV in major vessels. Each of these has associated problems and the use of large vessels to provide estimates of 100% CBV is particularly problematic since the relationship between signals in large and small vessels is heavily dependent of the image acquisition technique. Indeed many workers deliberately use spin echo techniques in order to specifically suppress signal contributions from contrast in large vessels.

The measurement of CBF also requires accurate estimation of MTT, which is extracted from the width of the contrast bolus in each voxel (CALAMANTE et al. 1999, 2000; SORENSEN and REIMER 2000). The width of the contrast bolus is actually affected by a combination of three factors. These are (1) the width of the bolus entering the voxel (the arterial input function or AIF), (2) changes in bolus width due to regional alterations in flow and relative blood volume and (3) physical bolus broadening due to dispersive effects which are unrelated to flow.

In practice the width of the bolus is strongly affected by individual variations in injection technique, contrast dose and cardiovascular function so that direct comparison of derived CBF measurements between individuals requires assumptions that these sources of variation have been minimised or removed (WEISSKOFF et al. 1993; REMPP et al. 1994).

One approach to this problem is to deconvolve data from each voxel with an input response function that removes such variability to produce an estimate of the contrast concentration time course in each voxel that approximates the changes that would be seen if the input were a bolus of infinitely short duration. This has been used as the basis of quantitative techniques for the absolute measurement of CBF (REMPP et al. 1994; OSTERGAARD et al. 1996, 1999; CALMANTE et al. 1999). The use of a deconvolution approach assumes that the input function to each voxel can be accurately measured, which is in actuality impossible. These techniques therefore measure a surrogate AIF from one of the major arteries in the basal cisterns, most commonly the middle cerebral artery. The use of a surrogate measure requires an assumption that no additional broadening of the contrast bolus occurs between the AIF measurement point and the voxel (OSTERGAARD et al. 1998; CALAMANTE et al. 1999). In fact it is clear that these effects do occur even in normal subjects (Fig. 24.13)

(OSTERGAARD et al. 1998; THACKER et al. 2000; LYTHGOE et al. 2000). Recent simulation studies have suggested that this error introduces significant underestimation of CBF and overestimation of MTT. Simulation studies suggest that additional broadening of the bolus by over 2.5 s overestimates MTT by 200% and underestimates CBF by 50% and this underestimation increases further as bolus broadening increases (CALAMANTE et al. 2000).

In practice a typical arterial bolus can be expected to broaden by 100–150% during its passage through the head. This means that the typical bolus width in draining veins will be in the region of 8–10 s, assuming an AIF bolus width of 4 s. Using deconvolution with the AIF we would estimate the MTT in such a vein as 4–6 s whereas the measured MTT in small veins is approximately 0.02 s (SEGEBARTH et al. 2000) and in major dural venous sinuses approximately 0.01 s (BEARDS et al. 1998). Estimations of venous perfusion using this approach can therefore be shown to have fractional errors between 20,000% and 60,000% of the true value. These values can be calculated confidently since direct measurement of the deconvolved bolus width and of the actual venous flow rates is straightforward. In addition to inevitable errors in large veins, small cortical veins will also be included as partial volume contributions in cortical pixels and will directly contribute to grey matter estimates of MTT.

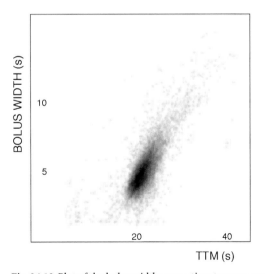

Fig. 24.13. Plot of the bolus width versus time to mean contrast arrival in a normal volunteer shows a striking linear relationship between the width and age of the bolus due to bolus dispersion effects

24.3.3
Clinical Applications of DSC-MR

The use of bolus tracking experiments appears to be very attractive and allows rapid collection of high-quality data concerning blood flow. Some of these data, specifically the contrast arrival time parameters, are unique to this technique and provide useful clinical information in a range of vascular disorders including carotid stenosis, arteritides and stroke (Figs. 24.14, 24.15). The measurement of CBV has clear clinical value in a number of areas, particularly in the study of neoplasm microvascular structure (Fig. 24.16). The quantitative measurement of CBF is far more complex than was originally expected. Attempts to produce quantitative measures must account for individual variations in bolus delivery and bolus width between patients, and the statistical variability in estimates of flow-related parameters between voxels must be addressed. However, even if these steps are taken the effects of bolus dispersion will produce very significant errors in any quantified estimation of blood flow and such measurements must be treated with extreme caution in clinical applications (Figs. 24.17, 24.18).

24.4
Measurement of Endothelial Permeability

In the presence of leaky capillary endothelial membranes intravascular contrast agents will leak into the interstitial space causing enhancement. The speed with which this leakage occurs will be governed by the surface area of leaky endothelium within the voxel, the permeability of the endothelium and the contrast agent concentration gradient across the vessel wall. The patterns of enhancement will therefore vary between different tissues and it has become evident that the permeability is a powerful indicator of the state of neovascular angiogenesis in pathologies such as tumours and inflammatory tissue. This has particular relevance in cancer, where inhibition of angiogenesis presents new therapeutic opportunities by targeting of the newly formed vessels or by inhibition of the angiogenic process itself. Since promotion of endothelial permeability is a prime effect of the cytokines which stimulate angiogenesis, such as vascular endothelial growth factor (VEGF), capillary leakage of contrast agents on MR provides an attractive possible approach for monitoring the effects of these drugs (DVORAK et al. 1995; BRASCH et

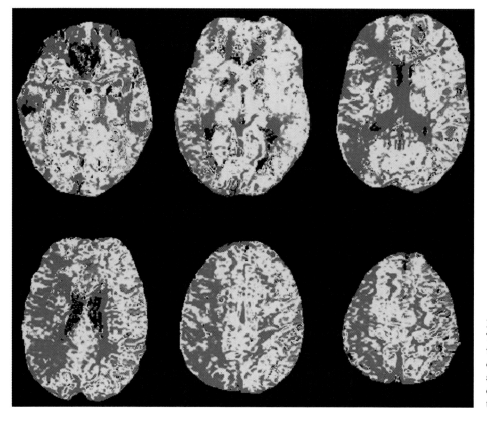

Fig. 24.14. Images of TTP in a patient with right-sided carotid stenosis showing delay of contrast arrival on the right side

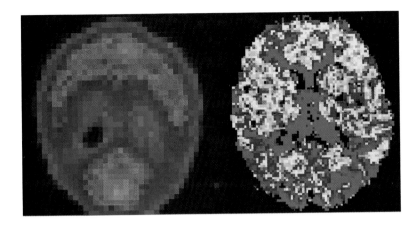

Fig. 24.15. Tc^{99m}-HMPAO map of cerebral perfusion *(left)* and TTP map in a patient with Alzheimer's disease showing reduced blood flow and delayed flow in the parietal areas bilaterally

al. 1997; AMOROSO et al. 1997; DELORME and KNOPP 1998; JENSEN 1998). Quantification of the enhancement effect can be performed using a variety of techniques which range from simple measures of the rate of enhancement to complex algorithmic analyses that apply pharmacokinetic models to the imaging data with the intention of measuring the transfer constant of contrast between the blood stream and the extracellular space (TOFTS 1997). In tissues where flow is adequate to deliver contrast to the tissues the transfer constant, $k_{(trans)}$, represents the product of the endothelial permeability and endothelial surface area.

24.4.1
Simple Analysis Techniques

The simplest approach to the quantification of enhancement is to compare directly the signal intensity curves from regions of interest. There are many measurements which have been suggested to allow

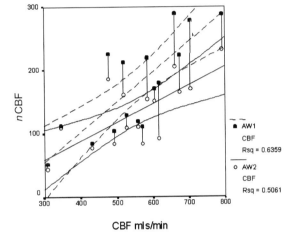

Fig. 24.17. The relationship between normalised blood flow from DSC-MR (*n*CBF) and true CBF measured from carotid and basilar phase contrast angiography. The points show measurements from the anterior watershed area in patients with severe carotid stenosis. The *filled* points are contralateral to the worst stenosis and the *open points* ipsilateral

this type of analysis. The simplest of these is a measurement of the time taken for the tumour tissue to attain 90% of its subsequent maximal enhancement (T90) (STACK et al. 1990). Another measures the maximum rate of change of enhancement (maximal intensity change per time interval ratio, MITR) (FLICKINGER et al. 1993). Each of these is designed to minimise the variation which will occur between patients as a result of variations in contrast dose, injection and scanning techniques and scanner type. A slightly more independent description of curve shape is provided by the approach of BRIX et al. (1991), which calculates a standardised slope of the enhancement curve, commonly referred to as k_{21},

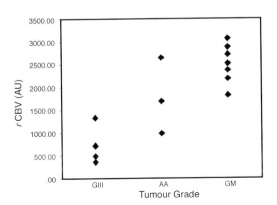

Fig. 24.16. The relationship between *r*CBV and tumour grade in glioma

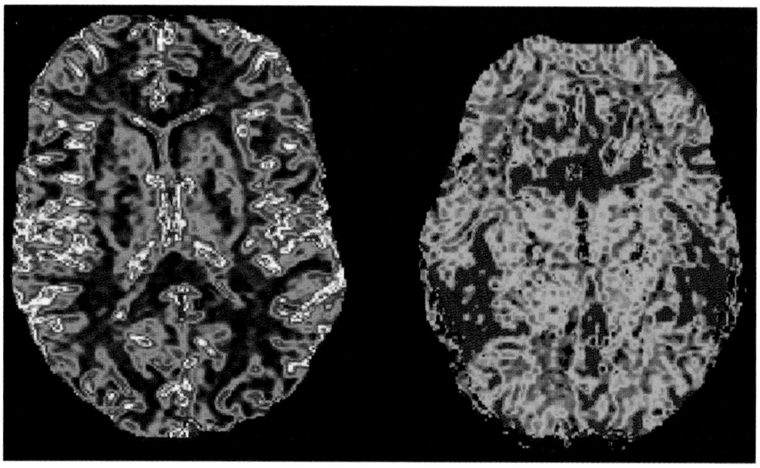

Fig. 24.18. Images of normalised CBF in a normal subject and a patient with Alzheimer's disease, showing decreased overall levels of blood flow in Alzheimer's disease

which should relate directly to endothelial permeability. Unfortunately most of these methods remain sensitive to variations between acquisition systems such as field strength and appear to have relatively poor reproducibility. Despite this, these approaches to analysis have demonstrated clear clinical utility in a number of areas and may provide the majority of information required in clinical use.

24.4.2
Pharmacokinetic Analysis Techniques

The poor reproducibility of techniques which describe the shape of the enhancement curve has led many groups to attempt to develop a quantitative technique which will be independent of scanner type, scanning technique or individual patient variations. This could be achieved if the data were used to calculate the endothelial permeability and the endothelial surface area, which are biological features independent of imaging approach. The product of the endothelial permeability and endothelial surface area represents the transfer coefficient, $k_{(trans)}$, which governs the leakage of contrast from the vascular to the extravascular compartment (Fig. 24.19). The leakage of contrast will have the form:

$$v_l \frac{dC_l}{dt} = k_{trans}(C_p - C_l)$$

where v_l is the proportion of the voxel into which contrast can leak (contrast distribution space), C_l is the concentration of contrast in the space and C_p is the concentration of contrast in the blood. From this simple equation we can calculate $k_{(trans)}$ if we have

accurate estimates of the change in concentration of contrast in the blood stream and in the tissue over time. The calculation of contrast concentration also requires knowledge of the initial T1 value of the tissues before contrast arrival ($R1_0$), which must therefore be measured before the dynamic imaging is performed.

The measurement of $k_{(trans)}$ therefore has six principal steps:

- Acquire images to allow the calculation of $R1_0$
- Acquire T1-weighted dynamic images of contrast enhancement which include the enhancing tissue and its major vessels
- Correct images for motion using co-registration techniques
- Calculate contrast agent concentration maps
- Identify and measure the AIF
- Calculate $k_{(trans)}$ for each voxel

The measurement of $R1_0$ can be performed in a number of ways but the use of gradient echo images with variable flip angles is quick and accurate. The dynamic series of images must be acquired at a temporal resolution adequate to allow accurate characterisation of the AIF, which will in turn depend on the injection technique. Many workers prefer the use of a bolus injection similar to the technique used for DSC-MR, which imposes a need for high temporal resolution (≤ 5 s) and restricts the coverage and spatial resolution which can be achieved. The dynamic imaging sequence must include pre contrast images and must collect data for a sufficient period to allow accurate estimation of the v_l and of the contribution of renal excretion. In practice this requires data collection over a period of 5–10 min. The data collection technique can use any T1-weighted approach and we

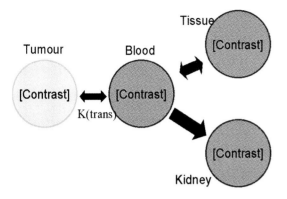

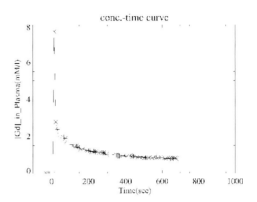

Fig. 24.19. Basis of the pharmacokinetic modelling approach for measurement of $k_{(trans)}$. Contrast injected into the blood pool equilibrates with the tumour and other tissues and is excreted by the kidney

Fig. 24.20. Changes in contrast concentration with time in the aorta following injection of contrast. Note the presence of the first-pass bolus and the second recirculation followed by gradually decreasing contrast due to renal excretion

routinely use a simple 3D gradient echo sequence with a spatial resolution of 128×128×25, TR of 4.3, TE of 1.1 and a flip angle of 35° which gives a temporal resolution of approximately 5 s. Measurement of the AIF is problematic and it is important to ensure that no inflow effects contribute to the signal change, which requires some form of presaturation of inflowing spins. This can be achieved using a presaturation slab (with the inevitable time penalty) or by using the slice select gradients of the imaging sequence to saturate inflowing spins where this is possible (Fig. 24.20). Once the images have been co-registered they can be used to calculate contrast agent concentration maps for use in the final pharmacokinetic model (Box 24.3). The calculation of $k_{(trans)}$ is then straightforwardly performed using the pharmacokinetic model shown in Box 24.4 (Fig. 24.21).

24.4.3
Problems with Measurement of $k_{(trans)}$

The measurement of $k_{(trans)}$ using the approaches described above has two major disadvantages. The first of these is the assumption that the signal change in each voxel of the target tissue can be attributed to contrast leakage. The second is that the measurement takes a considerable period of time, requiring imaging over at least 5 min.

Partial Volume Averaging Effects. The analysis technique we have described assumes that samples taken from voxels in blood vessels will represent blood concentration changes whilst voxels within the target tissue will represent extravascular contrast leakage. In practice this assumption is incorrect and voxels within the target tissue are actually likely to represent a mixture, some of which will have significant intravascular contrast content. This will result in overestimation of $k_{(trans)}$ in these voxels, which can be seen

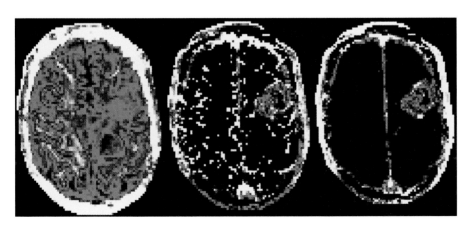

Fig. 24.21. Parametric images of $R1_0$ (*left*), $k_{(trans)}$ (*centre*) and v_l (*right*) in a patient with a glioblastoma

as areas of apparently high permeability in areas of normal brain (Fig. 24.21). The original approach to remove these erroneous measurements was to exclude any voxel which produced values over a certain threshold (1.2 min⁻¹) as being vascular in origin (Tofts 1997). Unfortunately, this approach does not completely remove contributions from intravascular contrast agent and can lead to exclusion of up to 50% of voxels from the image in enhancing tumours or other very vascular enhancing tissues. This problem has been approached by the development of more complex pharmacokinetic models which explicitly model the contribution of intravascular contrast to the signal change (Fig. 24.22). These techniques result in greater reproducibility and do not require the loss of any pixels containing significant intravascular contrast (Fig. 24.23) (Li et al. 2000).

Breath-hold Imaging Approaches. The need to collect data for 5 min or longer is a major problem with permeability imaging. In the head this is easily possible and results in little or no misregistration of data and can be easily corrected by data co-registration.

In other areas of the body, problems with movement are far greater. This is particularly true in areas affected by respiratory motion, where image acquisition during normal respiration leads to significant misregistration whereas respiratory gating techniques markedly limit the image acquisition strategy and the temporal sampling rate which can be achieved. One approach to this is to modify the pharmacokinetic model to examine the first pass of the contrast bolus. In these circumstances it is possible to assume that the concentration of contrast agent in the interstitium is negligible and this provides sufficient freedom in the model to estimate the $k_{(trans)}$ from data obtained during a breath-hold acquisition (Fig. 24.23) (Li et al. 2000). This technique also eliminates the problems with partial volume averaging described above and produces highly reproducible parametric maps of both $k_{(trans)}$ and CBV.

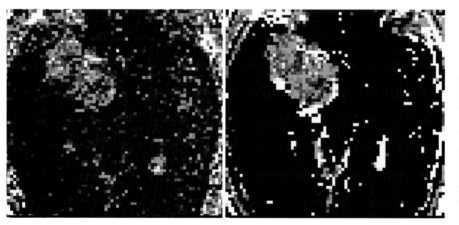

Fig. 24.22. Parametric maps of $k_{(trans)}$ acquired with (*left*) and without (*right*) correction for vascular partial volume averaging. Note the presence of inappropriate areas of high permeability corresponding to vessels in the right-hand image

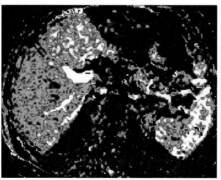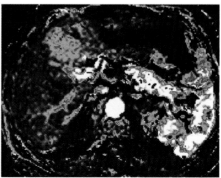

Fig. 24.23. Parametric images using a breath-hold acquisition technique of $k_{(trans)}$ (*left*) and CBV (*right*) in a patient with hepatic metastases from a colonic adenocarcinoma

Box 24.1
Correlation Analysis of fMR Data

The correlation methods used in block paradigm data analysis can be grouped into three alternative approaches:

1. A simple correlation measure with no explicit (fixed) normalisation.

$$C_j^1 = \sum_{t=1}^{T} S_j(t).W(t)$$

where W is a normalised correlation waveform $|W|^2 = 1$ and S_j is a mean subtracted temporal data set at voxel j. This correlation measure can be converted into a simple null hypothesis statistic by dividing by a pooled estimate of the standard deviation on the measure $\sqrt{(var(C))}$ and will behave in the same way as any measure which makes the basic assumption of constant uniform image noise, including Fourier approaches. Such a simple measure is unlikely to be used unmodified in serious fMR analysis but it is included here for completeness.

2. Correlation measure with individual voxel-based normalisation.

$$C_j^2 = \frac{\sum_{t=1}^{T} S_j(t).W(t)}{1/(T-1)\sqrt{\sum_t^T [S_j(t) - W(t).C_j^1]^2}}$$

where the numerator is the estimate of variation about the assumed model. Once again S_j is a mean subtracted temporal data set at voxel j. This technique will behave in the same way as any measure which estimates variance from the data, such as t-tests and Z-scores.

3. Finally a normalised correlation measure as used in programs such as in STIMULATE

$$C_j^3 = \frac{\sum_{t=1}^{T} S_j(t).W_t}{\sqrt{\sum_t^T S_j(t)^2}}$$

with parameters as described above.

Box 24.2
Calculation of Perfusion Parametric Maps and Scaled Fitting Error Maps

The contrast concentration $C(t)$ is proportional to the changes in the effective transverse relaxation rate $\Delta R2^*(t)$ · $R2^*(t)$ is calculated as:

$$C(t) \propto \Delta R2^*(t) = -\ln[S(t)/S_0]/TE$$

where S_0 is mean value of the base line signal intensity, $S(t)$ is the pixel intensity at time t in the T2*-weighted dynamic imaging series and TE is the echo time.

A Γ variate function is used to eliminate second-pass or recirculation effect (BELLIVEAU et al. 1989; ROSEN et al. 1991b):

$$\Delta R2^*(t) = Q(t-t_D)^r \exp[-(t-t_D)/b]$$

where Q, r, b and time offset t_D of the $\Delta R2^*(t)$ curve are fitting constants (ROSEN et al. 1990).

The area under the $\Delta R2^*(t)$ curve, representing relative cerebral blood volume (rCBV), is estimated as:

$$rCBV = q \cdot G(1+r) \cdot k^{(1+r)}$$

where $G(x)$ is the γ function (PRESS et al. 1992). Relative mean transit time, arrival time of contrast agent (t_0) and time to peak tracer concentration are also calculated pixel by pixel based on the fitting constants of $\Delta R2^*(t)$ curves.

Scaled fitting error (SFE) maps are calculated by comparing root mean square differences between the $R2^*(t)$ curves directly observed from the MR experiment and those reconstructed from the fitting constants of the fitted Γ variate. These values are subsequently scaled using the area under the theoretical $\Delta R2^*_{theoretical}(t)$ curve (derived from the curve fitting):

$$SFE = \sqrt{\frac{\sum_{t=P1}^{P2} [\Delta R2^*_{experimental}(t) - \Delta R2^*_{theoretical}(t)]^2}{\sum_{t=P1}^{P2} \Delta R2^*_{theoretical}(t)}} \times 100\%$$

where $P1$ is the arrival time of contrast agent (t_0), $P2$ is the onset time of re-circulation, $t_{recirculation}$, ($t_{recirculation} > TTP$ and $\Delta R2^*_{theoretical}(t_{recirculation}) = 0.5 \cdot \Delta R2^*(TTP)$, TTP denotes the time to peak of Gd-concentration. Hence, $\Delta R2^*(TTP)$ is the maximum T2* rate changes in tissue after bolus injection of contrast agent). $\Delta R2^*_{experimental}(t)$ is converted from MR signal intensities in dynamic scans using and $\Delta R2^*_{theoretical}(t)$ is reconstructed from fit constants Q, t_D, r, and b in the second equation in this box

Box 24.3
Calculation of $R1_0$ and Contrast Concentration Maps

Maps of proton density (M_0) and intrinsic longitudinal relaxation rate ($R1_0 \equiv 1/T1_0$) maps are calculated by fitting the steady state T1-FE signals $S(\alpha)$ with the Ernst formula (assuming TE<<T2*):

$$S(\alpha)=M_0\times\sin\alpha\times(1-E1_0)/(1-\cos\alpha\times E1_0)$$

where α is the flip angle and has three discrete values ($\alpha=2°, 10°, 35°$) and $E1_0=\exp(-TR\times R1_0)$.

Four-dimensional (X, Y, Z, T) longitudinal relaxation rate $R1(t)$ maps are then calculated for each dynamic phase using signal intensity data from pre- and post-contrast T1-weighted FE images [$S(t)-S(0)$]:

$$R1(t)=-(1/TR)\times\ln\{[1-(A+B)]/[1-\cos\alpha\times(A+B)]\}$$

where $\alpha=35°$, TR=4.3–7.0 ms, $A=[S(t)-S(0)]/(M_0\times\sin\alpha)$, $B=(1-E1_0)/(1-\cos\alpha\times E1_0)$.

These are then used to calculate contrast agent concentration maps:

$$C(t)=[R1(t)-R1_0]/\Re 1$$

where $\Re 1$ is the relaxivity of the contrast agent at 37 °C.

Box 24.4
Calculation of Permeability Maps

Maps of $R1_0$, $C(t)$ and the AIF are used to calculate the permeability surface area product per unit volume ($k_{(trans)}$) and contrast leakage space (v_l) on a pixel by pixel basis using the tri-exponential model described by TOFTS and KERMODE (1991):

$$C(t)=D\times\{b_1\times\exp(-m_1 t)+b_2\times\exp(-m_2 t)-(b_1+b_2)\times\exp(-k_{(trans)}\times t/v_l)\}$$

where $b_1=k_{(trans)}\times\alpha_1/(k_{(trans)}/v_l\times m_1)$ and $b_2=k_{(trans)}\times\alpha_2/(k_{(trans)}/v_l\times m_2)$.

References

Amoroso A, Del Porto F, Di Monaco C (1997) Vascular endothelial growth factor: a key mediator of neoangiogenesis. A review. Eur Rev Med Pharmacol Sci 1:17–25
Aronen HJ, Gazit IE, Louis DN (1994) Cerebral blood volume maps of gliomas: comparison with tumor grade and histologic findings. Radiology 191:41–51
Bandettini P, Jesmanowicz A, Wong EC (1993) Processing strategies for time course data sets in functional MRI of the human brain. Magn Reson Imaging 30:161–173
Baudendistel K, Schad LR, Friedlinger M (1995) Post-processing of functional MRI data of motor cortex stimulation measured with a standard 1.5 T imager. Magn Reson Imaging 13:701–707
Beards SC, Yule S, Jackson A (1998) Effect of anatomical variation on the source of jugular bulb blood samples. Anaesthesia 153:627–633
Belliveau JW, McKinstry R, Kennedy DN (1989) Functional imaging by gamma analysis of contrast enhanced NMR. Eighth annual meeting of the Society of Magnetic Resonance in Medicine, p 63
Benner T, Heiland S, Erb G (1997) Accuracy of gamma-variate fits to concentration-time curves from dynamic susceptibility-contrast enhanced MRI: influence of time resolution, maximum signal drop and signal-to-noise. Magn Reson Imaging 15:307–317
Boxerman JL, Weisskoff RM, Aronen H (1992) Signal to noise and tissue blood volume maps from dynamic NMR imaging studies. Eleventh annual meeting of the Society of Magnetic Resonance in Medicine, p 1130
Boxerman JL, Rosen BR, Weisskoff RM (1997) Signal-to-noise analysis of cerebral blood volume maps from dynamic NMR imaging studies. J Magn Reson Imaging 7:528–537
Brammer ML, Bullmore ET, Simmons A (1997) Generic brain activation mapping in functional magnetic resonance imaging: a non-parametric approach. Magn Reson Imaging 15:763–770
Brasch R, Pham C, Shames D (1997) Assessing tumor angiogenesis using macromolecular MR imaging contrast media. J Magn Reson Imaging 7:68–74
Brix G, Semmler W, Port R (1991) Pharmacokinetic parameters in CNS Gd-DTPA enhanced MR imaging. J Comput Assist Tomogr 15:621–628
Bullmore E, Brammer M, Williams SCR (1996) Statistical methods of estimation and inference for functional MR image analysis. Magn Reson Med 35:261–277
Bullock PR, Mansfield P, Gowland P (1991) Dynamic imaging of contrast enhancement in brain tumors. Magn Reson Med 19:293–298
Calamante F, Thomas DL, Pell GS (1999) Measuring cerebral blood flow using magnetic resonance imaging techniques. J Cereb Blood Flow Metab 19:701–735
Calamante F, Gadian DG, Connelly A (2000) Delay and dispersion effects in dynamic susceptibility contrast MRI: simulations using singular value decomposition. Magn Reson Med 44:466–473
Delorme S, Knopp MV (1998) Non-invasive vascular imaging: assessing tumour vascularity. Eur Radiol 8:517–527
Dvorak HF, Brown LF, Detmar M (1995) Vascular permeability factor/vascular endothelial growth factor, microvascular hyperpermeability, and angiogenesis. Am J Pathol 146:1029–1039

Flickinger F, Allison J, Sherry R (1993) Differentiation of benign from malignant breast masses by time-intensity evaluation of contrast enhanced MRI. Magn Reson Imaging 11:617–620

Friston KJ, Holmes A, Poline JB (1996) Detecting activations in PET and fMRI: levels of inference and power. Neuroimage 40:223–235

Gowland P, Mansfield P, Bullock P (1992) Dynamic studies of gadolinium uptake in brain tumors using inversion-recovery echo-planar imaging. Magn Reson Med 26:241–258

Hajnal JV, Young IR, Bydder GM (1997) Contrast mechanisms in functional MRI of the brain. In: Advanced MR imaging techniques in functional MR imaging, p 62–78

Jensen RL (1998) Growth factor-mediated angiogenesis in the malignant progression of glial tumors: a review. Surg Neurol 49:189–195

Jiang A (1995) Motion detection and correction in functional MR imaging. HBM 3:224–235

Kuhl CK, Bieling H, Gieseke J (1997a) Breast neoplasms: T2* susceptibility-contrast, first-pass perfusion MR imaging . Radiology 202:87–95

Kuhl CK, Bieling HB, Gieseke J (1997b) Healthy premenopausal breast parenchyma in dynamic contrast-enhanced MR imaging of the breast: normal contrast medium enhancement and cyclical-phase dependency. Radiology 203:137–144

Lange N (1996) Tutorial in biostatistics. Statistical approaches to human brain mapping by functional magnetic resonance. Imaging Stat Med 15:389–428

Levin JM, Kaufman MJ, Ross MH (1995) Sequential dynamic susceptibility contrast MR experiments in human brain: residual contrast agent effect, steady state, and hemodynamic perturbation. Magn Reson Med 34:655–663

Li K, Zhu X (1998) Scaled error mapping in MR perfusion imaging. Proceedings of the 2nd conference on medical image understanding and analysis, Leeds

Li K, Zhu X, Waterton J (2000) Improved 3D quantitative mapping of blood volume and endothelial permeability in brain tumours. J Magn Reson Imaging 12:347–357

Lythgoe DJ, Ostergaard L, William SC (2000) Quantitative perfusion imaging in carotid artery stenosis using dynamic susceptibility contrast-enhanced magnetic resonance imaging. Magn Reson Imaging 18:1–11

Maeda M, Male JE, Crosby DL (1997) Application of contrast agents in the evaluation of stroke: conventional MR and echo-planar MR imaging. J Magn Reson Med 7:723–728

Miyati T, Banno T, Mase M (1997) Dual dynamic contrast-enhanced MR imaging. J Magn Reson Imaging 7:230–235

Moonen C, Bandettini PA (2000) Functional MRI. Springer, Berlin Heidelberg New York

Ostergaard L, Sorensen AG, Kwong KK (1996) High resolution measurement of cerebral blood flow using intravascular tracer bolus passages. II. Experimental comparison and preliminary results. Magn Reson Med 36:726–736

Ostergaard L, Johannsen P, Host Poulsen P (1998) Cerebral blood flow measurements by magnetic resonance imaging bolus tracking: comparison with [015]H$_2$O positron emission tomography in humans. J Cereb Blood Flow Metab 18:935–940

Ostergaard L, Hochberg FH, Rabinov JD (1999) Early changes measured by magnetic resonance imaging in cerebral blood flow, blood volume, and blood-brain barrier permeability following dexamethasone treatment in patients with brain tumors. J Neurosurg 90:300–305

Presciutti O, Pell:iccioli GP, Tarducci (1997) New processing methods in functional MRI. Riv Neuroradiol 10:261–264

Press W, Teukolsky S, Vetterling W (1992) Numerical recipes in C: the art of scientific computing. Cambridge University Press, New York

Rempp KA, Brix G, Wenz F (1994) Quantification of regional cerebral blood flow and volume with dynamic susceptibility contrast-enhanced MR imaging. Radiology 193:637–641

Robson MD, Z J, Gore JC (1994) Errors associated with fitting dynamic susceptibility contrast images for cerebral perfusion calculations. Thirteenth annual conference of the Society of Magnetic Resonance in Medicine, p 972

Rosen BR, Belliveau JW, Vevea JM (1990) Perfusion imaging with NMR contrast agents. Magn Reson Med 14:249–265

Rosen BR, Belliveau JW, Aronen HJ (1991a) Susceptibility contrast imaging of cerebral blood volume: human experience. Magn Reson Med 22:293–299

Rosen BR, Belliveau JW, Buchbinder BR (1991b) Contrast agents and cerebral hemodynamics. Magn Reson Med 19:285–292

Sadato M, Ibanez V, Deiber M (1996) Frequency dependent changes of regional cerebral blood flow during finger movement. J Cereb Blood Flow Metab 16:23–33

Segebarth C, Delon-Martin C, Belle V (2000) Functional MR angiography using in-flow and phase contrast MR acquisition techniques. In: Moonen C, Bandettini P (eds) Functional MRI. Springer, Berlin Heidelberg New York, pp 83–89

Sorensen A, Reimer P (2000) Cerebral MR perfusion imaging: principles and current applications. Thieme, Stuttgart, p 152

Stack J, Redmond O, Codd M (1990) Breast disease: tissue characterization with Gd-DTPA enhancement profiles. Radiology 174:491–494

Thacker NA, Burton E, Lacey AJ (1999) The effects of motion on parametric fMRI analysis techniques. Physiol Meas 20:251–263

Thacker NA, Zhu X, Jackson A (2000) A new approach for the estimation of MTT in bolus passage perfusion techniques. Proceedings of the eighth annual meeting of the ISMRM, 2000, Denver

Tofts PS (1997) Modeling tracer kinetics in dynamic Gd-DTPA MR imaging. J Magn Reson Imaging 7:91–101

Tofts PS, Kermode AG (1991) Measurement of the blood-brain barrier permeability and leakage space using dynamic MR imaging: fundamental concepts. Magn Reson Med 17:357–367

Van Gelderen P, Ramsey NF, Liu G (1995) Three-dimensional functional magnetic resonance imaging of human brain on a clinical 1.5 T scanner. Proc Natl Acad Sci USA 92:6906–6910

Weisskoff RM, Chesler D, Boxerman JL (1993) Pitfalls in MR measurement of tissue blood flow with intravascular tracers: which mean transit time? Magn Reson Med 29:553–558

Woods RP, Mazziotta JC, Cherry SR (1993) MRI-PET registration with automated algorithm. J Comput Assist Tomogr 17:536–546

Woods RP, Grafton ST, Holmes CJ (1998a) General methods and intrasubject, intramodality validation. J Comput Assist Tomogr 22:139–152

Woods RP, Grafton ST, Watson JD (1998b) Automated image registration. II. Intersubject validation of linear and nonlinear models. J Comput Assist Tomogr 22:153–165

25 Basis and Principles of Virtual Reality in Medical Imaging

Nigel W. John

25.1 Introduction

This chapter provides an introduction to the technology behind medical virtual reality (VRe). The six main VRe technology components required are described: visual displays; tracking; input devices; haptics; audio; and computer hardware. Example uses in medical applications are provided. An overview of the medical areas where VRe is already being applied is then given, including training, diagnosis, planning and computer-augmented surgery.

The terms "virtual reality" and "virtual environments" are primarily used to describe a variety of computer interface technologies that have been designed to leverage our natural human capabilities. VRe technologies let you interact with (and often

be immersed in) real time three-dimensional (3D) graphics in an intuitive and natural manner. The goal is to enhance the user's ability to understand, learn, analyse, create, manipulate and communicate.

The use of VRe to model potentially dangerous and expensive procedures is not a new concept. The airline industry has been using flight simulators to train pilots for many years both in routine flying and critical incident handling. The use of VRe in medical applications is just as appropriate and there is huge potential for its application in this domain. The use of VRe technology here includes:

- allowing trainees to build up experience and confidence at no risk to patients,
- allowing experienced surgeons to plan and rehearse a procedure on virtual models created from patient-specific data,
- augmenting the traditional approach for carrying out a procedure with extra computer-generated information,
- providing innovative tools for patient education

Example applications from these and other medical areas are presented in Sect. 25.3. First, a brief overview of the terminology and equipment that may be found in a virtual environments is provided. The chapter ends with some predictions for the future of medical VRe.

25.2 Terminology

Whether intended for a medical application or not, a virtual environment will typically be built mostly from some combination of the six technology components described in this section. Vince (1998) also provides a comprehensive overview of the potential and techniques of VRe applied to a number of different application areas. Kalawsky (1993) provides a more technical reference guide aimed at the computer scientist.

N.W. John, PhD
Deputy Director, Manchester Visualisation Centre, University of Manchester, Oxford Road, Manchester, M13 9PL, UK

25.2.1
Visual Displays

Visual displays are the devices that present the 3D computer-generated world to the user's eyes. There are five general categories of visual displays, each providing a different degree of immersion, namely: desktop displays, head-mounted displays, arm-mounted displays, single-screen displays and surround-screen displays. Most are capable of producing wide-angle stereoscopic views of the scene, although monoscopic projection may also be used.

Head-mounted displays (HMDs) have been widely used in VRe systems. A HMD consists of a pair of display screens placed directly in front of the user's eyes. The screens are mounted on a helmet that the viewer wears whilst in the virtual world. HMDs have limited use in medical VRe as a typical surgeon does not want to be encumbered with a heavy helmet. An alternative is an arm-mounted display, which looks like a pair of binoculars mounted on an articulated arm. The user looks at the virtual environment through the lenses, having his or her movements constrained by the arm's length and motion range. Arm-mounted displays are appropriate for simulations involving a surgical microscope.

Single-screen projection displays include the Immersive Workbench products. Most of these displays use a tabletop metaphor, in which virtual objects appear to lie on the table's surface. They also make use of stereoscopic projection, typically using shutter glasses (Fig. 25.1). An interesting example of this type of display system is the BARCO Virtual Surgery Table, developed for medical and specialized industrial applications. It combines active with passive stereo to enable two viewers to work on the same data

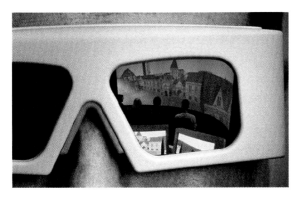

Fig. 25.1. Stereoscopic shutter glasses. The left eye and right eye images are projected in quick succession. This image projection is synchronized with the glasses, which black out the right eye when the left eye image is being displayed, and vice versa

simultaneously and independently, from either side of the table. Autostereoscopic displays (Fig. 25.2) are also becoming more common and are starting to be applied to medical VRe (JOHN et al. 2001b). In general, single-screen systems are good options for applications that require manipulation of objects located directly in front of the viewer.

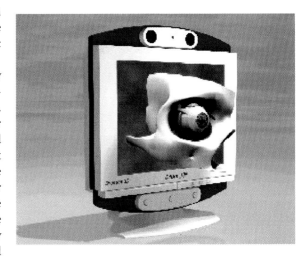

Fig. 25.2. Autostereoscopic display currently being applied to a project addressing planning of otolaryngology surgery. The user sees stereo images without having to wear special glasses. (The image of the D4D digital display is courtesy of Dresden 3D GmbH)

The Immersive Projection Theatre (Fig. 25.3) and CAVE are examples of surround-screen projection systems where stereoscopic images are projected onto a cylindrical or cube configuration of display screens. The viewer explores the virtual world by moving around inside the immersive environment.

25.2.2
Tracking Systems

Tracking is a critical component of any immersive environment. The measurements of the user's head position and orientation are particularly important because they allow the correct perspective of the world to be calculated from the user's point of view. Computing a viewer-centred perspective lets users explore virtual environments in the same way they would explore real environments. Usually, one or both of the user's hands are also tracked to provide interaction, e.g. the position of the surgical tool in the virtual environment is often required.

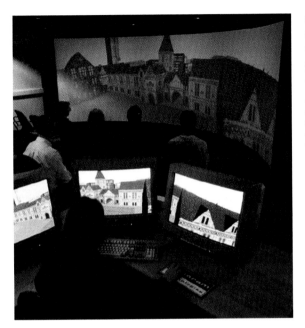

Fig. 25.3. The Immersive Projection Theatre at the Manchester Visualisation Centre

There are six tracking technologies in use today: (1) electromagnetic; (2) mechanical – rigid structures with several joints; (3) acoustic – using ultrasonic sound; (4) optical – a combination of markers such as light-emitting diodes (LEDs), video cameras and image processing techniques; (5) inertial systems – using gyroscopes; and (6) image processing – using video cameras.

25.2.3
General Input Devices

Input devices allow the user to interact with the virtual world, and there are a large variety of options available. Common examples include the data glove, 3D joysticks and wands, and even voice recognition systems. Many custom devices are also in use, and some medical systems use the same instrument that would be used in the real procedure, e.g. a needle and catheter for a vascular access simulator (URSINO et al. 1999).

25.2.4
Haptic Devices

Haptic devices are input and output devices that can measure the position and forces of the user's hand

and other body parts when manipulating a virtual environment, and can apply force feedback to the user to simulate the corresponding sensation of the feel of the objects being manipulated. The application of this technology to a virtual environment can significantly enhance the experience. STONE (2000) provides a valuable overview of how this technology has been employed to good effect in several application areas, including medicine.

25.2.5
Sound (Sonification) Systems

Sound systems in VRe require localization, i.e. the ability to generate 3D dimensional sound. Localized sounds can be attached to objects or can be used to enhance the sense of immersion in the environment. Humans use audio cues to acquire information about their surroundings, in addition to what is being provided by visual channels. Therefore, if used correctly, sonification can greatly enhance the sense of immersion provided by the visual displays. A medical example has been developed by WEGNER and KARRON (1998) who use audio to guide biopsy needle placement.

25.2.6
Graphics and Computing Hardware

The hardware used to deliver a surgical (or other medical) simulation must typically be expected to perform the following tasks in real time:
– Collision detection between anatomical models and/or surgical instruments. This is usually simplified to schemes that detect object/point collisions or object/line segment collisions.
– Physically-based modelling for simulating soft tissue behaviour. Spring and damper models, and finite element models, are the most common approaches. The latter are more comprehensive but also more computer-intensive.
– Haptic rendering of deformable objects.

BASDOGAN (2001) provides a good tutorial on how to go about implementing these tasks. One generally agreed benchmark for medical simulation is the constraint for real time output to be at least 10–15 frames per second (WIET et al. 1996). From a system performance standpoint, real time image generation means that images are generated quickly enough to be displayed at a chosen frame rate, ideally 30–60 frames per second, while the delay between user input and the system response must be less than 100 ms and ideally less than 10 ms. The update of a haptic feedback device is even more demanding, typically at least 100 updates per second being required.

The processing power of graphics and computer hardware is a major factor in the growth of medical VRe. As the processing power of desktop computers continues to grow, then more of the applications described in the next section will become commonplace.

25.3
Medical Applications

The development of medical VRe applications is an extremely active area of research. Commercial solutions are beginning to appear but their take-up is at an early stage (SOFERMAN et al. 1998). Available systems tend to be expensive, and most surgeons are conservative about adopting new technology such as VRe. However, this situation is changing. A detailed survey is beyond the scope of this chapter; interested readers should refer to the conference proceedings from *Medicine Meets Virtual Reality (MMVR)* and *Medical Image Computing and Computer-Assisted Intervention (MICCAI)*. This section lists the different categories of VRe in medicine and provides a sampling of some of the current state-of-the-art applications.

25.3.1
Procedures Training

Currently, training in medical procedures (e.g. surgical training) is based almost entirely on close supervision on the apprenticeship model. A variety of mannequin simulators do exist to supplement training, but these are often expensive, not widely available, and do not always provide realistic simulations. VRe simulators have the potential to revolutionize the training process, allowing the clinician to practice and train on a virtual patient.

DAWSON and KAUFMAN (1998) identified three criteria for surgical simulators: they must be realistic, they must be affordable, and they must be validated. It is only by satisfying all these criteria that a surgical simulator will become an accepted tool in the training curriculum, and provide an objective measure of procedural skill. Creating a medical simulation that

satisfies these criteria is not a trivial challenge, especially when considering the demands of motion and object interaction. Good examples are the simulators developed by Immersion Medical for endoscopy procedures (bronchoscopy, sigmoidoscopy and colonoscopy), and endovascular procedures (angiography and angioplasty). Another successful product is the minimally invasive skills trainer (MIST), originally developed by Virtual Presence (Fig. 25.4). MIST abstracts the surgical task through a software environment in which the user manipulates simple geometric objects (spheres, cubes, etc.) represented on a standard two-dimensional (2D) monitor. The object manipulation is performed by a hardware interface, which emulates endoscopic surgical devices. The repeated tasks are simple in concept but difficult to execute, and have proven successful in increasing student facility (TAFFINDER et al. 1998).

Low-fidelity simulators also have their role to play as training tools. For example, the WebSET project (JOHN et al. 2001a) is delivering training tools for procedures such as ventricular catheterization (PHILLIPS and JOHN 2000) and lumbar puncture using Web-based technologies (Fig. 25.5). This solution is extremely cost-effective, as the clinician needs only to assess a Web browser on a standard personal computer. Work is in progress to provide the validation results for this approach.

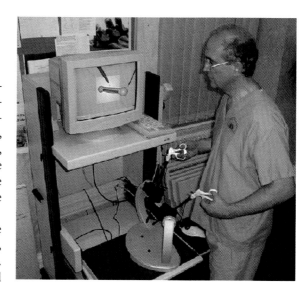

Fig. 25.4. The MIST/VR simulator in use at the Wolfson Centre, Manchester Royal Infirmary. (Image courtesy of MUSE Virtual Presence Limited)

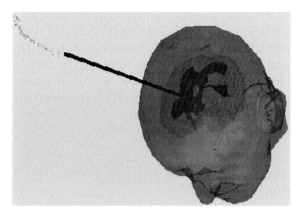

Fig. 25.5. The Ventricular Catheterization Simulator from the WebSET project

25.3.2
Diagnosis

This book contains many examples of how medical data scans can be rendered in three dimensions. The resulting volume visualization can provide the clinician with extra insights for diagnostic and other purposes. For example, Fig. 25.6 shows how today's emerging 3D ultrasound systems can be used to aid in diagnosis.

Virtual endoscopy is another good example. This is a VRe application that is meant to provide an alternative to the unpleasant real endoscopy procedure. Virtual endoscopy can be exploratory or diagnostic without any data manipulation. Patient data are used from CT, MR imaging or ultrasound to reconstruct anatomical models of organs specific to that patient. In surgical endoscopy the model is manipulated and deformed. The virtual endoscopy software will then allow the clinician to "fly-through" the organ and, for example, enable him or her to identify polyps along the colon wall. Chapter 6 gives more details of this technique.

25.3.3
Pre-operative Planning

The ability to interact with 3D data in a virtual environment facilitates the development of sophisticated pre-operative planning tools. A surgeon can view a volume rendered image of data from the patient, and rehearse the operative procedure beforehand. At Manchester, we are working to develop such a system for surgery of the petrous bone (JOHN et al. 2001b). The patient-specific data are segmented to

identify and reconstruct the anatomy surrounding the petrous bone. This data are then fed into a physics-based simulator that allows the surgeon to drill into the petrous bone to perform a virtual mastoidectomy. Haptic feedback devices are used to enhance the simulation by providing the surgeon with tactile feedback.

SHAHIDI et al. (1998) has presented a variety of other examples of pre-operative planning applications.

25.3.4
Computer-Augmented Surgery

The use of computer graphics techniques to assist a surgeon in the operating theatre is an application of computer-augmented reality (AR). The essence of AR is the combination of a view of the real world with computer-generated objects. AR can enable a surgeon to perceive hidden structures derived from pre-operative images without having to look away from the surgical scene. AZUMA (1997) provides a useful survey of AR, and there continues to be much work in this field. There are two main methods employed: the use of an optical combiner and video technology. The optical combiner uses a semi-trans-

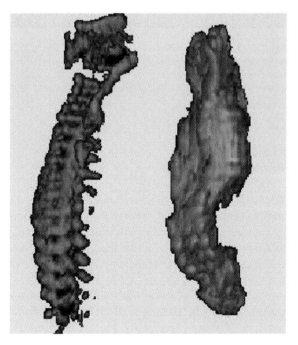

Fig. 25.6. Fetal spines: the *left* spine is normal, the *right* spine is showing symptoms of spina bifida. Images were obtained using the SONOReal system for 3D ultrasound. (Images courtesy of BIOMEDICOM, Israel)

parent mirror on a video display, allowing the real world to be seen through the mirror whilst a computer-generated image is simultaneously reflected on to it. The second approach consists of viewing the outside world via a video camera fixed on a HMD. The video image is combined digitally with the computer graphics image and displayed on the HMD (possibly in stereo). A conventional monitor or surgical microscope can be used instead of a HMD. The work of STATE et al. (1996) with ultrasound-guided needle biopsies, and of KING et al. (2000) in their microscope-assisted guided interventions (MAGI) system (Fig. 25.7) for use with surgical microscopes in neurosurgery procedures, demonstrates the enormous potential of AR applications in medicine.

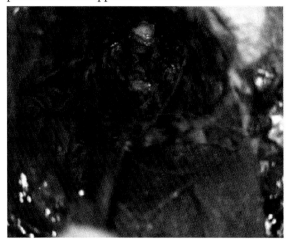

Fig. 25.7. A surgeon's view of the scene through the microscope in the MAGI system, including overlays of hidden blood vessels. (Image courtesy of D. Hawkes, A. King and E. Edwards, Computational Imaging Sciences Group, Guy's Hospital, London, UK)

25.3.5
Telemedicine and VRe

Telemedicine involves the electronic transmission of radiological images and reports from one location to another. It is usual to include collaboration tools to allow the clinician to discuss a patient's case with colleagues remotely. Telemedicine has been in use for well over 10 years and there are several commercial solutions available. The radiological images transmitted will be 2D images (from CT or MR scanners), or in some cases video streams (such as 2D ultrasound data). Few solutions exist today that allow 3D data to be used in telemedicine. Exceptions are the TeleInViVo workstation (KONTAXAKIS et al. 2000) that facilitates the transmission of volumetric models

created from 3D ultrasound data, and the Web-based solution from the NOVICE project (JOHN et al. 2000) that utilizes a multi-user 3D Web environment. The next step is to extend the collaboration into an immersive environment. This is an area of current research and applications will appear in the next 2–3 years.

25.4
Conclusions

There is no doubt as to the huge potential of using VRe technology to provide added value to medical applications. The applications described in this chapter are just a starting point for what is to come. The ever-increasing power of computer graphics hardware is making real-time simulation of medical processes possible on affordable processing platforms. The main challenges ahead will be focused on better interface peripherals, and on improving the application software.

Future developments will require more interdisciplinary research in order to bridge the gap between computer science and everyday clinical practice. This will deliver answers to many of the challenges associated with image segmentation, such as extracting meaningful content from data sets, and the correlation of information to produce efficient interpretations.

References

Azuma RT (1997) A survey of augmented reality. Presence: Teleoperators Virtual Environ 6:355–385

Basdogan C (2001) Simulation of instrument-tissue interactions and system integration. Tutorial notes from Medicine Meets Virtual Reality 2001. http://eis.jpl.nasa.gov/~basdogan

Dawson SL, Kaufman JA (1998) The imperative for medical simulation. Proceedings IEEE 86:479–483

John NW, Riding M, Sadarjoen A (2000) Bringing 3D to teleradiology. Proceedings of the international conference on information visualisation (IV2000), London

John NW, Riding M, Phillips NI (2001a) Web-based surgical educational tools. Proceedings of Medicine Meets Virtual Reality 2001. IOS Press, Amsterdam, pp 212–217

John NW, Thacker N, Pokric M (2001b) An integrated simulator for surgery of the petrous bone. Proceedings of Medicine Meets Virtual Reality 2001. IOS Press, Amsterdam, pp 218–224

Kalawsky RS (1993) The science of virtual reality and virtual environments. Addison-Wesley, Wokingham

King AP, Edwards P, Maurer CR (2000) Stereo augmented reality in the surgical microscope. Presence: Teleoperators Virtual Environ 9:360–368

Kontaxakis G, Walter S, Sakas G (2000) EU-TeleInViVo: 3D ultrasound telemedical portable workstation. Proceedings of the MEDNET 2000 5th world congress on the internet in medicine, Brussels

Phillips N, John NW (2000) Web-based surgical simulation for ventricular catheterisation. Neurosurgery 46:933–937

Shahidi R, Tombropoulos R, Grzeszczuk RP (1998) Clinical applications of three-dimensional rendering of medical data sets. Proceedings IEEE 86:555–568

Soferman Z, Blythe D, John NW (1998) Advanced graphics behind medical virtual reality: evolution of algorithms, hardware, and software interfaces. Proceedings IEEE 86:531–554

State A, Livingston MA, Garrett WF (1996) Technologies for augmented reality systems: realizing ultrasound-guided needle biopsies. Computer graphics proceedings, annual conference series, 1996. ACM SIGGRAPH, pp 439–446

Stone RJ (2000) Haptic feedback: a potted history from tele-presence to virtual reality. Proceedings of the 1st international workshop on haptic human-computer interaction, Glasgow

Taffinder N, Sutton C, Fishwick RJ (1998) Validation of virtual reality to teach and assess psychomotor skills in laparoscopic surgery: results from randomised controlled studies using the MIST VR laparoscopic simulator. Proceedings of Medicine Meets Virtual Reality 1998. IOS Press, Amsterdam, pp 124–130

Ursino M, Tasto JL, Hguyen BH (1999) CathSim: an intravascular catheterization simulator on a PC. Proceedings of Medicine Meets Virtual Reality 1999. IOS Press, Amsterdam, pp 360–366

Vince J (1998) Essential virtual reality fast. Springer, Berlin Heidelberg New York

Wegner K, Karron DB (1998) Audio-guided blind biopsy needle placement. Proceedings of Medicine Meets Virtual Reality 1998. IOS Press, Amsterdam, pp 90–95

Wiet GJ, Strendney D, Yagel R (1996) Cranial base tumor visualization through high performance computing. Proceedings of Medicine Meets Virtual Reality 1996. IOS Press, Amsterdam, pp 43–59

26 Head and Hand Tracking Devices in Virtual Reality

Enrico Gobbetti, Riccardo Scateni, Gianluigi Zanetti

CONTENTS

26.1 Introduction

This short introduction to head and hand tracking devices summarizes the characteristics of some of the technologies most relevant to medical application and presents the configuration chosen in three representative test beds.

The ability to track human movement is an essential requirement for many virtual reality systems. More than 30 years have passed since research activity in this field began (Sutherland 1968). Nowadays, almost any virtual medical application that allows the user to interact actively with the scene needs to know where the user is looking, and, often, which are the hands movements. There are many different tracking scenarios and technologies. The selection among the several different technologies that can be used to implement a tracking device is obtained by weighting factors that range from technical requirements of specific applications to the cost of specific systems.

In this introduction to the subject, we will limit ourselves to the description of some of the techniques and systems that are specifically relevant to medical applications. For a general discussion see Meyer et al. (1992), Azuma (1993), Bar-Shalom and Li (1993), Bhatnagar (1993), Kalawsky (1993), Burdea and Coiffet (1994), Sturman and Zeltzer (1994), Durlach (1995) and Youngblut et al. (1996).

26.2 Tracker Technologies

The evolution and the diffusion of virtual environment applications has spurred the development of many different kinds of tracking systems. Their characteristics are expressed in terms of the following parameters:

- Accuracy: the measure of the error in position and orientation reported by the tracker.
- Resolution: the smallest change in position and orientation that can be detected by the tracker.
- Frequency: the rate at which position and orientation measurements are reported by the tracker to the host computer.
- Latency: the delay between a change in position and/or orientation and the notification of the change to the computer.
- Working volume: the volume within which the tracker can measure position and orientation with its specified accuracy and resolution.

An ideal tracker should have high accuracy, fine resolution and high frequency. Its latency should be as low as possible and it should work over wide areas, possibly scalable at will. It should also not need any specialized environment for operation and the wearable parts of the tracker should be small and lightweight, for user comfort.

The purpose of a tracker is to report to a computer changes in the position of selected reference

E. Gobbetti, PhD, R. Scateni, MD, G. Zanetti
CRS4 – Centre for Research, VI Strada Ovest, ZI Macchiareddu, CP 94, 09010 Uta (CA), Italy

points. Depending on the tracking technology used, these changes may be known either in terms of relative motion or with respect to some external, fixed reference system. For instance, gloves with piezo-resistive flex sensors are able to report on the relative motion of the fingers but not on the global movement of the hand. On the other hand, in medical applications it is usually important to be able to describe the motion of the tracked part, e.g., the surgeon's hand in a surgical simulator system, with respect to a fixed reference frame. From a technological point of view this may be obtained either by having a sensor that is attached to the tracked body and able to report its position by measuring the intensity of a location-dependent field, or by having a detection system that it is able to measure, e.g., distances from some external reference points to some specific targets attached to the tracked body.

It is possible to summarize these considerations in the following classification categories (see MULDER 1994):

- Inside-in systems are defined as those which employ sensor(s) and source(s) that are both on the body (e.g., a glove with piezo-resistive flex sensors), thus allowing for an unlimited working volume. The sensors are generally small and are therefore especially suitable for tracking small body parts, but they are only able to provide relative motion information.
- Inside-out systems employ sensor(s) on the body that sense artificial external source(s) (e.g., a coil moving in an externally generated electromagnetic field), or natural external source(s) (e.g., a mechanical head tracker using a wall or ceiling as a reference or an accelerometer moving in the Earth's gravitational field). Although these systems provide position information with respect to a fixed reference frame, their working volume and accuracy are generally limited due to use of the external source.
- Outside-in systems employ an external sensor that senses artificial source(s) or marker(s) on the body, e.g., an electro-optical system that tracks reflective markers or a natural source on the body (e.g., a video camera based system that tracks the pupil and cornea). These systems generally suffer from occlusion, and a limited workspace.

The most common tracking technologies are: electromagnetic trackers, acoustic trackers, optical trackers, mechanical trackers, and inertial trackers. For a selected number of systems we included references to the Web documents containing further specifications.

26.2.1
Electromagnetic Trackers

Electromagnetic trackers use orthogonal electromagnetic (EM) fields to determine the relative location of a receiver with respect to a known transmitter. The receiver is typically attached to the object to be tracked, while the transmitter is at a fixed reference position. Electromagnetic tracker systems (ETS) are widely used in virtual reality because they are relatively inexpensive, and provide a fairly good resolution in a reasonably large workspace. Moreover, ETS do not suffer from optical occlusion. The main drawback of ETS is that the EM fields used could be seriously degraded and distorted by the presence of metallic structures and stray fields from other sources. Modern ETS, e.g., Flock of Birds (ASCENSION 2001), use pulsed magnetic fields to avoid the perturbation introduced by diamagnetic and paramagnetic materials (e.g., aluminum, stainless steel), but they cope with difficulty with ferromagnetic materials due to their high magnetic susceptibility. A single EM tracking system can pack up to 32 receivers (Star*Trak) (POLHEMUS 2001) processing full-body movements with a frequency as high as 120 Hz, allowing them to catch even a human performer's fast-pace dancing.

26.2.2
Acoustic Trackers

Acoustic trackers use ultrasonic waves to determine the position of the target object. They can be classified into two categories: time-of-flight (TOF) trackers and phase-coherent trackers.

TOF trackers compute position and orientation of the target object by measuring the time taken by ultrasonic pulses to travel from a set of transmitters to a set of receivers. A typical system might consist of three transmitters and three receivers. The transmitters are mounted on the target object and the receivers are arranged at known fixed positions in the environment.

Phase-coherent trackers track position and orientation by comparing the phases of emitted acoustic waves with the phase of a reference wave. Transmitters of acoustic waves are mounted on the target object and receivers are set up at fixed positions in the environment. The receivers periodically measure the phase difference between the waves emitted by the transmitters and a reference wave.

Acoustic trackers suffer from occlusion and are disturbed by large air movements in the working volume.

An example of an acoustic tracker is the 6 degrees-of-freedom (DOF) Head Tracking System by FakeSpace Labs Inc. (FAKESPACE 2001). It consists of a transmitter, helmet-mountable receiver and control box. The transmitter contains three speakers which emit ultrasonic signals and the receiver contains three miniature microphones to sense these signals. The tracker works at 50 Hz, in a cone-shaped working volume 150 cm long, 100° wide.

26.2.3
Optical Trackers

A wide variety of technologies is used for optical trackers. Most can be classified as beacon trackers, but there are some types, like the laser ranging trackers, which do not belong to this category.

Beacon trackers use a set of optical beacons which may be either active (emitters of light) or passive (reflectors of light). A set of sensors such as cameras or photodiodes is used to track them (INMOTION SYSTEMS 2001). This arrangement is extremely reliable and accurate and particularly suited for medical applications such as computer-aided surgery (CAS). In CAS the optical beacons, usually light-emitting diodes (LEDs), are mounted on rigid bodies such as surgical tools and/or bone fragments (FlashPoint 5000) (IMAGE GUIDED TECHNOLOGIES 2001). The main drawback of optical tracking systems is that they require a free line of sight between the LED and the cameras, and this could be too great a limitation in an actual surgical setting.

Using low-cost infrared LED arrays as a reference frame, compact optical trackers can be used for coverage of very large areas (hundreds of square meters) while maintaining a good level of accuracy: less than 1 mm in location, less than a prime in orientation (3rdTECH 2001).

26.2.4
Mechanical Trackers

Mechanical trackers measure the position and orientation of a target object that is attached to the end of a movable mechanical arm. The arm is anchored at a fixed point of reference and is made up of several sections that can rotate and move at the joints. The rotations and movements are measured by gears, potentiometers or optical encoders and are used to compute the position and orientation of the target object relative to the fixed point of reference. Due to the

relatively small working volume they are mainly used as very accurate probing systems (FARO 2001; FAKESPACE 2001).

When coupled with motors giving force feedback to the user's movements, they are basic components for virtual simulators (SENSABLE 2001).

26.2.5
Inertial Trackers

Inertial trackers use accelerometers and gyroscopes to compute changes in position and orientation from measurements of acceleration and velocity. These trackers tend to accumulate error over time and need to be updated periodically by some external source. On the other hand they can be very light, small and cheap to be use in emerging markets such as head-mounted displays for video games (INTERSENSE 2001). Apart from this, their main use is to complement EM trackers by providing a mechanism to compensate for EM field distortions.

26.3
Tracking in Medical Applications

Medical applications have very specific tracking requirements: typically, accuracy and resolution have to be high, since very precise movements have to be followed; frequency and latency depend on the type of application (they are low in telesurgery, and higher in surgical simulation); the working volume is generally restricted to tens of centimeters.

Another important challenge is provided by the medical environment: tracking technology for surgical applications has to follow the same sterility standards as the other surgical instruments; also the medical machinery should not interfere with the tracking systems and vice versa. For all these reasons it is impossible to define the most appropriate technologies for a generic medical application; the choice has to be made on a case-by-case basis, after the analysis of specific application requirements.

In the following, we provide a short description of the tracking technology used in three recently developed applications.

26.3.1
Ultrasound-Guided Breast Biopsy

The system for ultrasound-guided breast biopsy developed at the Department of Computer Science at the University of North Carolina at Chapel Hill (STATE et al. 1996) merges rendered live ultrasound data and geometric elements with stereo images of the patient acquired through head-mounted video cameras, and presents these merged images to the physician in a head-mounted semi-transparent display: augmented reality (AR). This application is of great interest because the physician is able to see a visualization of the ultrasound data directly under the ultrasound probe, properly registered within the patient and with the biopsy needle. Although it is still experimental, the system has already provided useful clinical results, allowing a physician to successfully insert a needle into an artificial tumor within a training phantom of a human breast.

Accurate tracking is crucial for precise registration of real and synthetic imagery, especially in a medical application where surgical intervention is to be performed under AR guidance. In this system double tracking is required: the physician's head and the hand-held ultrasound probe.

The prerequisites for the head tracking system were that it should be lightweight and a minimal encumbrance for the physician, so a magnetic tracker appeared to be an ideal choice. Since the metallic structures in the laboratory interfered with EM tracking accuracy the developers combined magnetic tracking with vision-based landmark tracking for improved registration.

In addition tracking of the ultrasound probe had to be very precise for correct registration of ultrasound slices. Two registration tasks need to be performed: a slice-to-slice registration leading to a reconstruction of the volume of data, and an alignment of the visualized volume with the patient, seen through the semi-transparent visor. The probe usually has a small working and tracking volume and is already tethered to the ultrasound machine. The solution of choice was, then, to track the probe with a 6 DOF FARO mechanical tracker (FARO 2001), even though it hinders probe motion to a certain extent.

The data reported by the authors about task precision are very demanding: the physician may be required to place a thin needle – for example, 0.7 mm diameter for cyst aspiration, 2.1 mm diameter for biopsy – into a 3 mm cyst. Since no commercially available tracker had the accuracy and precision required for this medical application the system was set up combining a mechanical tracker with a magnetic tracker (Flock of Birds) (ASCENSION 2001) corrected by a lookup table, and vision-based tracking to achieve improved registration of real imagery (patient, ultrasound probe, biopsy needle) and synthetic imagery (ultrasound slices, rendered visual and occlusion cues).

26.3.2
Catheter Insertion

The insertion of a catheter into a vessel (artery or vein) is one of the most common procedures in clinical practice. Precise catheter insertion requires a perfect knowledge of the three-dimensional architecture of vessels and a high level of dexterity during vessel puncture, which is only attainable after considerable practice. If badly performed, catheter insertion can result in undue harm to the patient, and inadequate training in this technique is a leading cause of hospital-acquired infections (ZORCOLO et al. 2000a).

The first part of the operation, needle insertion, is difficult to learn, and requires a combination of visual and tactile skills, to identify the needle insertion point and control needle position and orientation during penetration. It is thus important for a training system to provide co-registered visual and haptic responses. The system enhances touch perception with visual perception by using head-tracked stereoscopic viewing and a custom-made display system which provides hand-immersed interaction. The user looks into a mirror through shutter glasses and perceives the virtual image within the workspace of a PHANToM haptic device which controls needle insertion. By co-registering physical and virtual spaces beforehand and using stereoscopic projections that dynamically follow head movements, the virtual patient is made to appear at a fixed physical position on a virtual surgical table. This produces, without resorting to a head-mounted display, a combined haptic and stereoscopic view of a virtual volume in which users can manipulate the needle with their hands without obscuring the display.

As visual feedback and force feedback have different frequency requirements dictated by the human perceptual system, computation and tracking threads work in parallel and different tracking technologies are integrated in the same application.

Force feedback computation has to work at 1 kHz, 6 DOF hand position tracking requires about 100 Hz, while stereo visual feedback guided by head tracking has to be provided at 10–20 frames per second (ZOR-

COLO et al. 2000b). To achieve these goals the system combines a PHANToM haptic device (SENSABLE 2001) for hand position sensing (6 DOF: X, Y, Z, yaw, pitch, roll) and force feedback (3 DOF: X, Y, Z) with an ultrasound Logitech tracker mounted on SGI CrystalEyes (CRYSTALEYES 2001) stereo goggles for hand tracking and stereo image presentation.

26.3.3
Mastoidectomy Simulation

The most superficial and common surgery of the petrous bone is mastoidectomy, which consists of the removal of the air cavities just under the skin behind the ear.

A virtual reality system for simulating surgical procedures on the petrous bone is a human-computer interface tool that puts the user in the loop of a real time simulation mimicking a realistic synthetic operating environment. The surgical simulator receives external input driving the positioning of surgical instruments.

Such a system is being designed and developed in the framework of the EU IST-1999–12175 IERAPSI project (JOHN et al. 2001). The project began with a detailed user task analysis of surgeons carrying out the procedures being targeted. Subjective analysis of video records, together with in situ observations, highlighted a correlation between drilling behaviors and type and depth of bone (STONE 2000).

The system needs to track both the dominant hand (controlling the burr) and non-dominant hand (controlling the sucker). The work volume for both hands is in the order of 5 cm. The range of motion for the dominant hand varies from 2–4 cm sweeps to static drilling while maintaining minimal surface pressure. The accuracy of the tracking must accommodate both rapid lateral strokes and polishing motion quality. The parameters for the non-dominant hand are less demanding. High-quality force feedback is required for the dominant hand (sensing the tissue variations) while only collision detection is required for the non-dominant one.

The task analysis identified that the only commercially available system capable of replicating the qualities required for the dominant hand is Sensable Technologies' PHANToM with stylus encoder. For the non-dominant hand cheaper force feedback systems are available (e.g., Haptech/Immersion Corporation PenCAT Pro) (IMMERSION 2001).

Careful consideration must be given to the head tracking and display-control technology used in the

training system for temporal bone surgery. The surgeon sees the patient through a surgical microscope. The size of his movements are not great: typically, the minimum requirements are as follows:

Translation left and right (relative to center of surgeon's face):	±10 cm (approx.)
Translation up and down:	±5–10 cm
Translation in and out:	±5 cm
Rotation of eyepiece unit (in pitch – away from and back to surgeon's face):	±30°–45°

Magnetic tracking devices are not well suited to the application because of the interference of force feedback motors. Mechanical tracking systems would perfectly match these requirements. However, since the training application does not have stringent accuracy requirements ultrasound devices, which are much cheaper, or hybrid devices could be successfully integrated.

26.4
Conclusions

In this short introduction to head and hand tracking devices, we have summarized the characteristics of some of the technologies most relevant to medical application and presented the configuration chosen in three representative test beds.

Acknowledgement. This work was partially supported by the Sardinian regional authorities.

References

Ascension (2001) http://www.ascension-tech.com
Azuma RT (1993) Tracking requirements for augmented reality. Communications of the ACM 36:50–51
Bar-Shalom Y, Li XR (1993) Estimation and tracking: principles, techniques, and software. Artec House, Boston
Bhatnagar DK (1993) Position trackers for head mounted display systems: a survey. Technical report TR93–010. University of North Carolina at Chapel Hill, Chapel Hill
Burdea G, Coiffet P (1994) Virtual reality technology, 1st edn. Wiley, New York
CrystalEyes (2001) http://www.stereographics.com
Durlach N (1995) Position tracking and mapping. In: Durlach N, Mavor AS (eds) Virtual reality: scientific and technological challenges. National Academy Press, Washington, DC, pp 188–204

FakeSpace (2001) http://www.fakespacelabs.com

FARO (2001) Faro arm. http://www.faro.com/products

Image Guided Technologies (2001) http://www.imageguided.com

Immersion (2001) http://www.immersion.com

InMotion Systems (2001) CODA mpx30. http://www.inmotionsystems.com

Intersense (2001) http://www.isense.com

John NW, Thacker N, Pokric M (2001) An integrated simulator for surgery of the petrous bone. In: Westwood JD (ed) Medicine meets virtual reality 2001. IOS, Amsterdam

Kalawsky RS (1993) The science of virtual reality and virtual environments. Addison-Wesley, Wokingham

Meyer K, Applewhite H, Biocca F (1992) A survey of position trackers. Presence 1:173–200

Mulder A (1994) Human movement tracking technology. Technical report TR 94–1. School of Kinesiology, Simon Fraser University

Polhemus (2001) http://www.polhemus.com/home.html

Sensable (2001) http://www.sensable.com/haptics/products.html

State A, Livingston MA, Garrett WF (1996) Technologies for augmented reality systems: realizing ultrasound-guided needle biopsies. Proceedings of the SIGGRAPH 96, New Orleans, LA, 4–9 Aug 1996, pp 439–446

Stone RJ (2000) A human-centred definition of surgical procedures. IERAPSI (IST-1999–12175), Work package 2, deliverable D2 (part 1)

Sturman DJ, Zeltzer D (1994) A survey of glove-based input. IEEE Comput Graph Appl 14:30–39

Sutherland IE (1968). A head-mounted three dimensional display. Proceedings of the 1968 Fall Joint Computer Conference, AFIPS conference proceedings. Thompson Books, Washington, DC, 33:757–764

3rdTech (2001) http://www.3rdtech.com

Youngblut C, Johnson RE, Nash SH (1996) Tracking interfaces. Review of virtual environment interface technology. IDA Paper. Institute for Defense Analyses, Alexandria, Va 3186:47–77

Zorcolo A, Gobbetti E, Zanetti G (2000a) Catheter insertion simulation with co-registered direct volume rendering and haptic feedback. In: Westwood JD, Hoffman HM, Mogel GT, Robb RA, Stredney D (eds) Medicine meets virtual reality 2000 – envisioning healing: interactive technology and the patient-practitioner dialogue. IOS, Amsterdam, pp 96–98

Zorcolo A, Gobbetti E, Zanetti G (2000b) A volumetric virtual environment for catheter insertion simulation. In: van Liere R, Mulder J (eds) EGVE2000. Lecture notes in computer science. Springer, Berlin Heidelberg New York

27 Computer-Aided Surgery in Otolaryngology

Stefano Sellari Franceschini, Stefano Berrettini, Reto J. Bale

CONTENTS

landmarks are altered or absent (as in neoplasms and revision operations), in the presence of bleeding or rare anatomical variations such as sphenoethmoidal cells (Onodi cells) or infraorbital ethmoid cells (Haller cells), as well as in orbital decompression, optic nerve surgery, the draining of abscesses (orbital and epidural) and resection of tumours of the skull base (Anon et al. 1997; Fried et al. 1997; Anon 1998). Particular assistance in these conditions is given by frameless stereotactic systems, which enable visualization of the actual spatial location of the surgical instrument on preoperatively acquired images.

27.1
Introduction

Endoscopic surgery of the paranasal sinuses is increasingly employed for the treatment of nose and sinus pathologies. However, despite the wide availability of excellent optical systems and high-resolution computed tomography, serious complications related to this surgical technique have been reported. May et al. (1994) reported an incidence of 0.85% for major complications and 6.9% for less serious ones. The major negative consequences include orbital damage (disturbances of vision and eyeball motility or position) and intracranial complications (haemorrhage, meningitis, anosmia, carotid or optical nerve lesions), while the reported minor complications are epistaxis and ecchymosis and/or periorbital emphysema. To reduce these risks, the techniques of image-guided neurosurgery are also being applied in the field of otorhinolaryngology. This type of surgery is particularly useful in cases where the anatomical

27.2
Methodology

Computer-aided surgery makes use of preoperative computed tomography or magnetic resonance imaging. All navigation systems are composed of a three-dimensional (3D) digitizer (coordinate detection or tracking system) interfaced with a computer workstation that shows the actual position of the probe with respect to cross-sectional images of the preoperative data set. However, they differ in the way the stylus is tracked in 3D space and in the way they achieve patient-to-image registration, both of which have effects on accuracy. The three main types of tracking systems are based on electromechanical, optical and electromagnetic principles. Basically, the software capabilities and the registration algorithms of the commercially available navigation systems are comparable to each other.

S. Sellari Franceschini, MD, S. Berrettini, MD
Otolaryngologic Unit, Department of Neuroscience, University of Pisa, Via Savi 10, 56126 Pisa, Italy
R. J. Bale, MD
Department of Radiology I, University Hospital, University of Innsbruck, Anichstrasse 35, 6020 Innsbruck, Austria

27.3
Electromechanical System (Viewing Wand)

The Viewing Wand (Leggett et al. 1991; Freysinger et al. 1998) is a 6 degrees-of-freedom articulated mechanical arm (FARO Technologies Inc., Lake Mary, Fl.) connected to a computer with a high-resolution monitor. The arm is equipped with a detachable, sterilizable point probe at its extremity. Technically, this type of arm is called an electrogoniometer, that is, an electrical detector that measures the angle between incoming radio signals. Each of the arm's six joints carries a high-resolution transducer that electrically measures rotations of the articulation with a precision of 0.05°. The tracking precision of the electrogoniometer is 0.25 mm.

Because the mechanical arm's spatial system is entirely self-referential, rigid fixation of both the patient's head and the arm is an important prerequisite for successful implementation of the arm. In addition, due to its bulkiness the following optical and magnetic systems have replaced the Viewing Wand.

27.4
Active Optical Systems (Medivision, Philips, Medtronic, Zeiss, Radionics)

The equipment for active optical systems includes a probe with infrared light-emitting diodes, two or three (depending on the navigation system) infrared position sensor cameras that are mounted on a trolley-stand (Fig. 27.1) and a dynamic reference frame (DRF).

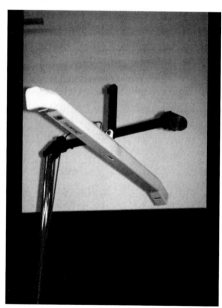

Fig. 27.1. Active optical system: the equipment includes a probe equipped with infrared light-emitting diodes, two or three infrared position sensor cameras that are mounted on a trolley-stand and a dynamic reference frame

Instruments and anatomical structures are assumed to be rigid bodies. DRFs, originally developed for spinal surgery, are used to track the actual position of the patient in space by providing a spatial coordinate system relative to the patient's anatomy. The DRF must be rigidly attached to the patient. Once registration of the patient has been carried out, the patient (with the tracker) and the camera can be moved with respect to each other without losing spatial information. In spinal surgery the DRF is clamped to a spinal process. In frameless stereotactic neurosurgery the tracker is usually attached to the head fixation device. The DRF may be attached directly to the patient's head, so that even if the patient's head moves, the system compensates for such movement, thus avoiding the need for re-calibration. Attachment has been achieved by means of a Neoprene band placed around the patient's head on which six infrared diodes are fastened by means of a plastic support (Tebo et al. 1996). However, the displacement of the DRF due to skin movement may lead to serious inaccuracies.

To avoid displacement of the DRF with respect to the patient Ryan intraoperatively mounted the DRF on the patient's skull by means of a bone screw, while Hauser et al. (1997) and Bale et al. (1997) used a non invasive dental cast. Caversaccio uses his device only for attachment of the tracker; registration is performed using the skin surface. Bale's and Hauser's devices act as accurate registration tools as well (Bale et al. 1997; Hauser et al. 1997).

27.5
Passive Optical Systems (Medtronic, Brainlab)

In contrast to active optical systems the instruments of passive systems are equipped with reflective markers. Light signals emitted by two cameras are reflected by the markers and detected by the same cameras. The computer calculates the actual spatial position of the markers (instruments) on the basis of the angles of the incoming reflected light. The precision of passive instruments is comparable to that of mechanical and active optical systems. DRFs are also equipped with passive markers. In contrast to active infrared systems the instruments are wire-less, which improves the surgeon's flexibility. The camera used by the Medtronic system can simultaneously detect active and passive instruments.

27.6
Electromagnetic System (Instatrack)

One major drawback of navigation systems based on optical technology is the requirement of a "line of sight" between the tracker, the pointer and the camera, which is not necessary with electromagnetic navigation systems.

FRIED et al. (1996, 1997) have reported their experience with the electromagnetic image-guided surgical device called Instatrak (Visualization Technology, Boston, Mass.). The system is based on two electromagnetic sensors, to provide positional information during surgery. One sensor is incorporated into the instrument and the second is located on a headset that the patient wears during both the preoperative CT scan and the surgical procedure. The headset, which fits in the ear canals and on the bridge of the nose, serves two functions: it provides automated registration and compensates for head movements during surgery. One major drawback of the system is that large metallic objects (such as are found in operating rooms) influence the accuracy of the system.

27.7 Procedure

27.7.1
Preoperative Step

Usually 1 mm or 3 mm axial contiguous CT slices of the patient's head are obtained. Most authors use so-called fiducial markers applied to the patient's skin during CT or MR imaging; these must remain in place until surgery. CT images are transferred to the navigation system via optical disc, magnetic tape or network. The CT data set is then reconstructed to generate a 3D data set.

27.7.2
Intraoperative Step

After intubation the DRF is rigidly attached to the patient by means of an immobilization device. If the Viewing Wand is used the patient has to be rigidly immobilized with respect to the operating table. If a DRF is used it has to be rigidly attached to the patient's head. Various instruments including forceps, suction tube and endoscopes are calibrated. The critical step is the so-called registration process, during which the spatial configuration of the patient's head, positioned on the operating table, is correlated with the CT or MR images of the patient's head itself. This procedure is performed by indicating the reference points (skin fiducials) on the patient using the probe of the navigation system and co-registering the respective points on the data set. Patient preparation and the complete registration process generally takes about 10 min. The mean accuracy of this fiducial registration based system is 1.88 mm, with a minimum error of 1.00 mm and a maximum of 4.00 mm. Once the registration process has been completed, the tip of the probe is displayed in real time on the computer monitor. Once registered, the tracking system guides the surgical manoeuvres intraoperatively. The position of the instrument's tip appears on the screen within various reconstructed images of the surgical area, thereby enabling the surgeon to follow the exact position of the instrument even in endoscopically inaccessible regions.

27.8
Alternative Registration Methods

The simplest registration method is the use of anatomical landmarks. Clearly defined external (nasion, spina nasalis, tragi, medial canthi) and/or internal landmarks are touched with the probe and correlated with their locations in the imaged CT or MR data set. The advantage of using landmarks is that the retrospective data set can be used, thus necessitating an additional scan. Identification of the landmarks in both the patient and the imaged data set is difficult and to a certain extent subjective. Generally, these methods are inaccurate and they require time and an experienced operator. Surface matching, which is done by touching about 40 points of the patient's skin or bone, can be used to refine anatomical registration. In conclusion, all registration methods which are based on the skin surface are sensitive to skin shift, which may lead to inaccuracies.

The most accurate registration can be achieved with markers implanted into the skull. They cause major patient discomfort and should not be left in place for an extended period.

Reproducible external reference frames (BALE et al. 1997; HAUSER et al. 1997; FRIED et al.1997) in combination with DRFs provide the opportunity for registration of the patient in his or her absence the day before surgery. In addition they allow DRFs to be attached non-invasively to the patient for tracking the patient's movement during surgery. The patient has to wear the frame during the CT scan, the data from which are processed by computer software in order to obtain and display the three two-dimensional scans (axial, coronal and sagittal), as well as a 3D reconstruction of the surgical field. These data are then transferred to a computer workstation in the operating room that can be connected, depending on the type of methodology to be used, to an electromechanical arm, infrared optical instrument or electromagnetic instrument. The three main types of instrumentation used in image-guided surgery, therefore, are electromechanical, optical and electromagnetic systems. The critical step for each is the so-called registration process, a type of calibration during which the spatial configuration of the patient's head, positioned on the operating table, is correlated with the CT/MR images of the patient's head itself. In practice, some reference points on the patient's head are chosen, touched with the tip of a probe, and the position is localized on the images in order to record their coordinates. As we shall see, such markers may be either anatomical, that is, some particular landmarks of the cranium facial skeleton, or fiducial, that is, points on which small radiopaque adhesive markers are applied prior to CT or MR imaging; they can therefore be easily located both on the images and on the patient's head. Once this registration process has been completed, the tip of the probe is displayed in real-time on the computer monitor.

Image-guided surgery, therefore, makes use of a computerized system and a coordinate-detection or tracking system. The computer system builds a model of the anatomy of the skull using the CT or MR images acquired preoperatively. The tracking system then guides the surgical manoeuvres intraoperatively. The position of the instrument's tip appears on the video within the reconstructed images of the skull, thereby enabling the surgeon to follow the exact position of the instrument even in endoscopically inaccessible regions (Fig. 27.2).

HAUSER et al. (1997) have developed a dedicated frame with fiducials which is anchored to the external auditory canals, the nose and the upper dental arch. During surgery, the same frame is once again placed on the patient's head and then fitted with a further support bearing infrared light-emitting diodes, which yield the relative coordinates between the position sensor and the patient's head.

The headset of the Instatrak system, which fits in the ear canals and on the bridge of the nose, provides external reference points also, and compensates for head movements during surgery. In addition the system automatically detects the markers in the headset. FRIED et al. (1997) compared the precision attained through the automatic registration method with that of the traditional techniques of cutaneous fiducial markers: the results show that there are no statistically significant differences. A mean accuracy of automatic registration of 2.28 mm, a 95th percentile of 2.5 mm and a maximum value of 5.08 mm were reported (FRIED et al. 1996, 1997). However, should the headset inadvertently shift in relation to the patient's skull, the surgeon does not get any feedback from the system, so an accuracy check is required before each application of the guidance tool.

The Vogele-Bale-Hohner mouthpiece (GUNKEL et al. 1999) has successfully been used for immobilization and registration of the patient during more than 100 computer-assisted video endoscopic ENT (ear nose and throat) surgeries. In contrast to the other external reference frames, repositioning can be controlled by the amount of under-pressure on the vacuum scale. Should the required under-pressure not be attained, the mouthpiece is not precisely repositioned. A recently published study confirms the submillimetric repositioning accuracy of the Vogele-Bale-Hohner mouthpiece with respect to the patient's head, thus providing the most accurate non invasive external reference points (MARTIN et al. 1998). The mean localization accuracy of an optical navigation

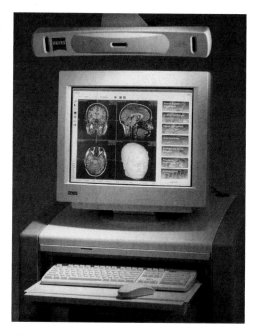

Fig. 27.2. The position of the instrument's tip within various reconstructed images of the surgical area appears on the screen, enabling the surgeon to follow the exact position of the instrument even in endoscopically inaccessible regions

system using the Vogele-Bale-Hohner mouthpiece for registration with 3 mm axial CT slices was 1.47±0.63 mm (standard deviation). One major drawback of the mouthpiece is its dependency on a minimum of two intact teeth.

27.9
Conclusions

The techniques of image-guided surgical systems enable surgical procedures to be performed with greater precision, thereby permitting more radical resections and reducing the risk of complications. This type of surgery is particularly useful in cases in which the landmarks are altered or absent (as in neoplasms and revision operations), in the presence of bleeding or rare anatomical variations such as spheno-ethmoidal cells (Onodi cells) or infraorbital ethmoid cells (Haller cells), as well as in orbital decompression, optic nerve surgery, the draining of abscesses (orbital and epidural) and resection of tumours of the skull base (ANON et al. 1997; FRIED et al. 1997; ANON 1998,). In addition, they represent excellent teaching aids.

By examining the various types of localization systems, it can be seen that each has different drawbacks, especially in terms of difficulty of application. The first navigation system, the Viewing Wand, has been replaced by optical and magnetic systems. All these systems have similar software capabilities and precision. Research must therefore be aimed at eliminating, or at least limiting, the disadvantages inherent in each of these methods.

The reported mechanical accuracy of navigation systems is in the range of 0.3–0.7 mm. However, clinical accuracy does not equal bench accuracy. The reported application accuracies of the different navigation systems are in the range of 1–10 mm. Every surgeon using image-guided surgical systems must be aware of possible sources of error, including slice thickness, movement artefacts during CT/MR imaging, registration method, movement of skin markers, the distribution of the markers and the shift in the

DRF in relation to the volume of interest. One universal problem remains, however: that of the precision with which the radiographic images render the patient's head. Reports from those with the greatest experience in using the various systems seem to indicate that systems with sensors anchored to the patient's head provide the greatest tracking accuracy.

References

Anon JB (1998) Computer-aided endoscopic sinus surgery. Laryngoscope 108:949–961

Anon JB, Klimek L, Mosges R (1997) Computer-assisted endoscopic sinus surgery: an international review. Otolaryngol Clin North Am 30:389–401

Bale RJ, Vogele M, Freysinger W (1997) Minimally invasive head holder to improve the performance of frameless stereotactic surgery. Laryngoscope 107:373–377

Freysinger W, Gunkel AR, Bale RJ (1998) Three-dimensional navigation in otorhinolaryngological surgery with Viewing Wand. Ann Otol Rhinol Laryngol 107: 953–958

Fried MP, Hsu L, Topulos GP (1996) Image-guided surgery in a new magnetic resonance suite: preclinical consideration. Laryngoscope 106: 411–417

Fried MP, Kleefield J, Gopal H (1997) Image-guided endoscopic surgery: result of accuracy and performance in a multicenter clinical study using an electromagnetic tracking system. Laryngoscope 107: 594–601

Gunkel AR, Vogele M, Martin A (1999) Computer-aided surgery in the petrous bone. Laryngoscope 109: 1793–1799

Hauser R, Westermann B, Probst R (1997) Noninvasive tracking of patient's head movements during computer-assisted intranasal microscopic surgery. Laryngoscope 107: 491–499

Leggett WB, Greenberg MM, Gannon WE (1991) The Viewing Wand: a new system for three-dimensional computed tomography-correlated intraoperative localization. Curr Surg 48:674–678

Martin A, Bale RJ, Vogele M (1998) Vogele-Bale-Hohner mouthpiece: registration device for frameless stereotactic surgery. Radiology 208:261–265

May M, Levine HL, Mester SJ (1994) Complications of endoscopy sinus surgery: analysis of 2108 patients. Incidence and prevention. Laryngoscope 104:1080–1083

Tebo SA, Leopold DA, Long DM (1996) An optical 3D digitizer for frameless stereotactic surgery. IEEE Comput Graph Appl 16: 55–64

28 Computer-Aided Brain Surgery: Present and Future

WIESLAW L. NOWINSKI

28.1
Introduction

The traditional practice of surgery, built upon learning, reading, observation, performing under guidance and practicing, has remained relatively unchanged over many years. Rapid advancement in information technology, and thus the way knowledge is gathered, disseminated and absorbed, threatens the stability of this model. Technology affects the way in which surgery is practiced. Advances in computers, medical physics, applied mathematics, diagnostic imaging and biomedical engineering have enabled continual growth in minimally invasive techniques in surgery. Computer-aided surgical systems enable neurosurgeons to treat their patients more rapidly and with greater precision than before, without the traumatic overexposure formerly required. In addition, the advent, growth and development of computer-aided technologies as adjunctive educational, training and certification modalities in surgery will likely affect surgical practice in ways that are difficult to predict.

W.L. NOWINSKI, DSc, PhD
Medical Imaging Laboratory, Kent Ridge Digital Labs, 21 Heng Mui Keng Terrace, Singapore 119613, Singapore

This chapter gives a short overview of the state of the art in technological advancement and features three high-tech brain intervention applications developed in our laboratory for: (1) atlas-assisted stereotactic and functional neurosurgery, (2) simulation of endovascular procedures, and (3) virtual reality-enhanced neurosurgery. In addition, we present our vision of how these applications could contribute to the neurosurgical system of the future.

28.2
Technological Advancement

Technology is the major driving force in surgery. Technology has become available to build displays that approximate actual vision, physical models that are increasingly realistic, and haptic simulators that produce actual physical feedback at increasing speeds that give these developments practical utility in the operating room. We give below a short overview of the state of the art in technological advancement in some selected areas.

28.2.1
Information Technology and the Internet

Information technology is transforming the way we live, work and learn. Advances in microprocessors, memories, storage, software and communication make it possible to build computers that are increasingly affordable and to develop increasingly powerful systems at reasonable cost. The wide acceptance of Internet standards and technologies is instrumental in building global computer networks capable of connecting everything and reaching everyone at any time. Computer-aided surgery with Internet-based video is used to demonstrate surgical procedures to others. Telemedicine applications are commonplace, with the use of videoconferencing and telesensing to interview and examine patients who may be hundreds of kilometers away. Powerful systems provide expert advice based on analysis of a huge amount of medical data. Patients are empowered in making decisions about their own care through new ways of interaction with their physicians and increasing access to biomedical information via digital medical libraries and the Internet. Within the next two decades, computer networks will penetrate our society more than any previous network, including the telephone, radio, television, transportation, and electric power distribution networks. And information technology will continue to lead to dramatic changes in healthcare and surgery.

28.2.2
Visualization

The recent developments in multidetector CT, faster MR acquisition techniques and rotational X-ray angiography result in the routine acquisition of large, high-resolution volumetric data sets of human anatomy, function and disease. Traditionally these data sets have primarily been interpreted as cross-sectional images; however, their effective interpretation requires the use of volume visualization. Furthermore, as therapy evolves to minimally invasive approaches, visualization of these data sets is becoming a critical step in planning and performing therapeutic interventions. The processing capabilities, memory capacity and relatively low cost of present-day computers enable the fast visualization and analysis of large data sets. Numerous techniques have been developed for volume visualization, including multiplanar reconstruction, maximum intensity projection, virtual endoscopy, surface rendering and volume rendering.

28.2.3
Modeling

Modeling focuses on the construction and use of human body models that provide the means to predict, evaluate, simulate, validate and enhance the outcomes of diagnostic and surgical procedures. Modeling techniques include geometric and physical modeling. A fundamental issue that arises when using anatomical models is that these models must be adapted to the individual anatomy of the patient. Information that is inherent in these models is then automatically mapped to the patient-specific data. This process is achieved via registration, which in its

simpler form is rigid and in a more complex form is deformable.

28.2.4
Virtual Reality and Augmented Reality

The term "virtual reality" is usually understood as a human-computer interface simulating a realistic environment while enabling user interaction. Virtual reality offers a solution to the problem of abundant medical information by creating integrated and intuitive interfaces which allow the neurosurgeon to focus on performing the operation on the patient rather than on the instrumentation. Surgeon-computer interaction may be multimodal, including speech, touch, and gesture recognition and synthesis. The user is immersed in a virtual world that models the real world to a varying degree, realized in real time when possible. A typical tool is the head-mounted display (HMD), a visual display system worn on the user's head usually as goggles or a visor. The user either sees only what is being fed into the HMD from outside inputs, such as video cameras or animations generated by the computer, or may see the real world with computer-generated images superimposed on the natural viewing field, so-called augmented reality. The advantage of augmented reality systems is that they allow the user to have real structures and anatomy as visual reference points, while supplementing them with useful clinical information such as presurgical scans and models.

28.2.5
Surgical Simulation

Simulation is well established in the training of civilian and military pilots and astronauts. The similarities between the activities of a pilot and a surgeon are striking: both must be ready to manage potentially life-threatening situations in dynamic and unpredictable environments. The successful use of flight simulators has inspired their application to surgical training. Advances in computer graphics, tissue modeling, haptic instrumentation and computer capabilities have enabled the development of computer-based surgical simulators. Before performing a neurosurgical procedure on a real patient, the neurosurgeon will be able to practice on high-fidelity computer models of patient-specific data to simulate the intervention. In this way, the safest and most effective surgical approach can be planned, requiring less time in an operating room.

A computer surgical simulator is an interactive computer virtual environment used to improve human performance and outcomes of surgical procedures. Computer-based surgical simulation is useful for education, training, preoperative planning and skill assessment. Virtual reality-based surgical simulators have only recently become available due to the complexity of anatomy and the demanding performance requirement to interact directly with volumetric, usually multimodal, images. A virtual reality simulator should be able to simulate surgical procedures, such as cutting, drilling, grasping, sucking, suturing and knot-tying. Requirements for this type of simulator include: realism to represent the accurate and detailed shape of the patient's organ; real-time interaction; quantitative deformation; haptic feedback; and simulation of various operations such as the pushing, pinching, picking, incising and excising of tissue models in a virtual environment.

28.3
Applications

We illustrate the use of some of these technologies in three systems developed in our laboratory for brain intervention. Each system allows the patient-specific data to be visualized, quantified and, most importantly, interacted with. The major difficulty in their development has been in maintaining high fidelity of the modeled and visualized data while providing a real-time response to the physician's actions, such as inserting an electrode, advancing a catheter or simulating removal of tumor.

28.3.1
Atlas-Assisted Stereotactic and Functional Neurosurgery

Deformable body models along with warping techniques provide a means for analysis of medical images, and deformable brain atlases, in particular, are suitable for analysis of brain scans. A deformable brain atlas is useful for image-guided procedures including functional neurosurgery, biopsy, gene therapy, radiosurgery and localized drug delivery.

Electronic brain atlases are commonly used in stereotactic and functional neurosurgery (NOWINSKI 2001a; NOWINSKI and BENABID 2002). Our Cerefy brain atlas (see Chap. 9) has become the standard in stereotactic and functional neurosurgery. It has

already been integrated with major image-guided surgery systems including the *StealthStation* (Medtronic/Sofamor-Danek), *Target* (BrainLAB), *SurgiPlan* (Elekta), *SNN 3 Image Guided Surgery System* (Surgical Navigation Network) and the neurosurgical robot *NeuroMate* (Integrated Surgical Systems). One of the simplest atlas-assisted approaches is to use *The Electronic Clinical Brain Atlas* on CD-ROM (NOWINSKI et al. 1997a). This allows individualized atlases to be generated without loading the patient-specific data, an ability which is useful for anatomical targeting. The planning procedure for stereotactic and functional neurosurgery by using this CD-ROM was proposed in NOWINSKI et al. (1998). The atlas is conformed to the patient's scan by means of a two-dimensional (2D) local deformation done by matching the atlas rectangular region of interest to the corresponding data region of interest. This deformation can be repeated in multiple orientations, increasing the accuracy of targeting and the neurosurgeon's confidence. This application displays the individualized atlas along with the marked stereotactic target and its coordinates.

The *NeuroPlanner*, another system developed by us for stereotactic and functional neurosurgery, supports preoperative planning and training, intraoperative procedures and postoperative follow-up (NOWINSKI et al. 2000). It comprises all mutually co-registered atlases from the Cerefy brain atlas database, including their three-dimensional (3D) extensions (NOWINSKI et al. 1997b). The *NeuroPlanner* provides four groups of functions: data-related (data interpolation, reconstruction, image processing); atlas-related (atlas-to-data interactive 3D warping, 2D and 3D interactive multiple labeling); atlas-data exploration-related (interaction in three orthogonal views and one 3D view, continuous data-atlas exploration); and neurosurgery-related (targeting, path planning, mensuration, simulating the insertion of a microelectrode, simulating therapeutic lesioning) (Fig. 28.1).

For atlas-to-data registration, the Talairach transformation (TALAIRACH and TOURNOUX 1988) is used with the Talairach landmarks specified in the data interactively. Alternatively, the placement of the landmarks can be done automatically (NOWINSKI and THIRUNAVUUKARASUU 2000). There are several problems associated with the original Talairach landmarks (see Chap. 9). To overcome them, a new, equivalent set of landmarks was introduced called *Talairach-Nowinski landmarks* (NOWINSKI 2001b). The new landmarks are defined in a more constructive way than the original Talairach landmarks. In addition, their automatic identification is easier.

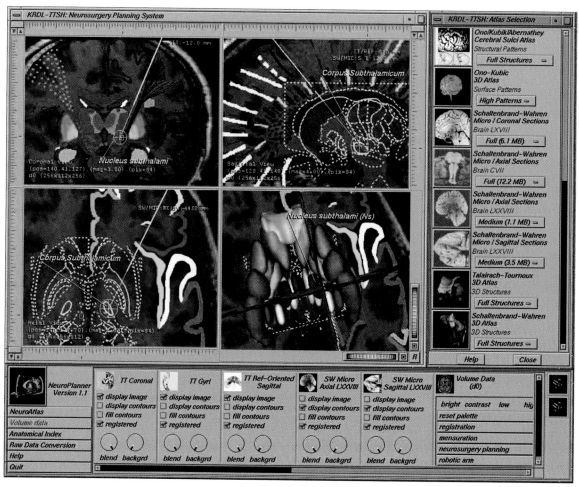

Fig. 28.1. The *NeuroPlanner. Center*: Main window with four resizable views. These views contain the orthogonal (axial, coronal and sagittal) data sections registered with 2D atlases and data-atlas triplanar registered with 3D atlases. The views are smoothly and continuously resized by dragging their common corner, allowing the neurosurgeon to balance the 2D and 3D presentations. The following atlases, presented as contours, images or polygonal models, are displayed: with subcortical structures and gyri in the axial view, with gross anatomy in the coronal view, with subcortical structures and brain connections in the sagittal view, and with subcortical structures in the 3D view along with the atlas triplanar. The stereotactic trajectory (*thin line*) along with the current position of the microelectrode (*thick line*) are displayed. The target structure, i.e., the subthalamic nucleus, is highlighted and labeled in all views. *Right*: Atlas selection panel with multiple atlases in multiple resolutions. *Bottom*: scrollable control panel; each loaded atlas and selected operation has its own control module

The *NeuroPlanner* is empowered with several operations enhancing the original Talairach transformation and making the atlas-to-data registration more accurate, efficient and easy. These include global and local registrations, editable position of the Talairach grid in three dimensions, real-time interactive atlas warping feasible any time, targeting in multiple orientations, and targeting with multiple atlases. To warp the atlas against data, a two-step Talairach transformation was introduced with global and local steps (NOWINSKI 1998). The Talairach transformation scales the gross anatomy globally and does not compensate for the width of the third ventricle or

internal capsule. Local warping by means of the same piecewise linear deformation mechanism enhances the accuracy of registration in the region of interest for the previously globally selected atlas plates. When registering locally, any landmarks clearly visible in the data can be used to improve the delineation of the usually non-clearly visible target structure. In addition, real-time interactive warping applied to the atlas contours, images and polygonal models allows the neurosurgeon to fit any atlas to data and fine-tune the atlas-to-data match. The use of a brain atlas in multiple orientations enhances the accuracy of targeting, gives more flexibility in choosing local land-

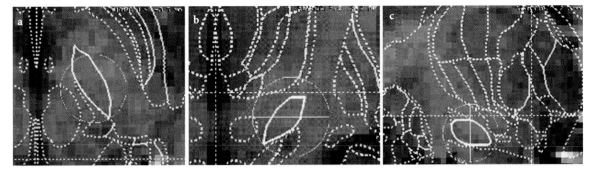

Fig. 28.2a–c. The *NeuroPlanner*: subthalamotomy targeted simultaneously in multiple orientations by using the atlas in contour representation: (**a**) axial; (**b**) coronal and (**c**) sagittal views. The point target is marked within the highlighted target structure by the cursor

marks, and provides an extra degree of confidence to the neurosurgeon. The global registration steps performed simultaneously in all three orthogonal planes were formulated in NOWINSKI (1998). The targeting steps and local registrations along with suitable landmarks for pallidotomy, thalamotomy and subthalamotomy were detailed in NOWINSKI (1998). In addition, the use of multiple brain atlases provides complementary information and overcomes some limitations of the individual atlases, which additionally enhances targeting (NOWINSKI et al. 2000). Fig. 28.2 illustrates the use of the atlas in multiple orientations for targeting in subthalamotomy. The target structure, i.e., the subthalamic nucleus, is delineated in all three orthogonal planes by the atlas contours

and the point target is set manually to lie within all three contours.

The *NeuroPlanner* provides numerous tools supporting surgery (Fig. 28.3). The stereotactic trajectory along with the current position of the inserted electrode is displayed in relation to the orthogonal views, triplanar and 3D structures. The list of atlas structures traversed along the stereotactic trajectory is calculated and displayed in the orthogonal views. In addition, the neurosurgeon is able to simulate electrode movement and therapeutic lesioning.

The major advantage of the *NeuroPlanner* is a potential saving in terms of cost, time and invasiveness. The initial validation shows (NOWINSKI et al. 2000) that the accuracy of the atlas-assisted approach

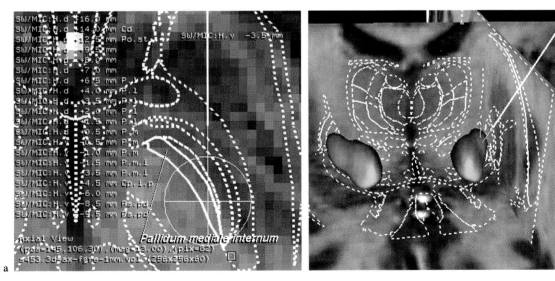

Fig. 28.3a, b. The *NeuroPlanner*: supporting tools for pallidotomy planning. **a** The target structure, the pallidum mediale internum, is delineated and labeled; the stereotactic trajectory (*thin line*) with the current position of the microelectrode (*thick line*) is shown; and the list of structures traversed along this trajectory is given. **b** Three-dimensional view of the microelectrode, target structure and the atlas-data triplanar

is superior to the non-atlas approach and that the functional target can usually be confirmed electrophysiologically with the first microelectrode used. As the number of tracts is typically from three to seven, this number can potentially be reduced to a single tract, resulting in an average saving of four tracts per surgery. This reduces the cost and invasiveness of the procedure as well as saving the time of the neurosurgeon, personnel and operating room.

The *NeuroPlanner*, licensed for trial to several commercial, clinical and research sites, has been playing an important educational role and influencing the design of the commercial systems that use the Cerefy brain atlas database.

The current computerized stereotactic atlases of the human brain have two major limitations. First, the original printed atlas plates are sparse and constructed from a few brain specimens only. Second, these atlases are anatomical, while the stereotactic targets are functional. The probabilistic functional atlas, the preliminary version of which has been constructed for the ventrointermedius nucleus, subthalamic nucleus, and globus pallidus internus, overcomes both limitations (NOWINSKI and BENABID 2002).

28.3.2
Simulation of Endovascular Procedures

The execution of endovascular procedures requires good eye-hand coordination, appreciation of fluoroscopic imaging in three dimensions and thorough knowledge of vasculature and pathological conditions. Pretreatment planning and training of endovascular brain intervention can be facilitated by using simulators. These procedures are particularly well suited for simulation because they already place the physician at a distance from the operative site while manipulating instruments and viewing procedures on video monitors.

The development of a computer simulator for endovascular brain intervention is a challenging task. This kind of simulator should have standard generic features such as realism, interactivity, user friendliness, resemblance to a stereotactic environment and numerous supportive tools. It also requires using various advanced methods for: filtration and enhancement of angiographic data, vasculature segmentation and feature extraction, quantification of normal and pathological vasculature, geometric modeling and meshing of vasculature, physical modeling of vasculature and interventional devices, hemodynamic

analysis, device-vessel interaction analysis, visualization, and haptic feedback. In addition, specific clinical procedures have to be simulated including angioplasty, stent placement and aneurysm coiling.

We have developed a real-time, interactive, simulation-based planning and training system for cerebrovascular disease treatment called *NeuroCath* (NOWINSKI and CHUI 2001). The *NeuroCath*: (1) supports extraction of vasculature from various imaging modalities and construction of a vascular model that represents the anatomy of patient in a computationally efficient manner, (2) models a physical behavior between the devices and the cerebral vasculature, and (3) contains the tactile apparatus that gives the clinician the sense of touch during intervention planning and training. The physical setup of the *NeuroCath* with dual-monitor display is shown in Fig. 28.4.

The *NeuroCath* contains a realistic visual interface with multiple, synchronized windows. The fluoroscopic display simulates views as in actual procedures while 3D and roadmapping displays enhance interpretation of the patient's anatomy. The usefulness of roadmapping is increased when it is combined with simultaneous 3D display of the vasculature and interventional devices.

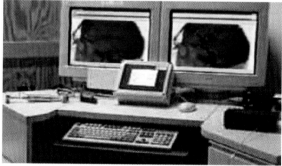
a

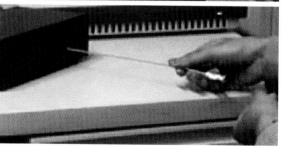
b

Fig. 28.4a, b. The *NeuroCath*. **a** Physical setup with two monitors, tactile apparatus (*right*), patient table manipulation unit (*center*) and simulated balloon inflation device (*left*). **b** Interventional device control by means of the tactile apparatus converting the physical movement of devices into their movement within a virtual patient. The device can be moved forward or backward and rotate to the right or left

a
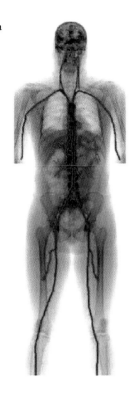

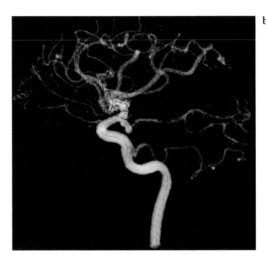
b

Fig. 28.5a, b. The *NeuroCath*: vascular models. **a** Complete human vasculature extracted from the Visible Human Data. **b** Patient-specific model with the central line extracted

Visualization and interaction with the vascular model and devices is a key feature of the *NeuroCath*. For training purposes, we have constructed a complete human vascular model derived from the Visible Human Data (Fig. 28.5). For pretreatment planning, patient-specific models have to be reconstructed (Figs. 28.5, 28.7). The vascular model is represented as a hierarchical structure of vascular segments connected by vascular branch junctions. Each segment is described by its central line, corresponding vessel cross-sections, and connections to other segments and/or junctions.

After loading the patient-specific data and extracting the vascular model, the clinician sets the size and shape of catheter and/or guidewire to be used for intervention. A library of interventional devices has been built into the *NeuroCath* for device selection, including catheters, guidewires, stents and coils from various manufacturers. Next, the clinician sets the insertion/entry point. Two methods are provided for catheter navigation. The clinician can control it from the user interface by clicking the direction buttons to advance the movement of catheter/guidewire. Alternatively, the tactile apparatus, an electromechanical device, can be used to control this movement (Fig. 28.4). This apparatus allows the clinician to translate and rotate the catheter the way he or she experiences during a real procedure. In addition, it provides tac-

tile feedback by controlling the friction of the catheter's movement. The amount of friction is calculated based on the interaction of a catheter, modeled as a flexible object, with a blood vessel.

The *NeuroCath* provides powerful and flexible visualization capabilities (Figs. 28.4–28.7). The hybrid volume and surface renderer gives insight into interior and exterior of the patient's vasculature. The 3D display combined with real-time manipulation of data, vascular model and devices saves time and cost, and potentially reduces the invasiveness of the procedure by decreasing the number of contrast agent injections and lowering the amount of X-ray radiation from fluoroscopy, X-ray rotational angiography and/or interventional CT.

The *NeuroCath* is able to simulate aneurysm coiling, ballooning and stent placement. Aneurysm coiling is simulated by navigating to the aneurysm and then replacing the wire with a coil wire. The coil is deployed by detaching it from the wire. Multiple coils can be deployed by repeating the detachment process with new coil wires. Ballooning and stent placement are simulated using a customized simulated balloon-inflation device (Fig. 28.4). The inflated balloon is modeled as a tank-like structure expanding uniformly and the stent deployed subsequently is displayed in fluoroscopic and 3D views (Fig. 28.7).

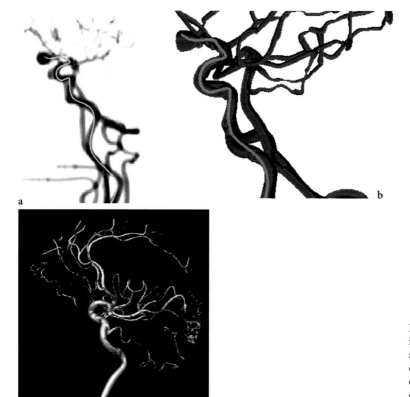

Fig. 28.6a–c. The *NeuroCath*: visualization. **a** Simulated fluoroscopic view showing the data and the catheter modeled as a flexible object. **b** Surface rendered vascular model along with the catheter. **c** Volume rendered patient-specific cerebral vasculature

The development of the *NeuroCath* is work in progress. Realistic modeling of pathology will be enhanced in visual and haptic senses. In addition, a hemodynamic model will be developed to credibly simulate the blood flow and its interaction with the devices.

28.3.3
Virtual Reality-Enhanced Neurosurgery

The current standard portal into medical information is the video monitor. Most monitors display monoscopic images, which makes it difficult for the surgeon to judge accurately the correct spatial relationships of objects. One of the most frequently used technologies to achieve 3D perception in surgical simulation is stereoscopic glasses containing shutters over each eye (Fig. 28.8). The glasses are synchronized to a computer monitor, which is able to generate left- and right-eye images. A stereoscopic effect is achieved by displaying images that are slightly different due to parallax. Emerging display technologies, such as HMD, digital holography or virtual reality projectors, may become alternative solutions to the video monitor.

Neurosurgical procedures involve not only 3D stereoscopic perception but also 3D manipulation with 6 degrees-of-freedom (i.e., three translations and three rotations). Therefore, to fully exploit the potential of stereoscopic medical images in a computer-aided surgery system, the user needs to explore them using 3D interaction. We have developed a 3D interface with stereoscopic display called *Dextroscope*[1] that is ideal for surgery planning and training. It is a virtual workbench device providing an immersive environment within which the user can visualize and interactively modify 3D multimodal volumetric images in real time. The *Dextroscope* consists of a mirror-based display system, 3D input device system and graphics workstation. A stereo virtual image is seen reflected in a mirror allowing the user wearing shuttered glasses to reach into the virtual space. The *Dextroscope* provides compatibility of the manipulating (physical) space and the visual (virtual) space, so that physical tools manipulate virtual objects in a hand-eye coordinated manner (Fig. 28.8). The *Dextroscope* overcomes some of limitations of the HMD, such as its size and weight that produce encumbrance and fatigue,

---

[1] The *Dextroscope*, along with the surgery planning software, is distributed by our spin-off, Volume Interactions.

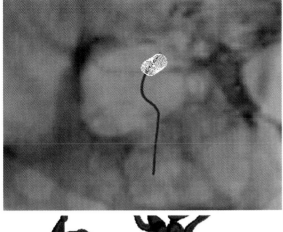

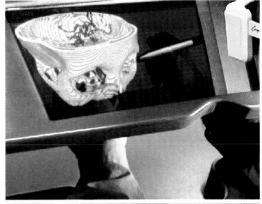

a

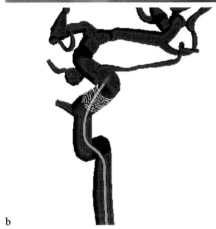

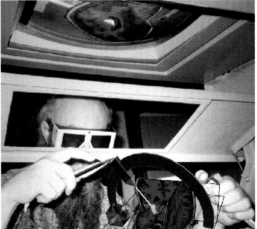

a

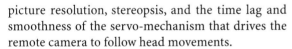

b

b

Fig. 28.7a, b. The *NeuroCath*: simulation of stent placement. **a** Fluoroscopic view. **b** Three-dimensional view

Fig. 28.8a, b. The *Dextroscope*. **a** The user reaches into the virtual head under the mirror, manipulates it using two hands, and perceives it stereoscopically by wearing shuttered glasses. A semi-transparent mirror is used to illustrate hand-eye coordination. **b** The virtual objects (in this case, the atlas, data and stereotactic arc of the *BrainBench*) placed in the space below the mirror as perceived by the user. The user's hands holding the sensors are invisible to the user and do not obscure the virtual objects

picture resolution, stereopsis, and the time lag and smoothness of the servo-mechanism that drives the remote camera to follow head movements.

We have developed several applications around this interface including two for neurosurgery: *Brain-Bench* for stereotactic and functional neurosurgery and *VIVIAN* (virtual intracranial visualization and navigation) for skull base and other complicated brain surgeries.

BrainBench (SERRA et al. 1997) is a surgical planning system for stereotactic frame neurosurgery. It contains a suite of neurosurgery-supporting tools and the Cerefy brain atlas (Figs. 28.8, 28.9). *BrainBench* allows the neurosurgeon to: prepare faster plans; have more accurate anatomical targeting; improve the avoidance of critical structures; have fewer suboptimal frame attachments and speedier, more effective planning and training.

VIVIAN (SERRA et al. 1998) is a system developed for preoperative neurosurgical planning and simulation. It uses hardware-accelerated multimodal volume rendering. Neurosurgeons use *VIVIAN* preoperatively to interact with multimodal images of the patient's skull, brain, tumor and blood vessels fused together and displayed as a single 3D virtual object (Fig. 28.10). The surgeon simulates bone and tissue removal in the image to plan the optimal entry path for tumor resection. The objective is to minimize the surgeon's "guess work", so that during surgery the pathological and anatomical landmarks are more easily identified and operated on. This leads to lower morbidity, shorter operations and faster recoveries. A variety of tools, activated simply by pressing virtual buttons on toolbars inside the virtual space, facilitate segmentation, registration, visualization, mensuration and simulation. The segmented structures can be manipulated, allowing the neurosurgeon to "pick" a tumor (or any other structure) (Fig. 28.9) and to look at it from any viewpoint, while its surrounding structures are revealed. The data can be displayed in an interactive triplanar mode or as a full volume which can be cropped by cutting planes in any angle (Fig. 28.10). With virtual measurement tools, intra- and extracranial dimensions can be measured and marked (Fig. 28.10). The virtual head can be positioned as in a real surgical approach and craniotomy performed by a virtual drill. In addition, virtual suction removes brain tissue, tumor and/or blood vessels from the volumetric image.

VIVIAN has already been used in more than 30 operations and our experience is reported in Kockro et al. (2000). *VIVIAN* was also instrumental in two successful landmark separations of craniopagus twins: Zambian twins in South Africa in 1997 (Carson 1999) and Nepalese twins in Singapore in 2001.

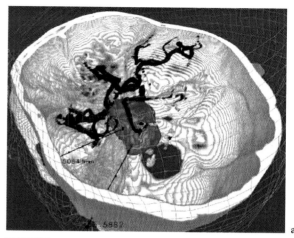

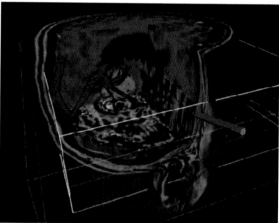

Fig. 28.10a, b. Multimodal visualization and 3D interaction by using *VIVIAN*. a CT and MR angiography data along with the segmented tumor displayed as a single image of the skull base region. Measurement of critical distances facilitates surgery. b Interacting with a multimodal volumetric image containing morphological, functional and angiographic MR data sets fused together

28.4
Summary

Over the past 30 years neurosurgery has been propelled by advances in the computational, biomedical and physical sciences. This chapter describes our contributions to the advancement in stereotactic and functional neurosurgery, endovascular brain intervention, and virtual reality-enhanced neurosurgery. In stereotactic and functional neurosurgery, the accuracy of atlas-assisted targeting is superior to that of non-atlas targeting and the number of tracts can be reduced, resulting in a lowering of the cost and invasiveness of the procedure as well as saving the time of the neurosurgeon, personnel and operating room.

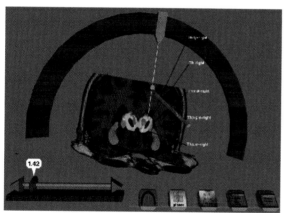

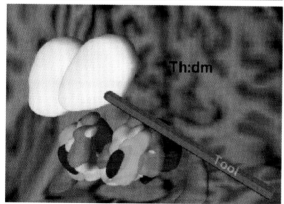

Fig. 28.9a, b. The *BrainBench*. a The stylus manipulates the stereotactic arc, stereotactic trajectory, 3D atlas, and data triplanar. Its behavior is controlled by the toolrack. b Picking an individualized cerebral structure for close inspection

Simulation of endovascular brain intervention reduces the cost of training and potentially improves the outcome of procedures. In addition, 3D real-time display and manipulation of data, vascular models and interventional devices save time and cost as well as reducing the invasiveness of the procedure by decreasing the number of contrast agent injections and lowering the amount of X-ray radiation from fluoroscopy, X-ray rotational angiography and/or interventional CT.

A virtual reality environment allows the neurosurgeon to manipulate the patient-specific multimodal data as a real object and to simulate bone and tissue removal in the volumetric image to plan the optimal entry path for tumor resection. This minimizes the surgeon's "guess work", leading to lower morbidity, shorter operations and faster recoveries. In particular, this makes a difference in difficult cases such as skull base tumors or craniopagus twin separation.

The current technological breakthroughs mark just the beginning of the prologue to computer-aided brain surgery. The pace of change in surgery will be accelerated dramatically by introducing new technologies such as molecular computing. This will offer the possibility of using molecules as microscopic switches to replace silicon in computers, and molecular computers will be orders of magnitude more powerful and far cheaper than today's machines. A key question that arises is what computer-aided surgery solutions will be developed beyond today's prologue. We believe that the advancements presented here and in Chap. 9 on electronic brain atlases may be important components of the neurosurgical system of the future. We also believe that technological progress should be accompanied by a paradigm shift from surgeon-centric to patient-centric.

Acknowledgements. Numerous individuals and institutions contributed to this work over many years. *The Electronic Clinical Brain Atlas* was a joint development with Prof. R.N. Bryan of Johns Hopkins Hospital, USA. The *NeuroPlanner* was developed within a joint project with Dr. T.T. Yeo of Tan Tock Seng Hospital/National Neuroscience Institute, Singapore. The construction of the probabilistic functional atlas is an ongoing joint work with Prof. A.L. Benabid, France. The *NeuroCath* is a joint development with Prof. J. Anderson of Johns Hopkins Hospital. The development of *BrainBench* and *VIVIAN* was done in collaboration with Singapore General Hospital involving Dr. P. Pillay (*BrainBench*) and Dr. C. Chan (*VIVIAN*). The developments of the *NeuroPlanner* and *Brain Bench/VIVIAN* were supported by grants from the National Science and Technology Board, Singapore. The key contributors to the development of applications described here were C.K. Chui, A. Fang, Q.M. Hu, R.A. Kockro, H. Ng, T. Poston, L. Serra, A. Thirunavuukarasuu, Y.P. Wang and G.L. Yang, among many others.

References

Carson B (1999) The big picture. Zondevand Publishing House, Baltimore

Kockro RA, Serra L, Yeo TT et al (2000) Planning and simulation of neurosurgery in a virtual reality environment. Neurosurgery 46:118–137

Nowinski WL (1998) Anatomical targeting in functional neurosurgery by the simultaneous use of multiple Schaltenbrand-Wahren brain atlas microseries. Stereotac Funct Neurosurg 71:103–116

Nowinski WL (2001a) Computerized brain atlases for surgery of movement disorders. Semin Neurosurg 12:183–194

Nowinski WL (2001b) Modified Talairach landmarks. Acta Neurochir (Wien) 143:1045–1105

Nowinski WL, Benabid AL (2002) New directions in atlas-assisted stereotactic functional neurosurgery. Advanced techniques in image-guided brain and spine surgery. Thieme, New York

Nowinski WL, Thirunavuukarasuu A (2000) Methods and apparatus for processing medical images. Patent application PCT/SG00/00185

Nowinski WL, Chui CK (2001) Simulation of interventional neuroradiology procedures. Proceedings of the medical imaging and augmented reality MIAR2001, Hong Kong, 10–12 June 2001. IEEE Computer Society Press, pp 87–94

Nowinski WL, Bryan RN, Raghavan R (1997a) The electronic clinical brain atlas. Multiplanar navigation of the human brain. Thieme, New York

Nowinski WL, Fang A, Nguyen BT et al. (1997b) Multiple brain atlas database and atlas-based neuroimaging system. Comput Aided Surg 2:42–66

Nowinski WL, Yeo TT, Thirunavuukarasuu A (1998) Micro-electrode-guided functional neurosurgery assisted by electronic clinical brain atlas CD-ROM. Comput Aided Surg 3:115–122

Nowinski WL, Yang GL, Yeo TT (2000) Computer-aided stereotactic functional neurosurgery enhanced by the use of the multiple brain atlas database. IEEE Trans Med Imaging 19:62–69

Serra L, Nowinski WL, Poston T et al (1997) The BrainBench: virtual tools for stereotactic frame neurosurgery. Med Image Anal 1:317–329

Serra L, Kockro RA, Chua GG et al (1998) Multimodal volume-based tumor neurosurgery planning in the virtual workbench. Proceedings of the medical image computing and computer-assisted intervention MICCAI '98, Cambridge MA, USA, 11–13 Oct 1998. Springer, Berlin Heidelberg New York, pp 1007–1016 (Lecture notes in computer science, vol 1496)

Talairach J, Tournoux P (1988) Co-planar stereotactic atlas of the human brain. Thieme, Stuttgart

29 Computer-Aided Surgery in Orthopaedics

Maurius Marcacci, Pier Francesco La Palombara, Laura Nofrini, Andrea Malvisti

29.1
Surgical Augmented Reality Navigation Systems

Recent advances in technology concerning image processing and computer visualization techniques have made more feasible the development and diffusion of augmented reality systems in several domains, including the medical field. Augmented reality system are systems based on a display technique that combines information taken from the real environment with data generated by the computer, augmenting the real scene with additional information and enhancing the user's perception of the world.

Surgical navigation systems are augmented reality systems that provides the surgeon with accurate visual and numerical information on the spatial relationship of the patient's anatomical structures and surgical tools during surgery, updated in real time. The augmentation can be carried out in several ways: some systems show in the virtual scene the three-dimensional (3D) model of the anatomy reconstructed either from a preoperative CT or MR study of the patient or by adapting existing generic models to the patient examination; other systems do not visualize the 3D model of the anatomy but show the model information required for the task with lines and points determined from direct measurement of

M. Marcacci, MD, P.F. La Palombara, MD, L. Nofrini, MD, A. Malvisti, MD
Istituti Ortopedici Rizzoli, Biomechanics Lab, Via Barbiano 1–10, 40136 Bologna, Italy

limb dynamics and the bone surface. In general, surgical navigation systems includes three main components (Nikou et al. 2000):

- An intraoperative position tracking system. This is the device used to monitor relevant objects in the operating field, collecting in real time the data relating to their location and orientation. Depending on the technology they use, these tracking systems can be mechanical, optical, electromagnetic or ultrasonic.
- A display device showing the virtual scenario, updated in real time.
- Control software that processes data collected by the tracking system to update the position of the objects in the virtual scenario and produces the images to be shown by the display device. These images have to be provided at a sufficient frame rate in order to avoid flicker. Moreover the system must be able to update the images as frequently as possible, because the longer the delay in processing the tracker's data to display new images, the worse is the accuracy of the virtual environment in reproducing the real world.

The use of augmented reality navigation systems in clinical practice potentially brings many benefits to orthopaedic surgery. First, these systems allow the preoperative or intraoperative planning of the surgery based on patient-specific information, permitting the simulation of different surgical strategies and the choice of the optimal one. In the case of preoperative planning, during the intervention the planned strategy can be displayed in the virtual scenario and integrated with the intraoperative information. During the intervention, by providing visual and numerical information on the position of surgical tools and the patient's anatomy updated in real time, these systems provide the surgeon with accurate visual feedback, guiding him towards the completion of the planned strategy. Furthermore, the capability of these systems to provide more visual information in the surgical field than is available to the naked eye, helps to solve the problems of visualization, especially in the case of minimally invasive surgery. It is well known that less invasive surgery contributes to better patient outcomes, but minimization of invasiveness generally reduces the surgeon's perception and dexterity. By showing the structural anatomy of the patient together with surgical tools, these augmented reality navigation systems allow the surgeon to accurately localize anatomical areas and reach predefined positions by watching the display device.

There is also a great potential to use these systems for surgical education and training – for example teaching the surgical strategy by simulating the intervention on dummies instead of real patients, and allowing trainees to perform the simulation. Several orthopaedic procedures lend themselves well to the use of augmented reality navigation systems. The most common tasks developed by existing navigation systems are:

- Joint replacement, where augmented reality systems can be used to guide the proper placement of the implant component, based on preoperative plans or intraoperatively collected data
- Arthroscopy surgery, where navigation systems are useful to provide the surgeon with a more global view of the joint and to display the position and the trajectory (field of action) of the surgical tools with respect to the patient's anatomy
- Treatment of fractures, for example intramedullary rod placement, where the rod insertion tool and drill guide can be tracked
- Spinal surgery, using real-time image-guided transpedicular screw insertion

As proposed in PICARD et al. (2000a), surgical navigation systems can be divided into:
- Systems using preoperative models
- Systems using intraoperative models

Preoperative models used by the systems of the first group can be either 3D anatomical models reconstructed from preoperative imaging studies (MR, CT or ultrasound) of the patient (patient-specific systems) or a generic anatomical model of the part under examination (non-patient-specific). A 3D patient-specific model can easily be derived from preoperative images such as CT or MR. In fact, these medical studies produce multiplanar images that can be combined spatially to create a volumetric data set; from this data set it is possible to reconstruct the 3D preoperative model of the anatomy that can be used both for preoperative planning of the intervention and for the visualization of the anatomy in the virtual scene.

An example of this type of system is HipNav (DI GIOIA et al. 1998b). HipNav is a navigation and guidance system for hip prosthesis implantation using optoelectronic tracking, developed by the Centers for Medical Robotics and Computer Assisted Surgery at Carnegie Mellon University and UPMC Shadyside Hospital. The system includes a preoperative planner, a range-of-motion simulator and an intraoperative navigation and guidance system. In the preoperative phase the surgeon plans the acetabular implant size and orientation on a 3D surface model of the pelvis derived from CT images of the patient and on three simulated orthogonal CT views (sagittal, coronal and transverse). For any chosen size, orientation and geometry of the implant components, the range-of-motion simulator dynamically predicts impingement for various leg motions; this prediction is based on estimates of the functional range of pelvic motion done on preoperative lateral standing and sitting radiographs of the pelvis. Using this information, the surgeon can optimize the plan of the implant in the individual case. Intraoperatively the navigation and guidance system helps the surgeon to achieve the planned implant: the pelvis, the data collection probe and the implant insertion tool are sensorized with securely affixed optical targets and, after the registration and calibration process performed using a particular procedure, they can be localized and tracked in real time.

The same principles have been employed for the development of a navigation and guidance system for total knee replacement surgery (KneeNav-TKR) and for anterior cruciate ligament (ACL) reconstruction (KneeNav-ACL), not yet used in clinical practice. KneeNav-TKR uses the preoperative 3D surface model derived from CT images of the femur and tibia. In order to obtain intraoperative measurements of alignment and guidance information, the system utilizes a precalibrated plate probe tracker in the usual saw slot of TKR mechanical guides; the user interface shows the predefined mechanical axes and starting from this information the surgeon can decide the ideal orientation of the cutting guides. Once the guides are properly aligned, bone cuts are made using a traditional oscillating saw. KneeNav-ACL (PICARD et al. 2000b) is a CT-based surgical navigation system developed to orient the placement of a standard guide-pin assembly in order to improve the precision of graft positioning. This version of KneeNav also uses the preoperative 3D surface model derived from CT images of the femur and tibia. The positions of the bones and guide-pin assembly are monitored simultaneously by means of an optical tracker and the surgeon place the femoral and tibial tunnels under computer guidance on the 3D bone models instead of arthroscopic views. This computer-assisted ACL reconstruction system, which is still under development, will allow accurate and reproducible positioning of the ACL tunnels according to a preoperative plan.

Another system using preoperative models is Navitrack (Amiot et al. 1995), developed by Orthosoft, Inc., Montreal, Canada. It is similar to HipNav and uses a preoperative model of the patient based on CT or MR images; the main difference is that it uses an electromagnetic tracking system. This has the advantage of allowing tracking of instruments even inside the body, and avoids the line-of-sight limitations of optical trackers The main drawback of this technology is that if used in the presence of ferromagnetic objects, the accuracy in localizing the tracked object deteriorates significantly.

Mitech Lab, Scuola Superiore S. Anna, Pisa in collaboration with Biomechanics Lab, Istituti Ortopedici Rizzoli, Bologna, Italy, have developed a navigation system for computer-assisted arthroscopic surgery (Dario et al. 2000); its adaptation for unicompartmental knee arthroplasty is still under development (Marcacci et al. 2000). It is based on the use of a 3D model of the joint reconstructed from a preoperative CT/MR data set. A 3D model and two-dimensional projections of the patient's joint and models of the arthroscope and other sensorized surgical instruments are shown. The positions of all sensorized objects, including the patient's anatomy, are tracked in real time by an optoelectronic localizer and reproduced in the virtual scene. The field of view of the arthroscope is dynamically highlighted on the 3D model of the joint, which is matched to the actual anatomy by means of an ICP-based non-fiducial registration algorithm.

A very interesting idea is the concept of image overlay systems. These (Blackwell et al. 1998a) are augmented reality navigation systems which use a particular computer display technique to intraoperatively superimpose the real patient's anatomy and the corresponding 3D model reconstructed from preoperative images; the virtual image is positioned such that it appears to lie within the patient around the region in which the surgeon is working, providing the surgeon with a sort of X-ray vision. In such systems the display device is semi-transparent, enabling the merging of computer-generated information with the real-world images. Examples are a standard flat-panel liquid crystal display with the back light removed, or the technique used by Blackwell et al. (1998b),

based on a standard computer display monitor coupled with a half-silvered mirror or beam splitter glass; the surgeon looks directly at the patient's anatomy while simultaneously seeing a reflection of the computer display from the glass. The tracking system employed has to be capable of tracking the viewer's eye position, the display, the patient and the most relevant surgical instruments used. The software must correlate the 3D virtual model with the corresponding patient's anatomy positions (registration module) and be able to transform images so that they appear to the eye exactly as they existed in their virtual spatial location, correctly sized when observed at any distance (e.g. if the eye gets closer to the image, the object must appear to grow larger).

Potential medical applications of image overlay systems include:

Intraoperative guidance. Image overlay is used in conjunction with the HipNav system to properly position the acetabular and femoral prosthetic components. It can be used also for the reduction of fractures and, in general, for intervention involving rigid bony anatomy.

Simulation for surgical education. Systems using intraoperative models include those that use intraoperatively acquired medical images to determine the model (image-based) and those that use models derived from information determined by direct measurement of the bone surface or limb dynamics (non-image-based). The first class includes the group of systems using generic models of the anatomy. These models can also be a statistical atlas of the relevant anatomy, including geometrical and physical properties that can be fused via registration with the real patient anatomy.

One example of a system belonging to this group is that for ACL reconstruction described in Fleute et al. (1999), which makes use of a generic model of the anatomy built using data derived by statistical analysis of a given bone population. The system uses a 3D optical tracker. During surgery, using the localizer, the surgeon collects points on tibial and femoral surfaces, and statistical information about the shape variation of the femur is used to interpolate the data points. Then, through the registration process, the system produces the ideal fit between acquired points and the generic model. Using a statistical method to build the model has the advantage of requiring fewer data points to obtain sufficient interpolation accuracy, thus reducing the intraoperative time required for data acquisition.

Another group of navigation systems using intra-operative images is those based on fluoroscopic images. The position and orientation of the surgical tools and of the patient's anatomy in the virtual scene are initialized by processing one or more single-shot C-arm images; then, using the tracking device, the navigation system tracks the movement of the surgical instruments and represents their position on the acquired images as though they were being imaged using constant C-arm control. One example of this type of navigation system is the system for ACL reconstruction proposed by KLOS et al. (1998). Fluoroscopic images are intraoperatively acquired and then digitized using a frame grabber. Surgical instruments within the fluoroscopic images are sensorized and tracked by the system, generating graphic overlays on the images that provide the surgeon with visual feedback on the position of the wire placement and of the surgical instruments with respect to the patient's anatomy, in real-time. Moreover the system visualizes the ideal locations of graft placement, determined using an overlap template coinciding with the lateral fluoroscopic view. NOLTE et al. (2000) describe a fluoroscopy-based navigation system developed for spine surgery.

Among systems using a patient's model derived from direct measurement of the bone surface and of limb dynamics is Orthopilot (LEITNER et al. 1997), which is a navigation system developed by Aesculap, Tuttlingen for the total knee replacement procedure. Orthopilot uses an optoelectronic tracking system and infrared transmitters positioned at predetermined points on the limb and on the cutting guide. Identifying hip, knee and ankle centres by tracking and recording the leg position during fixed movements, the system determines the ideal limb mechanical axis. Then the system-user interface shows the optimal cutting orientation with respect to the mechanical axis and the actual cutting guide orientation updated in real time, telling the surgeon when the saw cutting guide is in the best position in order to achieve optimal prosthesis implantation. Finally the surgeon secures the jigs and cuts the bone using a traditional oscillating saw.

Another example of a non-image-based system is that described in DESSENNE et al. (1998) for ACL reconstruction. The system is used to optimize the placement of the femoral tunnel. It includes an optical tracker and four rigid bodies with infrared diodes fixed on the femur, the tibia, the surgical drill and a pointer to collect 3D data points. The surgeon collects points on femoral and tibial surfaces, and points obtained by moving the knee. Using these data, the system computes the relative position between femur and tibia in order to define an isometric map, and to guide the surgeon in obtaining an optimal placement of the graft (minimal graft anisometry).

Even though recent technological advances have made medical applications of augmented reality more feasible, and these augmented reality navigation systems have shown great potential for providing a wealth of useful information, some problems have still to be solved. First, the accuracy of the navigation system must be suited to the task. Tracking systems are fundamental to the accuracy of augmented reality systems. Depending on the features of each task, the most suitable tracking system needs to be chosen: optical trackers are very precise but require a direct line of sight during the course of the procedure, and this line of sight can easily be interrupted by tools, or by the medical staff; magnetic trackers avoid the problem of the line of sight and are very useful for tracking of instruments even inside the body, but their accuracy deteriorates if used in the presence of metallic tools; mechanical systems, on the other hand, are not limited by occlusion and are very precise, but can be difficult to handle. Moreover, another problem is the difficulty in attaching tracking targets to every independently moving object in the field of interest. The degree of accuracy achievable by these systems depends also on other factors. The accuracy of preoperative models based on images of the patient depends both on the protocol used for image acquisition (e.g. slice thickness) and on the algorithm used for segmentation and reconstruction of the 3D model. Moreover systems using preoperative models require a registration phase to correlate the model with the intraoperative patient's anatomy, and it is well known that registration is still one of the principal causes of inaccuracy in computer-aided surgical techniques, particularly in the case minimally invasive surgery.

Systems using generic models have the advantage of avoiding the need for preoperative patient images, but their use is highly dependent on the accuracy required by the task; moreover they still do not eliminate the need for a registration phase to match the generic model with the real patient's anatomy. Among systems using intraoperative images, fluoroscopy-based systems, which carry a reduced radiation dose to both patient and surgical staff, provide the surgeon with a real-time updated virtual scene representing the operating field without the need for obtaining new views while the operation is in progress. Moreover, fluoroscopy-based navigation systems have the advantage that fluoroscopes are available in any orthopaedic applications; however, a good image quality of the fluoroscope is mandatory for a safe and precise system.

The main problem of systems based on the use of mechanical analysis is the lack of accuracy in determining geometrical features of the model and consequently in providing the surgeon with accurate indications to correctly perform the intervention.

Finally, to be accepted by surgeons, equipment has to be small, unobtrusive, user-friendly, safe and compatible with the surgical environment. Introducing any equipment into the operating room increases the risk of infection, so any part of the system that comes into contact with the sterile field must be easily sterilizable or draped.

29.2
Image and 3D Data Registration in Computer-Assisted Orthopaedic Surgery

Successful implementation of computer-aided surgery (CAS) protocols in orthopaedics requires a consistent integration of spatial data originating from a broad variety of imaging, sensing and actuating devices, each embodying its own coordinate frame. This is why an accurate estimation of the geometric relationships existing between different coordinate frames and 3D data sets, which is normally referred to as registration, plays a crucial role in virtually all CAS applications (SIMON 1997). The perceivable result of registration is often the determination of a link between medical images and the patient in the operating room (Fig. 29.1). Other more complex tasks involve establishing connections between models derived from medical images, the patient anatomy and independent devices, such as sensorized surgical instruments, image intensifiers, tracking systems and

robotic tools. Some inherent characteristics of bone, such as its relative rigidity and well-differentiated visualization in standard diagnostic imaging, can be exploited to simplify the registration procedure. That is one of the reasons why orthopaedics has been one of the earliest and most successful fields of application for CAS systems. Yet, when deformable objects (ligaments, tendons, fibrocartilaginous structures, etc.) are to be dealt with the above-mentioned advantages are lost.

Most CAS systems used in orthopaedics employ pre- or intra-operative medical images. The reason for this is the reduction of the operational field associated with modern minimally invasive surgical procedures and the fact that unaided visibility is limited to the surface of the exposed anatomy. Images and image-derived models are therefore employed to extend the field of view beyond the operational field and exposed anatomical surfaces. Both images and models usually need to be registered to the patient anatomy and/or to sensorized surgical tools. Popular imaging modalities used in orthopaedic CAS systems are conventional radiography, fluoroscopy (JOSKOW-ICZ et al. 1998; HOFSTETTER et al. 1999, 2000; BROW-BANK et al. 2000; MERLOZ et al. 2000; NOLTE et al. 2000; SLOMCZYKOWSKI et al. 2001; FOLEY et al. 2001), CT (MERLOZ et al. 1998; KAMIMURA et al. 1999; ELLIS et al. 1999; MARTELLI et al. 2000), ultrasound (CARL et al. 1997; TONETTI et al. 2001), and MR imaging (MARTEL et al. 1998; WOODARD et al. 2001). By examining the imaging modalities on which the existing systems are based, one can identify two antithetic trends. The first one is technology-oriented and tends to exploit the most advanced devices and techniques to reach excellent quality standards. CT- and MR-based systems generally go in this direction and are very powerful, accurate and expensive. The other trend is focused on simplicity and accessibility. Conventional radiography- and fluoroscopy-based systems are often less accurate, but affordable for most potential users.

The choice of a specific imaging modality is frequently linked with that of a particular registration approach. Registration is probably the most critical step in a CAS protocol and several issues must be addressed when implementing a registration procedure. The first concern is accuracy. Many applications need an overall accuracy level around 1°/1 mm. This requirement sets an important constraint on the registration accuracy, which has to be kept below 1°/1 mm (SIMON et al. 1995; ELLIS et al. 1996; VIANT 2001). A second issue is invasiveness. As the prevailing trend is towards a minimization of surgical invasiveness,

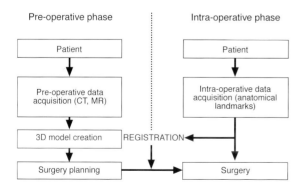

Fig. 29.1. The role of registration in computer-aided surgery: a conceptual scheme

the registration procedure should comply with this (La Palombara et al. 1997). A third problem is complexity. This problem is twofold and includes procedural and computational complexity. Procedural complexity is related to the actions the surgeon has to take, before and during the intervention, in order to make registration possible. Computational complexity, on the other hand, refers to the algorithm that constitutes the core of any registration procedure. Both procedural and computational complexities have a direct impact on time requirements, a critical parameter in any surgical intervention. In addition, procedural complexity influences the user's perception of the system and can negatively affect the system usability. In fact, the registration phase is generally perceived as an unclear and time-consuming step by users who are familiar with traditional surgical techniques (Simon and Lavallée 1998). An ideal registration procedure should be accurate, non-invasive and simple, but these requirements are usually in conflict. To be successfully implemented in a marketable system a registration routine must be fast and uncomplicated. That is why, despite the tremendous progress made in registration techniques in recent years, commercial CAS systems tend to follow simple, though sometimes dated, registration strategies. Several approaches have been proposed for registration (Lavallée 1995; Simon and Lavallée 1998). Most of these can be clustered in the following groups:

Paired point registration methods. The simplest way of registering two reference frames is seeking the linear transformation that links the coordinates of at least three points in space. Though simple from a computational viewpoint, this approach requires picking up the same points in different modalities/ environments and with different tools. A typical example is locating specific landmarks on a CT-derived preoperative model using graphical tools on a personal computer and retrieving the same points on the patient in the operating room using a precision digitizer. The inaccuracy intrinsically associated with such task propagates to the transformation estimated (Fitzpatrick et al. 1998; West et al. 2001).

Fiducial-based methods. To make landmark recognition easier, artificial markers can be attached to the patient. Markers, also called fiducials, are easily identifiable both on medical images and on the patient anatomy in the operating room. Habitually they are small metal beads, which can be either stuck on the skin or surgically implanted in the bone before the intervention. Unfortunately skin motion artefacts

lead to registration errors, so that the latter technique, though more invasive, is normally preferred (Ellis et al. 1996; Maurer et al. 1997). Fiducial-based registration is computationally simple and can be very accurate when implantable markers are employed. Fiducial implants increase, however, both the invasiveness and the procedural complexity of the intervention. Well-known and commercially available CAS systems such as RoboDoc (Integrated Surgical Systems, Davis, Calif., USA) and *CASPAR* (URS.-ortho, Rastatt, Germany) employ fiducial-based registration procedures.

"Non-fiducial" methods. "Non-fiducial" registration techniques do not employ artificial markers. Landmarks are, in this case, either anatomical or geometric. Anatomical landmarks are points that are easily locatable on the subject anatomy, be it on a model or "in vivo" (Amiot et al. 1995). Geometric landmarks are points that possess characteristic geometric properties and are usually automatically computed from more complex representations of the anatomy (segmented images, 3D models, digitized surfaces etc.). Both approaches are non invasive, but usually less accurate than fiducial-based methods.

ICP-based registration methods. Several CAS systems include a registration module relying on the ICP algorithm (Besl and McKay 1992) or on ICP-derived algorithms. Though based on a paired point matching routine, the ICP algorithm owes its success to the fact that it does not require two sets of corresponding points. As the algorithm works on sets of unpaired points, which nevertheless describe the same object, the user does not need to identify the same points in different modalities/environments and the inaccuracy and complexity associated with such a task are eliminated. ICP-based registration procedures are prone to problems affecting all optimization algorithms, such as the risk of getting stuck in local minima, which can considerably degrade the system accuracy. Several solutions have been proposed to overcome such problems (Simon et al. 1995; Cuchet et al. 1995; La Palombara et al. 1997). CAS systems such as HipNav (Di Gioia et al. 1998b) and the Rizzoli TKA system (Martelli et al. 2000) use the above-described registration approach.

Surface- and volume-based registration methods. Surface- and volume-based registration approaches employ surfaces and other geometric entities extracted from segmented images or features directly derivable from 3D image voxels. These approaches can deal with deformable structures, but their use, though common in image-to-image registration, is limited in orthopaedic CAS systems.

29.3
Surgical Robots

Robotics in surgical environments are becoming an increasingly common research area (Kwoh et al 1988; Glucksberg et al. 1994; Rabischong 1997; Charles et al. 1997; Kobayashi et al. 1998; Shoham et al. 1998) and a clinical reality. New standards and new results are expected from this branch of robotic application and the goal is to develop new surgical instrumentation for orthopaedic applications (Radermacher et al. 1994; Delp et al. 1998; Di Gioia et al. 1998a; La Palombara et al. 1998; Marcacci et al. 1999; Roffman et al. 1999) that could prevent the erroneous positioning of components – one of the major causes of surgical failure – and improve the overall quality and safety of the intervention. Robotic systems are those in which an active manipulator is used (Troccaz et al. 1997; Stoianovic et al. 1998) in some aspect of the surgical procedure. These innovative devices come into direct contact with the patient and must necessarily employ patient-specific models.

Several robotics systems have been developed for use in orthopaedic surgery, especially in knee and ankle surgery. Robotic devices can be loosely classified in two categories: automatic robotics systems and semi-automatic robotic systems. Automatic robotics systems are those in which an active manipulator performs the operation and the surgeon interacts with the system only with a human-machine interface (HMI). Semi-automatic robotic systems are those in which the robot places a dedicated end effector at the correct orientation and position in space, and the surgeon executes the operation. The end effector generally constrains the motion to a subregion (i.e. a plane).

The use of mechanically active devices in the operating room introduces new parameters and complex problems, from both the surgical and the robotic points of view, and requires new solutions. Because the robot is in direct contact with humans (i.e. the patient and surgical staff) it must therefore be equipped with reliable safety and fault tolerance mechanisms. Any possible problem must be prevented or intercepted, since an uncontrolled failure of the system would result in irreparable damage to

patient, staff or surgical equipment. Therefore robotic systems must be provided with an appropriate link and joint design, highly reliable control software, new hardware and powerful surgical tools. The main specification of the surgical robot is generally its precision in reaching the working position specified by the surgeon. In order to satisfy this apparently simple requirement, the following constraints must be satisfied:
- high degree of reliability and safety: the first issue is to preserve the surgical environment;
- accuracy: a fundamental feature in orthopaedic interventions;
- high degree of rigidity: an essential requirement, especially in cutting operations when considerable force is applied to the patient's limb.

The *RoboDoc* system has been developed for machining of femoral bones in hip surgery. The robot is a SCARA-based architecture in which workspaces have a relatively limited interaction with the surgical field. In the RoboDoc system the robot control subsystem performs an extensive safety check and monitors cutting force to ensure that unnecessary force cannot harm the patient. It uses force to allow the surgeon to guide the robot into the proximity of the surgical site, after which the robot performs the surgery autonomously. The robot works in the fields of primary total hip replacement, revision hip replacement and total knee replacement.

The *CRIGOS* (Compact Robot for Image-Guided Orthopaedic Surgery) project was set up for the development of a compact surgical robot system (Brandt et al. 1997, 1999) for image-guided orthopaedic surgery based on user requirements. The modular system comprises a compact parallel robot and a software system for planning of the surgical interventions and for supervision of the robotic device. The robot is provided with special interface designs and input devices all tested in the surgical procedure with a complete risk-analysis techniques. *ACROBOT* is a robot specially designed (Davies et al. 1991, 1997) for transparent cooperation with a human user, while nevertheless using an actuated joint. *ACROBOT* uses back-drivable motors and transmissions, whereas conventional robots are usually made strong and stiff at the expense of the back-drivability. All the motors are actively driven to comply with the user's force. As the user approaches and the robot contacts a constraint surface defined in the preoperative plan, the motors are actuated to gradually increases its resistance until, at the edge of the permitted region, it prevents further motion by the operator. The robot has been tested in total knee replacement in vitro experiments.

KNEEROB (Biomechanics Laboratory, Istituti Ortopedici Rizzoli, Bologna in collaboration with Scienzia Machinale, Pisa) is a custom-made 5 degree of freedom manipulator with a sliding short arm mounted on the wrist. The robot (MALVISI et al. 2000) is specifically designed for knee replacement surgery. The last joint of the robot holds an end effector consisting of a milling tool mounted on a passive sliding mechanism which constrains the tool to move in a fixed plane. The cutting plane is determined by the position of the other joints of the manipulator, which effectively acts as a programmable fixture for the milling tool. The tool is operated manually by the surgeon, who has full control on the actual cutting operation. The complete system can be easily cleaned and sterilized, since all mechanisms are protected and cables are routed inside flexible pipes or inside the robot structure. The prototype has been successfully tested on cadaver limbs.

CASPAR (Computer Assisted Surgical Planning And Robotics, by orto MAQUET, Germany) consists (KOBER and MEISTER 2000; PETERMANN et al. 2000) of an industrial robot (based on PUMA architecture) mounted on a mobile base, a milling tool and a calibration unit. The system assists the surgeon in carrying out orthopaedic interventions such as hip surgery or total knee replacement. On the basis of patient data, the placement of a hip prosthesis is simulated. All contours for a perfect fit are precisely milled under surgical supervision. *CASPAR* has been widely tested in operating rooms in total knee replacement and hip surgery.

References

Amiot LP, Labelle H, DeGuise JA (1995) Computer-assisted pedicle screw fixation: A feasibility study. Spine 20:1208–1212

Besl P, McKay N (1992) A method for registration of 3-D shapes. IEEE Trans Pattern Anal Machine Intell 14:239–256

Blackwell M, Morgan F, Di Gioia AM (1998a) Augmented reality and its future in orthopaedics. Clin Orthop354:111–122

Blackwell M, Nikou C, Di Gioia AM (1998b) An image overlay system for medical data visualization. In: Proceedings of medical image computing and computer-assisted intervention – MICCAI 1998, pp 233–240

Brandt G, Radermacher K, Lavallée S (1997) A compact robot for image guided orthopedic surgery: concept and preliminary results. In: Fourth international symposium on medical robotics and computer assisted surgery (CVRMed-MR-CAS'97), Grenoble, France, pp 767–776

Brandt G, Zilmolong A, Carrat L (1999) CRIGOS: a compact robot for image-guided othopaedic surgery. IEEE Trans Inf Technol Biomed 3:252–260

Browbank I, Bouazza-Marouf K, Schnabler J (2000) Robotic-assisted internal fixation of hip fractures: a fluoroscopy-based intraoperative registration technique. Proc Inst Mech Eng 214:165–179

Carl AL, Khanuja HS, Sachs BL (1997) In vitro simulation: early results of stereotaxy for pedicle screw placement. Spine 22:1160–1164

Charles S, Das H, Ohm T (1997) Dexterity-enhanced telerobotics microsurgery. In: Eighth international conference on advanced robotics (ICAR97), Monterey, Calif, USA

Cuchet E, Knoplioch J, Dormont D (1995) Registration in neurosurgery and neuroradiotherapy applications. J Image Guid Surg 1:198–207

Dario P, Carrozza MC, Marcacci M (2000) A novel mechatronic tool for computer assisted arthroscopy. IEEE Trans Inform Technol Biomed 4:15–29

Davies BL, Hibberd RD, Neg WS (1991) A surgeon robot for prostatectomies. In: Fifth international conference on advanced robotics (ICAR'91), Pisa, Italy, pp 871–875

Davies BL, Harris SJ, Lin WJ (1997) Active compliance in robotic surgery: the use of force control as a dynamic constraint. Proc Inst Mech Eng 211:285–292

Delp SL, Stulberg SD, Davies BL (1998) Computer assisted knee replacement. Clin Orthop 354:82–91

Dessenne V, Lavallée S, Julliard R (1998) Computer assisted knee anterior cruciate ligament reconstruction: first clinical tests. In: Nolte LP, Ganz R (eds) Computer assisted orthopaedic surgery CAOS. Hogrefe & Huber, Göttingen, pp 190–197

Di Gioia AM, Jaramaz B, Colgan BD (1998a) Computer assisted orthopaedic surgery, image guided and robotic assistive technologies. Clin Orthop 354:8–16

Di Gioia AM, Jaramaz B, Blackwell M (1998b) The Otto Aufranc Award. Image guided navigation system to measure intraoperatively acetabular implant alignment. Clin Orthop 355:8–22

Ellis R, Toksvig-Larsen S, Marcacci M (1996) Use of a biocompatible fiducial marker in evaluating the accuracy of computed tomography image registration. Invest Radiol 31:658–667

Ellis RE, Tso CY, Rudan JF (1999) A surgical planning and guidance system for high tibial osteotomy. Comput Aided Surg 4:264–274

Fitzpatrick JM, West JB, Maurer CR Jr (1998) Predicting error in rigid-body point-based registration. IEEE Trans Med Imaging 17:694–702

Fleute M, Lavallee S, Julliard R (1999) Incorporating a statistically based shape model into a system for computer-assisted anterior cruciate ligament surgery. In: Medical image analysis. Oxford University Press, Oxford, pp 209–222

Foley KT, Simon DA, Rampersaud YR (2001) Virtual fluoroscopy: computer-assisted fluoroscopic navigation. Spine 26:347–351

Glucksberg MR, Colgate JE, Grace KW (1994) Robotic micromanipulator for ophthalmic surgery. In: First international symposium on medical robotics and computer assisted surgery (MR-CAS'94), Pittsburgh, Pa, pp 204–210

Hofstetter R, Slomczykowski M, Sati M (1999) Fluoroscopy as an imaging means for computer-assisted surgical navigation. Comput Aided Surg 4:65–76

Hofstetter R, Slomczykowski M, Krettek C (2000) Computer-assisted fluoroscopy-based reduction of femoral fractures and antetorsion correction. Comput Aided Surg 5:311–325

Joskowicz L, Milgrom C, Simkin A (1998) FRACAS: a system for computer-aided image-guided long bone fracture surgery. Comput Aided Surg 3:271–288

Kamimura M, Ebara S, Itoh H (1999) Accurate pedicle screw insertion under the control of a computer-assisted image guiding system: laboratory test and clinical study. J Orthop Sci 4:197–206

Klos TVS, Banks AZ, Banks SA (1998) Computer assisted anterior cruciate ligament reconstruction. In: Nolte LP, Ganz R (eds) Computer assisted orthopaedic surgery CAOS. Hogrefe & Huber, Göttingen, pp 184–189

Kobayashi E, Masamune K, Dohi T (1998) A new laparoscope manipulator with an optical zoom. In: Proceedings of medical image computing and computer assisted interventions (MICCAI'98) pp 207–214

Kober R, Meister D (2000) Total knee replacement using the CASPAR-system. In: Fifth international symposium on computer assisted orthopaedic surgery (CAOS'2000), Davos, Switzerland, pp 16–22

Kwoh YS, Jonckheere E, Hayati S (1988) A robot with improved absolute positioning accuracy for CT guided stereotactic surgery. IEEE Trans Biomed Eng: 35:153–160

La Palombara PF, Fadda M, Martelli S (1997) Minimally invasive 3D data registration in computer and robot assisted total knee arthroplasty. Med Biol Eng Comput 35:600–610

La Palombara PF, Fadda M, Martelli M (1998) Computer and robot assisted total knee arthroplasty. In: Proceedings of the first European symposium on biomedical technology and medical physics, Patras, Greece

Lavallée S (1995) Registration for computer-integrated surgery: methodology, state of the art. Computer-integrated surgery:technology and clinical applications. MIT Press, pp 77–97

Leitner F, Picard F, Minfelde R (1997) Computer assisted knee surgical total replacement. In: Proceedings of CVRMed-MRCAS'97, pp 629–638

Malvisi A, Vendruscolo P, Morici F (2000) Bone milling: comparison of the temperature elevation and clinical performances during cutting. In: Proceedings of the millennium symposium on computer assisted orthopaedic surgery (CAOS 2000), Davos,Switzerland

Marcacci M, Martelli S, Nofrini L (1999) Computer and robot assisted total knee replacement. In: Proceedings of the international medical imaging and instrumentation technology conference (IMIIT'99), Kuala Lumpur, Malaysia

Marcacci M, Tonet O, Megali G (2000) A navigation system for computer assisted unicompartimental arthroplasty . In: Proceedings of medical image computing and computer-assisted intervention – MICCAI 2000, pp 1152–1157

Martel AL, Heid O, Slomczykowski M (1998) Assessment of 3-dimensional magnetic resonance imaging fast low angle shot images for computer assisted spinal surgery. Comput Aided Surg 3:40–44

Martelli M, Marcacci M, Nofrini L (2000) Computer and robot-assisted total knee replacement: analysis of a new surgical procedure. Ann Biomed Eng 28:1146–1153

Maurer CR Jr, Fitzpatrick JM, Wang MY (1997) Registration of head volume images using implantable fiducial markers. IEEE Trans Med Imaging 16:447–462

Merloz P, Tonetti J, Pittet L (1998) Computer-assisted spine surgery. Comput Aided Surg 3:297–305

Merloz P, Huberson C, Eid A (2000) Computer-assisted surgical navigation using fluoroscopy: first clinical use in spine surgery. In: Proceedings of the fourth annual North American program on computer assisted orthopaedic surgery (CAOS/USA '00), Pittsburgh, Pa

Nikou C, Di Gioia AM, Blackwell M (2000) Augmented reality imaging technology for orthopaedic surgery. Oper Techn Orthop 10:82–86

Nolte LP, Slomczykowski MA, Berlemann U (2000) A new approach to computer-aided spine surgery: fluoroscopy-based surgical navigation. Eur Spine J 9 [Suppl 1]:78–88

Petermann J, Schierl M, Heeckt PF (2000) The CASPAR-system in the reconstruction of the ACL: first follow-up results. In: Fifth international symposium on computer assisted orthopaedic surgery (CAOS'2000), Davos, Switzerland, pp 23–29

Picard F, Moody J, Jaramaz B (2000a) A classification proposal for computer-assisted knee systems . In: Proceedings of medical image computing and computer-assisted intervention (MICCAI 2000), pp 1145–1151

Picard F, Moody J, Martinek V (2000b) A computer-assisted ACL reconstruction system: assessment of two techniques of graft positioning in ACL reconstruction. In: Proceedings of medical image computing and computer-assisted intervention (MICCAI 2000), pp 1136–1143

Rabischong P (1997) Robots for surgeons or surgeons for robots? Comput Aided Surg 2:3–4

Radermacher K, Staudte HW, Rau G (1994) Computer assisted orthopaedic surgery by means of individual templates: aspects and analysis of potential applications. In: First international symposium on medical robotics and computer assisted surgery (MRCAS'94), Pittsburgh, Pa, pp 42–48

Roffman M, Borenstein E, Elber G (1999) Robot-assisted total knee arthoplasty. In: 72nd Annual Meeting, Japanese Orthopaedic Association, Yokohama, Japan

Shoham M, Ben-Horin R, Djerassi S (1998) Kinematics, dynamics and construction of a planarly actuated parallel robot. Robotics Comput Integrated Manuf 14:163–172

Simon DA (1997) What is "registration" and why is it so important in CAOS? In: Proceedings of the first annual North American program on computer assisted orthopaedic surgery (CAOS/USA '97), Pittsburgh, Pa, pp 57–60

Simon DA, Hebert M, Kanade T (1995) Techniques for fast and accurate intrasurgical registration. J Image Guid Surg 1:17–29

Simon DA, Lavallée S (1998) Medical imaging and registration in computer assisted surgery. Clin Orthop 354:17–27

Slomczykowski MA, Hofstetter R, Sati M (2001) Novel computer-assisted fluoroscopy system for intraoperative guidance: feasibility study for distal locking of femoral nails. J Orthop Trauma 152:122–131

Stoianovic D, Witcomb LL, Anderson JH (1998) A modular surgical robotic system for image guided percutaneous procedures. In: Proceedings of medical image computing and computer assisted interventions (MICCAI'98) pp 404–410

Tonetti J, Carrat L, Blendea S (2001) Clinical validation of computer assisted pelvic surgery using ultrasound: a percutaneous safe technique with low radiation exposure. Stud Health Technol Inform 81:515–520

Troccaz J, Peshkin M, Davies B (1997) The use of localizers, robots and synergistic devices in CAS. In: Fourth international symposium on medical robotics and computer assisted surgery (CVRMed-MRCAS'97), Grenoble, France, pp 727–735

Viant WJ (2001) The development of an evaluation framework for the quantitative assessment of computer-assisted surgery and augmented reality accuracy performance. Stud Health Technol Inform 81:534–540

West JB, Fitzpatrick JM, Toms SA (2001) Fiducial point placement and the accuracy of point-based rigid body registration. Neurosurgery 48:810–816

Woodard EJ, Leon SP, Moriarty TM (2001) Initial experience with intraoperative magnetic resonance imaging in spine surgery. Spine 26:410–417

Subject Index

List of Acronyms

2D	two-dimensional		EPI	echo planar imaging
2DFT	two-dimensional Fourier transformation		ERCP	endoscopic retrograde cholangiopancreato-graphy
3D	three-dimensional		ETS	electromagnetic tracker systems
3D CT	three-dimensional computed tomography			
3D US	three-dimensional ultrasound		FESS	functional endoscopic sinus surgery
3DFT	three-dimensional Fourier transformation		FISP	fast imaging with steady state processing
			FLASH	fast low angle shot
AC	anterior commissure		FLE	fiducial localization error
ACL	anterior cruciate ligament		fMR	functional magnetic resonance
AI	aorto iliac		fMR BOLD	functional MR blood oxygen level dependent
AIF	arterial input function		FNH	focal nodular hyperplasia
AIR	automatic image registration		FOBT	faecal occult blood testing
API	application programming interface		FOV	field of view
AR	augmented reality		FWHM	full width half maximum
ARA	accessory renal artery			
ATM	adaptive template moderated		GRE	gradient recalled echo
			GUI	graphical user interface
b-FOLD	blood flow oxygen level dependent			
BMS	bulk magnetic susceptibility		HA	hepatic artery
BOLD	blood oxygen level dependent		HCC	hepatocellular carcinoma
			HD	hepatic duct
CA	celiac artery		HMD	head-mounted display
CAS	computer-aided surgery		HMI	human-machine interface
CBD	common bile duct		HRCT	high-resolution computed tomography
CBF	cerebral blood flow			
CBV	cerebral blood volume		ICP	iterative closest point
CD	cystic duct		IEE	image-enhanced endoscopy
CE-MRA	contrast enhancement magnetic resonance angiography		IRB	institutional review board
c-FOLD	CSF flow oxygen level dependent		LED	light-emitting diodes
COLD	CSF oxygen level dependent		LHD	left hepatic duct
CPR	curved planar reconstruction		LI	linear interpolation
CRC	colorectal cancer		LIA	left iliac artery
CRT	conformational radiotherapy		LRA	left renal artery
CSF	cerebrospinal fluid			
CTA	CT angiography		MAGI	microscope-assisted guided interventions
CTVE	computed tomography virtual endoscopy		MinIp	minimum intensity projection
			MIP	maximum intensity projection
DCBE	double contrast barium enema		MIST	minimally invasive skills trainer
DOF	degrees-of-freedom		MITR	maximal intensity change per time interval ratio
DRF	dynamic reference frame		MOLD	motion oxygen level dependent
DSA	digital subtraction angiography		MPR	multiplanar reconstruction
DSC-MR	dynamic susceptibility contrast-enhanced MR imaging		MPVR	multiplanar volume reconstruction
DWI	diffusion weighted imaging		MR VE	magnetic resonance virtual endoscopy
			MRA	MR angiography
EGC	early gastric cancer		MRCP	magnetic resonance cholangiopancreatography
EM	electromagnetic		MRDCT	multi-row detector computed tomography
ENT	ear nose and throat		MRU	MR urography
			MSD	mean standard deviation

MTT	mean transit time
NES	nasal endoscopy simulator
PACS	picture archiving and communication system
PC	posterior commissure
PCI	personal computer interface
PD	pancreatic duct
PDW	proton density weighted
PET	positron emission tomography
PTC	percutaneous transhepatic cholangiography
PVR	perspective volume rendering
RAM	random accessible memory
RARE	rapid aquisition relaxation enhancement
RHD	right hepatic duct
ROI	region of interest
RRA	right renal artery
SFE	scaled fitting error
SMA	superior mesenteric artery
SNR	signal-to-noise ratio
SPECT	single photon emission computed tomography
SPGR	spoiled gradient recalled
SR	surface rendering

SSD	shaded surface display
SSFP	steady-state free precession
STM	statistical trained models
STS-MIP	sliding thin slab maximum intensity projection
SVC	spatially varying statistical classification
TBNA	transbronchial needle aspiration
TE	echo time
TKR	total knee replacement
TOF	time-of-flight
TR	repetition time
TSE	turbo spin echo
TTP	time to peak concentration
VA	virtual angioscopy
VB	virtual bronchoscopy
VE	virtual endoscopy
VEGF	vascular endothelial growth factor
VIVIAN	virtual intra-cranial visualization and navigation
VL	virtual laryngoscopy
VOI	volume of interest
VR	volume rendering
VRe	virtual reality
VRML	virtual reality modelling language
XLM	extensible mark-up language

List of Contributors

Werner Backfrieder, MS, PhD
Department of Biomedical Engineering and Physics
University of Vienna
General Hospital Vienna
Waehringer Guertel 18-20
1090 Vienna
Austria

Isabella Baeli, MD
Department of Radiology
University of Rome "La Sapienza"
Policlinico Umberto I
Viale Regina Elena n. 324
00161 Rome
Italy

Reto J. Bale, MD
Department of Radiology I
University Hospital
University of Innsbruck
Anichstrasse 35
6020 Innsbruck
Austria

Emese Balogh, MSc
Department of Applied Informatics
University of Szeged Àrpád tér 2
6720 Szeged
Hungary

Irene Bargellini, MD
Diagnostic and Interventional Radiology
Department of Oncology, Transplants,
and Advanced Technologies in Medicine
University of Pisa
Via Roma 67
56100 Pisa
Italy

Carlo Bartolozzi, MD
Professor and Chairman
Diagnostic and Interventional Radiology
Department of Oncology, Transplants,
and Advanced Technologies in Medicine
University of Pisa
Via Roma 67
56100 Pisa
Italy

Anna Vilanova Bartrolì
Institute of Computer Graphics and Algorithms
Vienna University of Technology
Karlsplatz 13/186/2
1040 Vienna
Austria

Stefano Berrettini, MD
Otololaryngologic Unit
Deparment of Neuroscience
University of Pisa
Via Savi 10
56126 Pisa
Italy

Elisabetta Bichi Secchi, MD
Department of Radiology
University Hospital "Umberto I°"
Via Conca
60020 Torrette di Ancona, Ancona
Italy

Wolfgang Birkfellner, MS, PhD
Department of Biomedical Engineering and Physics
University of Vienna
General Hospital Vienna
Waehringer Guertel 18-20
1090 Vienna
Austria

Alain Blum Moyse, MD
Professor, Service de Radiologie
Hôpital Central
29, avenue Maréchal de Lattre de Tassigny
54035 Nancy Cédex
France

Piero Boraschi, MD
2nd Department of Radiology
Pisa University Hospital
Via Paradisa 2
56124 Pisa
Italy

Darren Brennan, MB, BCh, MRCPI
Department of Radiology
Mater Misericordiae Hospital
Eccles Street
Dublin 7
Ireland

JOHN BRUZZI, MB, BCh, MRCPI
Department of Radiology
Mater Misericordiae Hospital
Eccles Street
Dublin 7
Ireland

GIUDITTA CAMPORI, MD
Diagnostic and Interventional Radiology
Department of Oncology, Transplants,
and Advanced Technologies in Medicine
University of Pisa
Via Roma 67
56100 Pisa
Italy

CARLA CAPPELLI, MD
Diagnostic and Interventional Radiology
Department of Oncology, Transplants,
and Advanced Technologies in Medicine
University of Pisa
Via Roma 67
56100 Pisa
Italy

DAVIDE CARAMELLA, MD
Diagnostic and Interventional Radiology
Department of Oncology, Transplants,
and Advanced Technologies in Medicine
University of Pisa
Via Roma 67
56100 Pisa
Italy

MONIKA CARTELLIERI, MD
Departmentof Otolaryngology
University Hospital of Vienna
Waehringer Guertel 18-20
1090 Vienna
Austria

CARLO CATALANO, MD
Department of Radiology
University of Rome "La Sapienza"
Policlinico Umberto I
Viale Regina Elena n. 324
00161 Rome
Italy

DANIA CIONI, MD
Diagnostic and Interventional Radiology
Department of Oncology, Transplants,
and Advanced Technologies in Medicine
University of Pisa
Via Roma 67
56100 Pisa
Italy

MARTIN CITARDI, MD
Department Ear Nose and Throat
Cleveland Clinic Foundation
9500 Euclid Avenue
Cleveland OH 44195
USA

ANNE COTTEN, MD
Professor, Service de Radiologie Ostéo-Articulaire
Hôpital R. Salengro –CHRU de Lille
Boulevard du Pr. J. Leclercq
59037 Lille Cédex
France

LAURA CROCETTI, MD
Diagnostic and Interventional Radiology
Department of Oncology, Transplants,
and Advanced Technologies in Medicine
University of Pisa
Via Roma 67
56100 Pisa
Italy

MASSIMILIANO DANTI, MD
Department of Radiology
University of Rome "La Sapienza"
Policlinico Umberto I
Viale Regina Elena n. 324
00161 Rome
Italy

HELEN M. FENLON, MD, BCh, MRCPI, FFRRSCI
Department of Radiology
Mater Misericordiae Hospital
Eccles Street
Dublin 7
Ireland

FRANCESCO FRAIOLI, MD
Department of Radiology
University of Rome "La Sapienza"
Policlinico Umberto I
Viale Regina Elena n. 324
00161 Rome
Italy

MARVIN P. FRIED, MD
Surgical Planning Laboratory
Department of Radiology
Brigham and Women's Hospital Boston
75, Francis Street
Boston, MA 02115
USA

CLAUDIA GIANNI, MD
Diagnostic and Interventional Radiology
Department of Oncology, Transplants,
and Advanced Technologies in Medicine
University of Pisa
Via Roma 67
56100 Pisa
Italy

ROBERTO GIGONI, MD
2nd Department of Radiology
Pisa University Hospital
Via Paradisa 2
56124 Pisa
Italy

Enrico Gobbetti, PhD
CRS4 - Center for Research
VI Strada Ovest, ZI Macchiareddu, CP 94
09010 Uta (CA)
Italy

Rudolf Hanel, MS
Department of Biomedical Engineering and Physics
University of Vienna
General Hospital Vienna
Währinger Gürtel 18-20
1090 Vienna
Austria

Franco Iafrate, MD
Department of Radiology
University of Rome "La Sapienza"
Policlinico Umberto I
Viale Regina Elena n. 324
00161 Rome
Italy

Riccardo Iannaccone, MD
Department of Radiology
University of Rome "La Sapienza"
Policlinico Umberto I
Viale Regina Elena n. 324
00161 Rome
Italy

Sandrine Iochum, MD
Service de Radiologie
Hôpital Central
29, avenue Maréchal de Lattre de Tassigny
54035 Nancy Cédex
France

Gary Israel, MD
Department of Radiology, Abdominal Imaging
NYU Medical Center
560 First Avenue
Suite HW 206
New York, NY 10016
USA

Alan Jackson, MD
Professor of Neurology
Imaging Science and Biomedical Engineering
The Medical School
University of Manchester
Oxford Road
Manchester M13 9PT
UK

Nigel W. John, PhD
Deputy Director
Manchester Visualisation Centre
University of Manchester
Manchester M13 9PL
UK

Ferenc A. Jolesz, MD
Director of MR Division
and Image Guided Therapy Program
Department of Radiology
Brigham and Women's Hospital Boston
75, Francis Street
Boston, MA 02115
USA

Joachim Kettenbach, MD
Department of Diagnostic Radiology
University Hospital of Vienna
Waehringer Guertel 18-20
1090 Vienna
Austria

Ron Kikinis, MD
Surgical Planning Laboratory
Department of Radiology
Brigham and Women's Hospital Boston
75, Francis Street
Boston, MA 02115
USA

Domagoj Kovacevic, MD
Department of Electronic Systems
and Information Processing
Faculty of Electrical Engineering Computing Zagreb
Unska 3
HR-10000 Zagreb
Croatia

Andrea Laghi, MD
Department of Radiology
University of Rome "La Sapienza"
Policlinico Umberto I
Viale Regina Elena n. 324
00161 Rome
Italy

Pier Francesco La Palombara, MD
Istituti Ortopedici Rizzoli, Biomechanics Lab
Via Barbiano 1-10
40136 Bologna
Italy

Riccardo Lencioni, MD
Diagnostic and Interventional Radiology
Department of Oncology, Transplants,
and Advanced Technologies in Medicine
University of Pisa
Via Roma 67
56100 Pisa
Italy

Mike E. Leventon, MS, PhD
Surgical Planning Laboratory
Department of Radiology
Brigham and Women's Hospital Boston
75, Francis Street
Boston, MA 02115
USA

SIMONE LODOVIGI, MD
Diagnostic and Interventional Radiology
Department of Oncology, Transplants,
and Advanced Technologies in Medicine
University of Pisa
Via Roma 67
56100 Pisa
Italy

SVEN LONCARIC, PhD
Department of Electronic Systems
and Information Processing
Faculty of Electrical Engineering Computing Zagreb
Unska 3
HR-10000 Zagreb
Croatia

WILLIAM E. LORENSEN, MD
GE Corporate Research and Development
Building KW Room C215, 1 Research Circle
Niskayuna, NY 12309
USA

MICHAEL MACARI, MD
Department of Radiology, Abdominal Imaging
NYU Medical Center
560 First Avenue
Suite HW 207
New York, NY 10016
USA

ANDREA MALVISTI, MD
Istituti Ortopedici Rizzoli, Biomechanics Lab
Via Barbiano 1-10
40136 Bologna
Italy

MAURILIO MARCACCI, MD
Istituti Ortopedici Rizzoli, Biomechanics Lab
Via Barbiano 1-10
40136 Bologna
Italy

LUIS MARTÍ-BONMATÍ, MD, PhD
Dr Peset University Hospital
Unidad de Resonancia Magnetica
Avenida Gaspar Aguilar 90
46017 Valencia
Spain

VIK M. MOHARIR, MD
Surgical Planning Laboratory
Department of Radiology
Brigham and Women's Hospital Boston
75, Francis Street
Boston, MA 02115
USA

ALESSANDRO NAPOLI, MD
Department of Radiology
University of Rome "La Sapienza"
Policlinico Umberto I
Viale Regina Elena n. 324
00161 Rome
Italy

EMANUELE NERI, MD
Diagnostic and Interventional Radiology
Department of Oncology, Transplants,
and Advanced Technologies in Medicine
University of Pisa
Via Roma 67
56100 Pisa
Italy

LAURA NOFRINI, MD
Istituti Ortopedici Rizzoli, Biomechanics Lab
Via Barbiano 1-10
40136 Bologna
Italy

WIESLAW L. NOWINSKI, DSc, PhD
Medical Imaging Laboratory
Kent Ridge Digital Labs
21, Heng Mui Keng Terrace
Singapore 119613
Singapore

LÀZLÒ G. NYÙL, MSc
Department of Applied Informatics
University of Szeged Àrpád tér 2
6720 Szeged
Hungary

KÁLMÁN PALÁGYI, PhD
Department of Applied Informatics
University of Szeged Àrpád tér 2
6720 Szeged
Hungary

MICHELA PANCONI, MD
Diagnostic and Interventional Radiology
Department of Oncology, Transplants,
and Advanced Technologies in Medicine
University of Pisa
Via Roma 67
56100 Pisa
Italy

VALERIA PANEBIANCO, MD
Department of Radiology
University of Rome "La Sapienza"
Policlinico Umberto I
Viale Regina Elena n. 324
00161 Rome
Italy

ROBERTO PASSARIELLO, MD
Department of Radiology
University of Rome "La Sapienza"
Policlinico Umberto I
Viale Regina Elena n. 324
00161 Rome
Italy

FEDERICA PEDICONI, MD
Department of Radiology
University of Rome "La Sapienza"
Policlinico Umberto I
Viale Regina Elena n. 324
00161 Rome
Italy

Marzio Perri, MD
Diagnostic and Interventional Radiology
Department of Oncology, Transplants,
and Advanced Technologies in Medicine
University of Pisa
Via Roma 67
56100 Pisa
Italy

Silvia Picchietti, MD
Diagnostic and Interventional Radiology
Department of Oncology, Transplants,
and Advanced Technologies in Medicine
University of Pisa
Via Roma 67
56100 Pisa
Italy

Helmut Ringl, MD
Department of Diagnostic Radiology
University Hospital of Vienna
Waehringer Guertel 18-20
1090 Vienna
Austria

Luca Salvolini, MD
Department of Radiology
University Hospital "Umberto I°"
Via Conca
60020 Torrette di Ancona, Ancona
Italy

Riccardo Scateni, MD
CRS4 - Center for Research
VI Strada Ovest, ZI Macchiareddu, CP 94
09010 Uta (CA)
Italy

Andreas G. Schreyer, MD
Department of Radiology
University Hospital Regensburg
Franz-Josef-Strauss Allee 11
93053 Regensburg
Germany

Stefano Sellari Franceschini, MD
Otolaryngologic Unit
Department of Neuroscience
University of Pisa
Via Savi 10
56126 Pisa
Italy

Ramin Shahidi, PhD
Image Guidance Laboratories
Stanford University
Stanford University Medical Center
Department of Neurosurgery
300 Pasteur Dr., Room S-006
Stanford, CA 94305-5327
USA

Erich Sorantin, MD
Department of Radiology
University Hospital Graz
Auenbruggerplatz 34
8036 Graz
Austria

Cheti Spinelli, MD
Diagnostic and Interventional Radiology
Department of Oncology, Transplants,
and Advanced Technologies in Medicine
University of Pisa
Via Roma 67
56100 Pisa
Italy

Marco Subasic
Department of Electronic Systems
and Information Processing
Faculty of Electrical Engineering Computing Zagreb
Unska 3
HR-10000 Zagreb
Croatia

Neil A. Thacker, PhD
Imaging Science and Biomedical Engineering
The Medical School
University of Manchester
Oxford Road
Manchester M13 9PT
UK

Paola Vagli, MD
Diagnostic and Interventional Radiology
Department of Oncology, Transplants,
and Advanced Technologies in Medicine
University of Pisa
Via Roma 67
56100 Pisa
Italy

Simon K. Warfield, PhD
Surgical Planning Laboratory
Department of Radiology
Brigham and Women's Hospital Boston
75, Francis Street
Boston, MA 02115
USA

Gianluigi Zanetti
CRS4 - Center for Research
VI Strada Ovest, ZI Macchiareddu, CP 94
09010 Uta (CA)
Italy

MEDICAL RADIOLOGY
Diagnostic Imaging and Radiation Oncology

Titles in the series already published

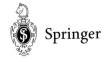 Springer

MEDICAL RADIOLOGY
Diagnostic Imaging and Radiation Oncology

Titles in the series already published

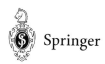 Springer

Printing and Binding: Stürtz AG, Würzburg